An Introduction to Intensive Short-Term Dynamic Psychotherapy

This book offers a comprehensive introduction to Intensive Short-Term Dynamic Psychotherapy (ISTDP), covering its theoretical foundations, core techniques, and practical applications.

The author first introduces six key psychodynamic concepts essential for ISTDP in an accessible, jargon-free way, then shifts focus to building strong conscious therapeutic alliances. Finally, core ISTDP techniques are clearly explained and demonstrated. Through clinical examples and real therapy transcripts, this book illustrates how to effectively integrate ISTDP to resolve unconscious conflicts by addressing feelings, anxiety, and defenses.

Whether you are a student or a beginner therapist new to ISTDP, or an experienced practitioner looking to revisit the fundamentals of this exciting method, this book serves as an accessible, relevant, and indispensable resource.

Jon Anders Lied is a psychologist and psychotherapist practicing, teaching, and supervising ISTDP and psychodynamic psychotherapy. He works at the Mental Health Service at Sit (the student welfare organization in Trondheim, Norway), maintains a small private practice, and has been teaching ISTDP and supervising students in the Clinical Program in Psychology at the Norwegian University of Science and Technology (NTNU) for several years. He also brings extensive experience from the public specialist healthcare service, both as a therapist and as a supervisor.

"This book is a must-buy for anyone who wants to learn how psychodynamic therapy works and why to do it. Clinical vignettes illustrate every concept and technique. As a result, the reader learns how clinical thinking leads to effective interventions that help patients achieve the changes they seek. Extremely practical and clearly written, this book will help all therapists develop greater empathy for their patients' conscious and unconscious struggles to form a more healing relationship. I strongly recommend this book to all psychotherapy instructors, students, and therapists."

Jon Frederickson, *Faculty, New Washington School of Psychiatry.*

"This volume presents a lively and accessible introduction to theory and practice of Intensive Short-term Dynamic Psychotherapy. In plain language, Lied leads the reader through the therapeutic process, illustrating each step with verbatim transcripts of a successful therapy. The author is refreshingly candid about the challenges and rewards of learning this complex but effective method of facilitating deep and lasting change. Highly recommended!"

Patricia Coughlin, *Ph.D.*

"I highly recommend Jon Anders Lied's new introduction to ISTDP! The book is illustrated with case material, is written in accessible and unpretentious language, and takes the time to explain basic psychodynamic ideas and phenomena without the use of psychodynamic jargon. It is also distinguished by placing great emphasis on the conscious part of the therapeutic collaboration, which is often neglected in ISTDP. This is also reflected in Lied's therapeutic style in the book, which is patient, pleasant and welcoming—a good new role model for new ISTDP therapists."

Mikkel Reher-Langberg, *Clincial Psychologist and President of the Danish Society for ISTDP.*

"With this book, Jon Anders Lied has accomplished something extraordinary. Every page of this book sings of an ISTDP deeply imbued with a humanism that places the real relationship at the heart of the therapeutic enterprise, while poignantly illuminating the core principles that make up the model."

Johannes Kiedling, *LCSW*

"Approachable, readable, and precise with clear explanations, this book provides a comprehensive introduction to ISTDP. Rich with transcriptions from real therapy sessions, it walks readers through both the theoretical foundation and the core techniques of the model. It is an invaluable resource, catering to both newcomers who are just starting their journey in ISTDP and seasoned practitioners who are seeking a deeper understanding of the basics of this dynamic and flexible therapy approach. Highly recommended!"

Tami Chelew, *LMFT, President of the International Experiential Dynamic Psychotherapy Association.*

"In his book, Introduction to ISTDP, Jon Anders Lied expertly illustrates through case examples how to apply integrative theory and techniques in psychotherapy. His approach to ISTDP is practical and to the point and he offers a refreshing perspective on how to empower your patients to experience the change they desire."

Kristin Osborn, *LMHC, Associate, Harvard Medical School President-Elect, Society for the Exploration of Psychotherapy Integration.*

"Jon Anders Lied's appreciation of the power of ISTDP is balanced by his willingness to acknowledge the challenges and pitfalls of learning to practice it. That, and his emphasis on the importance of building a collaborative working relationship with each patient, make this book a valuable contribution."

Nat Kuhn, *MD.*

An Introduction to Intensive Short-Term Dynamic Psychotherapy

Foundations of Clinical Practice

Jon Anders Lied

Routledge
Taylor & Francis Group

LONDON AND NEW YORK

Designed cover image: © Jo Waite

First published 2025
by Routledge
4 Park Square, Milton Park, Abingdon, Oxon OX14 4RN

and by Routledge
605 Third Avenue, New York, NY 10158

Routledge is an imprint of the Taylor & Francis Group, an informa business

© 2025 Jon Anders Lied

British Library Cataloguing-in-Publication Data
A catalogue record for this book is available from the British Library

ISBN: 9781032850382 (hbk)
ISBN: 9781032850375 (pbk)
ISBN: 9781003516217 (ebk)

DOI: 10.4324/9781003516217

Typeset in Times New Roman
by KnowledgeWorks Global Ltd.

Contents

Acknowledgments

Over the past ten years, the content of this book has evolved in my mind as I have studied and taught ISTDP. I have given lectures and have attended lectures. I have supervised and been supervised. I have practiced as an ISTDP therapist, and experienced ISTDP as a patient. I have read, discussed, and sought to understand. I am deeply grateful to everyone—patients, students, colleagues, teachers, supervisors, therapists, family, and friends—who has accompanied me on this journey.

Some of you deserve special thanks:

First and foremost, to Anne Lise, Oskar, and Aurora—thank you for all your patience and love. I know you love me, even if no one ends up reading this book.

I also want to express my deep gratitude to the Sweet Child, the Girl Who Wasn't a Princess, the Man Who Worried About His Heart, the Brain Exerciser, and the Pancake Maker for allowing me to include excerpts from your therapy sessions in this book. I have learned more from you than you can imagine, and your contributions are invaluable to aspiring therapists learning from this book.

Thank you to Patricia Coughlin for being my supervisor and mentor for many years, and for your invaluable advice on the English translation. So much of what is in this book is built upon what you have taught me. Without you, this book would not exist.

Thank you to Filip Myhre and Jonas Sharma-Bakkevig for introducing me to ISTDP and enduring all my critical questions. The two of you truly sparked my passion for ISTDP.

Thank you to Petter Møllenberg for nerding out with me about psychoanalysis and ISTDP, and for your valuable advice and comments.

Thank you to Heidi Trydal for your inspiring criticism, constructive advice, and thorough reading.

Thank you to my mother, "Modern" Sidsel Lied, and to Jan Kåre Hummelvoll, for your careful, critical, and supportive reading.

Thank you to Mariann Bakken at Scandinavian University Press for reading, supporting, and believing in my original Norwegian book project.

Thank you to Grace McDonnell at Taylor & Francis for your help and belief in the translated work.

Jon Anders Lied, September 2024

Introduction

If you are reading this book, it is likely that you are curious about Intensive Short-Term Dynamic Psychotherapy, commonly referred to as ISTDP (Davanloo, 1990). If that is the case, I invite you to delve into an exciting theoretical field, a transformative therapeutic approach, and a vibrant professional community that can be immensely fulfilling. If you happened upon the book merely by chance, I hope to inspire you and pique your curiosity about this exciting method.

ISTDP is a psychodynamic therapy method rooted in the psychoanalytic theory of unconscious conflict (Freud, 1920). It provides a structured yet flexible approach to effectively assessing and treating a broad range of patients over a short period of time. No matter if you work in private practice with well-functioning patients or in public health care with traumatized and fragile individuals, I am confident that ISTDP can boost both your effectiveness and your satisfaction in reaching therapeutic goals.

In my personal experience, the study and practice of ISTDP has yielded many rewards. ISTDP builds upon a *robust theoretical foundation* that draws from a psychoanalytic and psychodynamic understanding of mental suffering. Over the years, a series of *practical interventions* has been developed, making the integration of ISTDP into your practice an engaging and rewarding journey. As a learner of ISTDP you will become part of a *supportive professional community*: you can attend seminars and conferences, either in person or online, in order to gain valuable insight, and a wide array of experienced therapists are available to supervise you. When posting on the listserv of the International Experiential Dynamic Therapy Association (IEDTA, 2024), you will discover that your questions will often be answered by influential figures in the field. This fusion of strong *theory*, practical *application*, and communal *engagement* sets ISTDP apart from many other therapeutic approaches. In essence, it provides an environment in which ISTDP therapists can continuously evolve and embrace lifelong learning opportunities.

However, the extensive theoretical groundwork, technical advice, and myriad learning prospects do present a challenge. Many—myself included—have found learning and applying ISTDP to be rather demanding. ISTDP is a complex and multifaceted method which has proven effective for over 80% of patients in outpatient clinics (Abbass, 2002), yet achieving such results requires a comprehensive

DOI: 10.4324/9781003516217-1

understanding of numerous psychological phenomena and a range of different interventions. Amid the array of technical interventions showcased in video and audio lectures, books, and seminars, it is easy to feel overwhelmed. I'm sure I'm not the only one who has found themselves in the middle of a therapy session, staring at a patient, and thinking, "Oops, I can't remember the right thing to say in this situation!"

One of the hallmarks of ISTDP teaching is showing videotaped psychotherapy sessions. Learning by watching experienced therapists apply this method is inspiring and provides deep learning experiences. However, this can also be a mixed blessing: You have witnessed an expert demonstrate what appears to be the "correct" approach; the teacher typically selects emotionally charged material that exemplifies numerous psychological phenomena within a condensed timeframe. Upon returning to your office as an ISTDP novice, determined to emulate the experts, you may find yourself trying too hard to execute an intervention that you have not yet fully comprehended. In the pursuit of making use of new and compelling knowledge, it is possible to inadvertently lose sight of the fundamental goal of ISTDP.

I have personally witnessed and experienced unmistakable evidence of the effectiveness of the method, both as a therapist and as a patient in my own ISTDP therapy. When conducted respectfully and collaboratively, symptom relief, new insights, personal freedom, character change, and fulfilling, close relationships are within reach for most patients. Furthermore, my experience suggests that these outcomes can be achieved within a relatively short timeframe. There are, however, numerous accounts of negative experiences with ISTDP (Flåten, 2021). In my view, this scenario can arise when the therapist overlooks the fundamental theoretical principles upon which the therapy is built, neglects the development of a robust conscious working alliance and a collaborative case formulation, and rather becomes overly fixated on therapeutic techniques.

In writing this introduction to ISTDP, my intention is to promote more positive therapeutic experiences with the method for therapists and patients alike. The focus will be on the foundational aspects of the method that underpin every ISTDP session and intervention, including an understanding of the ways in which unconscious conflicts create and perpetuate symptoms and suffering. The text highlights how the therapist and patient can co-create a shared understanding of the mechanisms that are causing the patient's problems, and how to use this to build a strong working alliance with agreement on the therapeutic task and goal. On this basis, it also delves into how to conduct therapy within the framework of ISTDP. My hope is that by enhancing the fundamental comprehension of this method, a greater number of therapists will be able to harness the full potential of ISTDP in achieving ambitious therapeutic goals.

The principal purpose of this book is to help you, as a therapist, gain a clearer understanding of what you do, why you do it, and the ultimate objectives you aim to achieve in every session of ISTDP. As an introduction to the method, it assumes no prior knowledge of psychodynamic therapy or ISTDP. I sincerely hope that the book that you hold in your hands will positively impact how your therapy sessions are conducted, while inspiring you to delve deeper into the realm of ISTDP. There is a wealth of literature available for those interested in exploring ISTDP further, encompassing both theory[1] and technique.[2] Moreover, it is worth noting that an increasing body of research supports the effectiveness and cost efficiency of ISTDP across a broad spectrum of patients and symptoms (Abbass, 2021, 2022b; Abbass et al., 2012, 2021).

Notes

1 Recommended readings are Coughlin Della Selva (2004), Davanloo (1990), and Malan (1979).
2 Recommended readings are Frederickson (2013), Frederickson (2020), and Abbass (2015).

Part I

What Is Psychodynamic Therapy?

Intensive Short-Term Dynamic Therapy (ISTDP) is a psychodynamic therapy model (Coughlin Della Selva, 2004) developed by Habib Davanloo, a trained psychoanalyst, who based his understanding of what causes psychological distress on psychoanalytic theory.[1] After becoming increasingly frustrated with the results he obtained through classical psychoanalysis, particularly with patients who were resistant to change, he developed ISTDP. In his quest to condense and shorten[2] the therapy process, he encouraged his patients to confront their true feelings while simultaneously challenging their defenses and ensuring their anxiety was sufficiently regulated. He noticed that through his method, patients could more rapidly access memories that illuminated and helped resolve the dynamic roots of their conflicts, compared to traditional psychoanalysis.

To comprehend ISTDP, the therapist must first grasp the essence of what psychoanalytic/psychodynamic therapy is. Underpinning every course of ISTDP therapy is a psychodynamic understanding of the psyche, and without this, the interventions associated with ISTDP lack meaning. Thus, the therapist must understand the theoretical basis of the method in order to intervene effectively and to know *what* to do *when*.

Psychodynamic *therapy* is rooted in psychodynamic *theory*.[3] This theory provides a comprehensive theoretical foundation for the origins and perpetuation of psychological suffering, and it is upon this framework that ISTDP rests. Within this foundation, extensive literature exists on how to help patients solve their psychological conflicts. When, over a century ago, Freud launched the field of psychoanalysis (Freud, 1920), he triggered a deluge of theoretical development and sharing of therapeutic experiences.[4] This has resulted in the development of numerous psychodynamically oriented therapies of both short- and long-term formats. In this introductory text, I aim to elucidate only the most crucial aspects of this extensive field. Still, I hope to encourage you into further exploration of this captivating body of literature.

Most of the therapies grounded in psychodynamic theory are built upon a few common underlying principles, and many attempts have been made to distill the most essential of these. On the basis of some of these efforts (Gabbard, 2017; Shedler, 2006; Stänicke & Stänicke, 2014), I have elected to spotlight six

DOI: 10.4324/9781003516217-2

theoretical axioms and concepts within psychoanalysis and psychodynamic theory that one must comprehend when learning ISTDP. These are:

1 Human beings have an *unconscious* mental life.
2 Human beings harbor unconscious psychological *conflicts*.
3 *Transference* is at the core of all psychodynamic therapies.
4 Human beings use *defense mechanisms*.
5 Mental symptoms and problems hold psychological and phenomenological significance.
6 Mental disorders arise from an interplay between *developmental, genetic, and social factors.*

In this part, I elucidate these phenomena, providing an introduction to basic psychodynamic concepts and resource in comprehending what constitutes an effective course of ISTDP therapy. To exemplify these points I draw upon a patient I refer to as the Sweet Child. The Sweet Child will play a pivotal role in clarifying these fundamental psychodynamic therapy phenomena. She possessed a remarkable ability to articulate internal experiences, perhaps more lucidly than most individuals can. Consequently, she serves as an invaluable helper as I set about explaining the basics of psychodynamic therapy and theory. She also serves as a constant reminder of the importance of learning from the patient (Casement, 1985).

The Sweet Child

The Sweet Child was a woman in her late twenties who sought therapy as she approached the end of a master's program. The first session began like this:

T: With what can I help you?
P: *LAUGHS* Big question! I start crying every time I talk about it. But I calm down after a while…
T: Okay.
P: The thing is both my parents are sick. Dad has been ill for a very long time *CRIES*. He was diagnosed with early-onset dementia maybe ten years ago. And then we … uh … me, my mother, and my sister, who are the core of the family, have somehow learned to live with it. It affects him …. Well, physically he's in very good shape. But he has become a completely different person than he used to be.
T: That must trigger a whole bunch of emotions in you.
P: It's very painful *CRIES*. Well, we have somehow managed to learn to live with it.
T: Yes, I'm sure you have.
P: But during the last year my mother has also fallen ill. And so I feel that…
T: What was it again?

P: She's got severe rheumatism. A lot of pain. It's a disease that doesn't kill you, but it's terrible to live with.

T: How does it affect her?

P: She has severe inflammations in her knees. When I was at home this Christmas, it reached a whole new level where she has … she's sixty years old and needed help to get up from the sofa! Because she can't get up on her own!

T: Who helped her up, then?

P: It was me and Dad. So, this Christmas, both of us couldn't go out at the same time. Because if we were away and she had to go to the bathroom, she sort of wouldn't have been able to get up from toilet.

T: So how was it for you to leave home and come back here?

P: Both good and bad!

T: Yes, of course, of course.

P: Yes, that's what it feels like …. I struggle quite a bit with a guilty conscience. How am I supposed to take care of myself, in the middle of all this?!

T: Yes, right!

P: *SIGHS*

T: So, it triggers quite mixed feelings inside you?

P: Yes.

T: Is that what you're here to have a look at? These mixed feelings that give you such a guilty conscience?

P: That would be very nice …. Yes, figure it out a little …. Put it into words, sort through a few thoughts … um ….

T: So, you have a lot of thoughts, too.

P: Yes, quite a lot. And … I don't know. Sort of figure out how I still can be there for my family, but also take a little bit better care of myself.

From the beginning of therapy, the Sweet Child describes grappling with a guilty conscience and contemplating how to take care of herself. In the excerpt above she links these struggles to her parents' illnesses. Later in the session she explains that her difficulties emerged after working extensive hours at a part-time job at the same time as finishing her master's degree. She is a top student and has an exciting job opportunity lined up post-graduation. She also has a fulfilling social life and a loving boyfriend. In an attempt to take better care of herself she decided to quit her part-time job. To her surprise, her symptoms only got worse. She began feeling depressed, numb, and helpless once she had more time to herself. The Sweet Child found herself unable to appreciate and enjoy her social life and academic achievements as she once did.

Notes

1 See, e.g., Patricia Coughlin Della Selva's "blue book" (2004) for the history of ISTDP.

2 Shorten the therapy must be seen in the relation to the length of treatment in classical psychoanalysis, which was the dominant therapy when Davanloo developed ISTDP.

In traditional ISTDP, no predetermined time frames are set, but it is desirable to make the period of treatment as short as possible (McCullough Vaillant, 1997).

3 In this text the terms *psychoanalytic* and *psychodynamic* will be used interchangeably. This is because they are two forms of therapy that are built on the same theoretical foundation.

4 See, e.g., Mitchel and Black (2016) for a comprehensive review.

Chapter 1

The Unconscious

In my days as a student of psychology, I considered the unconscious to be old fashioned, outdated, and speculative, and a subject of interest only to Freud and his contemporaries. My belief was that it was of little relevance to modern psychology. I suppose the reason for this was partly due to the focus on cognitive and metacognitive therapies on the master program in clinical psychology at the Norwegian University of Technology and Science in Trondheim, Norway, where I trained. Little attention was paid in the program to psychodynamic theories and unconscious processes and I also found that the original psychoanalytic literature had an alienating effect on me. The texts were written in a way that confused me, and I found the content speculative and only tenuously relevant—and I don't think I was alone in viewing the literature this way.

When I voiced skepticism about the unconscious to Patricia Coughlin, ISTDP therapist, writer, and clinical educator, and also my mentor over the last decade, she broke into laughter and remarked that if anyone refuted the existence of the unconscious, it would be an intellectualizing psychologist. Patricia commented that every sales, real estate, and advertising professional understood the necessity of appealing to unconscious processes to reach their customers. These professions know that rational forces alone do not determine our preferences for cars, which homes to buy, or which shampoo to choose.

As therapists, our understanding of the significance of the unconscious is just as crucial to our ability to do our jobs. Psychological difficulties are not the product of rational and conscious processes. For instance, the Sweet Child could not simply be told to enjoy her successes and the good things in her life despite her parents' illnesses. She already knew she could! Despite her conscious understanding, this was incredibly challenging for her.

To further understand the unconscious, it is helpful to categorize unconscious processes into two: the normative unconscious and the dynamic unconscious (Weinberger & Stoycheva, 2019).

The Normative Unconscious

Understanding *the normative unconscious* and its processes is relatively straightforward. This aspect of the unconscious is thoroughly described within

DOI: 10.4324/9781003516217-3

cognitive theory and is called procedural memory (Lum et al., 2012). Procedural memory refers to the knowledge we possess but cannot consciously articulate. How do we actually maintain balance while cycling? We cannot rationally describe the intricate movements and shifts in weight that keep us on the bicycle. They occur automatically beyond our conscious awareness; they are *unconscious*. Hence, we do not rely on our conscious brain to observe and rationalize these actions.

Similarly, this applies to various skills we have automated, like handwriting, tying shoelaces, or navigating a roundabout with a car. Of course, it is not impossible to make these actions conscious, at least to a certain extent. If your goal is to learn a different way of tying shoelaces, you will probably succeed. First, you will need to become aware and *conscious* of how you do it today. Then you need to decide what to do differently. After this, you will need to pay close attention every time you are about to tie your laces in order to prevent reverting to the old, automatic pattern. With consistent practice, the new approach becomes automatic and, once again, unconscious.

This means that some actions we perform automatically and unconsciously can be made conscious and then changed, before again becoming automatized and unconscious. This is good news for psychotherapists as the same holds true with psychological phenomena. However, the automatic psychological processes causing mental challenges are seldom as easily altered as tying shoelaces. While some psychological processes may be modified and relearned through practice, for most patients, it is more complex than simply acquiring new knowledge or skills. Why is this? Why can't negative habits easily be changed and reprogrammed? This is where *the dynamic unconscious* comes into play.

The Dynamic Unconscious

The Sweet Child continues:

P: Mom is the second youngest of five siblings, and I'm her youngest child by far. So, when I was born, my mother was already taking care of her parents. And she has been doing this my whole life, because they were actually quite old. I've seen my mother in this caregiver role throughout my life, often visiting them with her, and it hasn't always been pretty. Among the five siblings, Mom shouldered most of the responsibility because the others had their own struggles. And she excelled in that caregiver role. Looking back, I realize that maybe she should have set more boundaries and taken better care of herself. I don't want to repeat what I grew up with, but it feels natural for me to do so!

T: Certainly, she's been a significant role model for you in how to handle these responsibilities. But again … mixed feelings. It sounds like there is a huge conflict in you.

P: Because she's almost always put everyone else first *CRYING*. While it's a nice trait, I believe she took it too far. I don't want to follow in her footsteps. So there's a balancing act, then.

The Sweet Child is a patient with plenty of resources and quite a clear understanding of herself, and she also acknowledges the risk of repeating her mother's behavior. Her mother dedicated her life to taking care of *her own* mother, doing so in a rather self-sacrificing way. The Sweet Child has grasped Freud's concept of repetition compulsion (Freud & Jones, 1922), wherein individuals repeat learned strategies to cope with life, even when these don't yield favorable results. Despite her logical and conscious desire to avoid such a repetition, the Sweet Child could quite possibly end up following a similar path.

Why doesn't she just do as she would if she wished to change the way she tied her shoelaces? Why not simply break out of this pattern? As a master's student with an enormous capacity for learning and an eagerness to face future challenges, why does she think she's incapable of managing this specific problem? Some people successfully navigate caring for sick parents while maintaining a balance, although many undoubtedly struggle. What sets them apart from each other? What is it that makes this particular challenge overwhelming for my patient?

Though there is much she understands, she still finds it difficult. It *feels so natural for her* to emulate her mother. The patient problems exist on an *unconscious* level. There are internal psychological forces that drive her toward actions she *consciously wishes to avoid*. Her attempts to prioritize her conscious desires trigger a guilty conscience. The Sweet Child finds it conflictual and uncomfortable to prioritize herself to the same degree that she prioritizes others.

Psychodynamic theory would suggest that this struggle is caused by *dynamic unconscious processes* (Freud, 1936, 1938). For the Sweet Child, there is something about putting herself before others that is particularly difficult. It goes beyond mere awareness of old habits and attempts to practice new behaviors—it involves dealing with something so painful, unpleasant, and anxiety-inducing that in order to avoid touching upon it she fears that she is willing to make the same sacrifice her mother did. So far, the specific unconscious psychological processes behind this remain unclear. However, certain themes are beginning to emerge: One is an inclination to go the extra mile for those around her. Another is a tendency to mimic her mother's actions.

In psychodynamic therapy, the therapeutic task would be to make the Sweet Child's unconscious struggles conscious (Carveth, 2013), and then process them. Following such a process, she would be free to utilize her abilities to discover new ways of coping with her parents' illnesses.

Hypotheses About the Unconscious

So how can this be achieved? The first step is to begin formulating hypotheses about what remains unconscious. Hypotheses are there to be tested, and they require data in order to be made more robust. In ISTDP, the data collected are the patient's responses to the therapist's interventions (Coughlin Della Selva, 2004). These responses indicate which hypotheses ought to be pursued.

The conversation with the Sweet Child continues. Being the helpful person that she is, she already has some theories about what lies at the bottom of her problems.

P: I realize that I most likely have a long life as a home carer ahead of me. Mom and Dad are both in their early sixties. This isn't something that's going to kill them, it's something that they have to learn to live with.

T: Right. Wow. It's actually pretty complicated what you're saying here, isn't it? Because on the one hand, it almost sounds easier if this was something that was going to kill them.

P: *WHISPERS* Yes.

T: But at the same time, it sounds like you care quite a lot about your parents.

P: *NEARLY CRYING* I do.

T: Right. So, in a way, you want them both dead and alive.

P: Sometimes I think that it would be easier if they were, in a way, seriously ill …. It *is* serious to a certain extent, but … I know that for them it will be perhaps thirty years at most, with decreasing quality of life. And then there's nothing you can do … stand on the sidelines … just … being there. And that, argh, well ….

While she explains, I try to formulate hypotheses about how this is all connected. I am aware that she is depressed, feels guilty about feeling good, and fears being unable to care for herself. She confirms that it would be easier if her parents had severe illnesses that would lead to their deaths. Perhaps if they died, she could live her life freely. But how does it feel to wish one's parents dead? She describes conflicted, contradictory feelings and desires of which she is partly aware. The question the psychodynamic therapist must then ask would be: How does the patient manage these conflicting desires? Is it acceptable for her to consider it easier if her parents would pass away? Or is this thought wrong, unacceptable, and shameful to her?

The Sweet Child acknowledges that for the next thirty years she will have to witness her parents' gradual decline. It is painful to watch loved ones suffer and become debilitated. She has already seen her mother go to great lengths to care for her grandparents in order to alleviate their pain. Could this be why the Sweet Child is uncertain whether she can continue living her own life? Putting her own life first would mean becoming less available for her parents, being less helpful, and rather pursuing things that make her happy. Her conflicts are becoming clearer: she desires to be present in her parents' lives to ease their pain, yet she also yearns to live a life of her own filled with joy and success. How does she navigate these conflicting desires?

Both Conscious and Unconscious

An important observation is that the Sweet Child is capable of discussing these phenomena, and thus she is *consciously* aware of the issues. At the same time, she encounters difficulties in managing her life and fears emulating her mother, despite wishing not to do so. In psychodynamic therapy it is assumed that this is due to *unconscious processes*.

We pick up the transcription again a few minutes later with the Sweet Child explaining that putting distance between herself and her family is by no means straightforward:

P: Anyway, I can't just cut them off; I have to deal with it.

T: Why can't you?

P: We're not that kind of family! *SIGHS* I could make things a little easier, though!

T: So, "we're not that kind of family" sounds like an external ... eh ... demand. Is there something internally that makes you hesitate to cut ties with your parents?

P: Yes.

T: What emotionally stops you from cutting ties?

P: I love them! Oh, I forgot to mention .... A year and a half before I was born, my mother and father lost my older brother to cancer.

T: Oh!

P: So, there were three of us. My older brother, the eldest ....

T: Mm.

P: Then my sister who was born three years after him.

T: All right, so big brother and sister three years older . . . . Was there another brother?

P: No, just the two of them. My brother died of cancer when he was twelve, and I was born a year and a half later.

T: So, you're some kind of a replacement, in some way?

P: Yes, that's what I mentioned during the assessment .... I have this memory from when I was young that my role is to make others happy. Because, like I said ... Mom is the youngest of five siblings. They've always been really close, so the extended group of cousins sort of acted like siblings. But I'm the only one in that generation who didn't lose a brother, a cousin, or a nephew. And then I came and was supposed to be everyone's "sunbeam."

T: And you have fulfilled that role?

P: Yes, always! *LAUGHS* I nailed it! And that's probably why ... I can't leave Mom and Dad. They've already lost one child; I can't inflict ....

Again, the Sweet Child is full of insights on how the different pieces fit together. Her older brother passed away before she was born, and she was born into a family in mourning. The Sweet Child, an empathetic and gifted child, realizes early on that she was born to fill a void, to be the "sunbeam" that would make everyone happy. I try to understand her unconscious: How is her perception of herself and her life mission affected when she feels responsible for others' happiness and with the knowledge that she possibly wouldn't exist if it hadn't been for her brother's death? Could this be affecting her ability to put herself first? Does she live with a complex, unspoken gratitude that she feels must somehow be repaid?

She is also consciously aware that her parents have lost one child and would not be able to bear the loss of another, and that distancing herself from them in order to live her own life would inflict on them another loss. This seems impossible for her: "I can't inflict …." The Sweet Child's thoughts circle around the possibilities of either making a sacrifice of her own life or sacrificing her relationship with her parents. But these are both unsatisfactory choices for her. Again, I try to hypothesize about her unconscious psychological processes. Does she perceive it as an either-or situation—being 100% with or 100% without her parents? Both alternatives will lead to complicated feelings. Could it be that she has become resigned and numb instead of accepting life's unfairnesses and complexities? In that case, no wonder she is depressed! The alternative to numbness and passivity (which she also sees as her problem) is to internalize a realistic view of the world. She must accept and mourn the loss of an uncomplicated life. She must live with her complex feelings and desires: She both wishes her parents were dead *and* she wants to help them.

American writer F. Scott Fitzgerald wrote, "the test of a first-rate intelligence is the ability to hold two opposed ideas in mind at the same time, and still retain the ability to function" (Fitzgerald, 1945, p. 73). This is the psychodynamic project in a nutshell. At its roots lies an assumption about unconscious psychological conflicts that are creating problems for the patient. The therapeutic goal is to make these processes conscious so that they can be handled in a more satisfactory way.

Chapter 2

Internal Conflicts

Central to all psychodynamic and psychoanalytic theories is the belief that humans harbor internal psychological conflicts (see, for example, Killingmo, 1989; Gullestad & Killingmo, 2019; Gabbard, 2017). Being human is inherently complex. We have needs, feelings, impulses, and potentials that do not always align. Yet, living a fulfilling life entails acknowledging and embracing these conflicting forces—the alternative is to use certain strategies to avoid these conflicts. These strategies, known in psychodynamic therapy as defense mechanisms, can quickly become a separate problem. At the heart of the psychodynamic understanding of mental suffering lies the assumption that the sufferer is somehow avoiding dealing with life's inherent conflicts. Hence, psychological difficulties arise as a result of the inadequate management of unconscious internal conflicts.

The existence of internal conflicts is evident when considering the number of people who engage in infidelity. Human beings naturally seek security, stability, and attachment through their relationships (Ainsworth et al., 1978). However, research from the General Social Survey (2012) suggests that a significant percentage of people in relationships—potentially as many as 20%—partake in infidelity. Alongside the pursuit of attachment and stability, individuals may harbor other needs, such as a desire for excitement and sexual exploration, which may not always be met within the confines of a committed relationship. In an attempt to have it all—both stability and excitement—some individuals cheat on their partner. However, infidelity often leads to subsequent problems for those involved: it may manifest psychologically through feelings of guilt and self-punishment, or relationally through the breakdown of the relationship with associated consequences. The endeavor to navigate the internal psychological conflict surrounding these desires can result in both psychological distress and relational problems.

Confronted with internal conflicts, exemplified by conflicting needs for stability and sexual exploration, people try to find solutions; however, not all solutions yield positive outcomes. In the scenario described earlier, the solution gives rise to additional problems and symptoms. The individual trying to balance the need for both stability and excitement through infidelity may experience guilt, marital breakdown, and subsequent feelings of depression and loneliness. Thus, the endeavor to solve the internal conflict inadvertently creates a new set of problems.

DOI: 10.4324/9781003516217-4

The Sweet Child

Multiple Internal Conflicts

In the previous chapter, excerpts from the Sweet Child's therapy sessions were used to elucidate the concept of the unconscious. Many of these excerpts also serve to illustrate the phenomenon of internal conflicts. Considering that psychodynamic therapy aims to address and resolve internal, unconscious conflicts, their dual nature is not unexpected:

P: ... I don't know. Sort of figure out how I still can be there for my family, but also take a little bit better care of myself.

The Sweet Child finds the act of finding a balance between attending to her family's needs yet still taking care of herself to be a complicated one. She is aware that this is related to having a mother who has been a less than ideal role model for managing the competing demands of self-care and familial responsibilities:

P: Because she (*mother*) has almost always put everyone else first *CRIES*. And that's a very good trait. But I think she took it a bit too far. And I don't want to completely follow in her footsteps—so it's about that balancing act.

The Sweet Child's mother went to great lengths to help her own parents, and perhaps went too far. The patient realizes that this has been destructive, but that it is nevertheless a positive quality and has been a part of their family culture. The outcome is a number of internal conflicts for the patient: One is a matter of balancing care for others with care for herself; another is about distancing herself from her family culture and finding her own way in life. The Sweet Child is adept at describing this challenge and conflict:

P: I don't want to repeat what I grew up with, but *it feels so natural for me to do so!*

For most individuals, it can be a challenge to break out of their family's established patterns: they are in our bones—we stay loyal to those closest to us—so it come so naturally to us to do what we grew up with.

The Sweet Child faces a tough balancing act. How can she take care of her mother and father at the same time as looking after herself? With her mother as a role model she has no desire to emulate, this has become even harder. And if she is honest with herself, as she was in Chapter 1, she must live with the insight that a part of her would find it easier if they were terminally ill. One part of her wants her parents, whom she is so fond of, to live and thrive. Another part wishes them dead. This internal conflict gives rise to a turbulent situation.

The Origin of Internal Conflicts

The challenge of breaking free from family patterns has already been discussed; however, for the Sweet Child, this challenge is even more complicated due to the loss of her brother before she was born (see Chapter 1).

P: And that's probably why … I can't leave Mom and Dad. They've already lost one child; I can't inflict ….

T: Right, so then the solution is to either stay close to them, or for them to die early. So that you can be freed.

P: So that's me, then!

T: Yes, that's your conflict.

The Sweet Child realized at an early age that she was destined to be the "sunbeam" that would make everyone happy and help the family through grief. Of course, her parents did not explicitly give her this task—but without her brother's death she would probably never have been born. She emerged into a family in mourning and it is easy to imagine that a cheerful and easy-going child would garner a lot of positive attention, providing desperately needed joy and relief. In this way the Sweet Child helped her family through their grief. Unfortunately, you can have too much of a good thing: This strategy made it challenging for her to address her own negative feelings and difficulties. Her parents already had more than enough emotional burdens in their life dealing with her brother's death. Having to deal with her negative emotions would be a lot more demanding for them than dealing with her positive ones. Subconsciously, the Sweet Child understood this and assumed the task of being a sunbeam.

P: Well, what I've been thinking is … I've always thought that we're a family that has talked a lot about feelings. But … I think we've talked a lot about other people's feelings! *CRYING* And not so much about mine! Because that was, in a way, my role. So the fact that I was supposed to be that sunbeam has probably meant that I, a lot of times … haven't told them how I really feel. So, I've talked about things if it's been in relation to my dead brother. I've also felt a kind of longing for him. So my feelings regarding that and the related sadness, I've been able to tell them about. But I probably haven't talked about a lot of other things. Because for me it implied giving Mom and Dad more worries and more to think about.

T: Okay …. How early did this start? How long have you been doing this? Protecting your mom and dad?

P: Ever since I was little a girl. That's what Mom and Dad say as well: I was a little girl who was really agreeable, never quarreled, and behaved nicely.

The conflict with its origin in her upbringing continues to affect her. She would like to talk to her mother about the role she was given as a child, but at the same time, this becomes emotionally difficult for both of them. The Sweet Child's solution, then, is to push it away and protect her mother:

P: I tried to put into words .... Well, I told my mother .... It was probably this fall sometime that we had quite a nice talk. About the memory I had; I guess I was four or five years old. That my function is to make others happy. But then Mom got so sad! It was terribly painful! That they didn't realize that was the role they imposed on me!

T: How is it for you to see .... How did your mother look, if you picture her face?

P: Mom started to cry and was very upset. She got really tense, and you saw it was hurting her. And I don't want to hurt others! So then we put it to rest, sort of.

T: Did you or she put it to rest?

P: Yeah, I kind of swept it away and just .... Don't be sad. It wasn't what I wanted to achieve by telling her!

Life Events Reawaken Past Conflicts

The Sweet Child has achieved a lot in life. She is well-liked, has a boyfriend she loves, has pursued higher education, engaged in rewarding volunteer work, and has an exciting job waiting for her. However, her problems arise when life events hit a tender spot, triggering her internal conflicts. A powerful force within her believes she should prioritize caring for others and be "the sunbeam." She would also like to live a life where she can focus solely on herself. While this has not hindered her to any significant extent so far in life, now that she has two sick parents, she must actively confront this internal conflict between self-care and caring for others.

P: I remember a conversation we had before Christmas—just before I was traveling home. I spoke to her on the phone, and it had been a really bad day for her.

T: So she told you about that?

P: I'm the one asking! *LAUGHS*

T: You ask about it. Okay!

P: It's my job to make inquiries! *LAUGHS*

T: It's your job to make inquiries! Into these things that you actually don't want to hear about. But that you ought to hear about. Okay.

The Sweet Child's conflict is once again evident. *She* is the one making inquiries, it's not her mother telling. Making inquiries is the Sweet Child's job.

P: Yes! So I asked her, and it had been a bad day. And she was in a lot of pain. And ... sometimes she is very unfiltered and honest. Other times I can tell that she's trying to protect me too.

T: Okay, so she tries.

P: Yes, sometimes. It depends on her current state and where she's starting off.

T: So it depends on her needs and not yours?

P: But sometimes …. Well, I actually think it's about my needs. But if she's having a really bad day, she doesn't have it in her to fake it.

T: So, on those occasions her needs are more important.

P: If it's a really bad day, I pick that up anyhow. But no matter what she does, it somehow feels wrong! Because if she tells the truth, then I'm left with a heavy conscience because I know my mother's in pain. And if she's trying to protect me, by not telling me about how it actually is, I feel like she's not telling me the truth. Then that's wrong too.

Again, it is clear how conflict-ridden the Sweet Child is. She feels guilty for not staying at home when she realizes how bad her mother is actually doing. She also wants to be in the city, studying, and have a good time on her own. At the same time, when her mother has the surplus to protect her, that also feels wrong:

P: I have a sister I talk to, from whom I also get a version. If there's my sister's and my mom's versions of how it has been don't match up … then I realize that, well ….

T: What happens then?

P: Sometimes that makes me feel that I'm being left out of the loop!

T: So if you don't get that information on how bad your mom feels …. If your mom actually manages to protect you and kind of understand that it would be painful for you to know: "She doesn't need this. She has enough to deal with for herself and her exams. I want her to enjoy herself." And you find out through your sister that she's been hiding stuff, then it's almost like she's shutting you out. Rejecting you.

P: Then it feels even worse to be far away!

Tolerating One's Internal Conflicts

As F. Scott Fitzgerald (1945) wrote, the test of a first-rate intelligence entails being able to live with conflicting ideas (that is, internal conflicts) and still maintaining the ability to function. Conversely, if we cannot reconcile conflicting ideas and conflicts, we are likely to encounter problems. This aligns with the psychodynamic theory's view of mental illness: When we refuse to accept and tolerate internal conflicts and instead avoid them, this avoidance often leads to the creation of new problems.

In psychodynamic therapy, practitioners diligently search for internal conflicts, as illustrated by Malan (1979) in his classic book *Individual Psychotherapy and the Science of Psychodynamics*. He presents a variety of cases that demonstrate the tension between external demands and individual freedom—jealousy and idealism, dependence and autonomy, and obedience and rebellion—as examples of the typical nature of internal conflicts explored in psychodynamic therapy.

As a psychodynamic therapist, you will hypothesize that a patient's difficulties stem from internal conflicts. Do you find evidence to support this hypothesis with your specific patient? If so, the goal of a psychodynamic therapy would be to assist the patient in learning to live with their conflicts without resorting to destructive avoidance or becoming overwhelmed by them. The patient then requires assistance in experiencing and tolerating the feelings that are associated with the conflict. As a therapist it is essential to create a therapy process that is emotionally manageable and not overly anxiety-provoking.

For the Sweet Child this would involve coming to agreement that the therapeutic task is to manage the balance between taking care of others and herself, which is one of the major conflicts in her life. An important theme would likely emerge: when she solely focuses on caring for others, she neglects her own well-being. I can help her understand that prioritizing either herself or others can be a way to avoid finding a balance between the two. Additionally, I can assist her grieve the loss of healthy parents, and perhaps help her deal with guilt-inducing anger toward her mother, whom she also loves deeply, but who has not been a model for this balance. She might also need help managing her ambivalence about continuing in her role as the family's "sunbeam." Through this process, the Sweet Child can gain both *understanding* and *insight* into the root cause of the problem, and she can undergo a corrective experience in which internal psychological conflicts are faced rather than avoided.

Chapter 3

Transference

In my review of key terms and phenomena that are crucial to understanding psychodynamic therapies like ISTDP, the focus now shifts to transference. This phenomenon is extensively discussed in psychoanalytic literature, as seen in works by Glen O. Gabbard (2017), and by Siri Erika Gullestad and Bjørn Killingmo (2019), former dean and professors, respectively, at the Faculty of Psychology at the University of Oslo, Norway.

Transference is a phenomenon that many find challenging to grasp. In my job as a teacher and supervisor at the master's program of clinical psychology at the Norwegian University of Science and Technology in Trondheim, Norway, I frequently encounter students who believe that transference is an outdated concept. They perceive this classical psychoanalytic phenomenon as irrelevant for modern psychologists practicing contemporary therapy. Inspired by such perceptions and also by Jonathan Shedler's (2006) text "That Was Then, This Is Now: Psychoanalytic Psychotherapy for the Rest of Us," I aim to emphasize the ongoing relevance of the term. Not only is transference still pertinent, it is also crucial for practitioners of psychodynamic therapy, such as ISTDP, to comprehend. At the heart of psychodynamic therapy is the exploration of thoughts, feelings, and ideas emerging in the therapist-patient relationship (Blagys & Hilsenroth, 2000). Consequently, ISTDP literature consistently emphasizes working in the transference (Abbass, 2015). But to prevent this from becoming merely a detached technique, it is essential to grasp the essence of transference.

The Automaticity of Transference

Imagine encountering a new person for the first time. Your past experiences will naturally influence how you perceive and understand this new individual. It's impossible to meet someone without being influenced by your previous encounters (Shedler, 2006). If you have been let down in the past, you may anticipate further betrayals. Similarly, if you have been surrounded by angry people, you may expect more anger from new acquaintances. An upbringing in a tribal community in Somalia would undoubtedly shape your worldview differently than growing up in bustling Manhattan. Likewise, being raised in a conservative family as opposed to

DOI: 10.4324/9781003516217-5

being part of a liberal community of hippies in the late 1960s could have a profound impact on your perception of sex and sexuality.

Human beings are inherently wired to utilize past experiences in order to anticipate and make sense of new ones. This instinctive process occurs automatically and inevitably (Shedler, 2006) and manifests whenever individuals engage with one another. Naturally, this uniquely human occurrence also takes place within the realm of psychotherapy in the therapy room—and psychoanalytic scholars have coined the term "transference" to describe the phenomenon (Gabbard, 2017). Through their previous relational experiences, patients have acquired a lot of knowledge. This knowledge shapes their perceptions of others and is *transferred* as expectations onto the therapist.

Definitions

Different theorists use slightly different definitions of transference. Jonathan Shedler (2006) defines transference like this:

> The term transference refers specifically to the activation of preexisting expectations, templates, scripts, fears, and desires in the context of the therapy relationship, with the patient viewing the therapist through the lenses of early important relationships.
>
> *(p. 23)*

Gullestad and Killingmo (2019) provide a more complex description of the phenomenon:

> Transference is a psychological process that takes place in several steps in the analytic space. The starting point is that unconscious attitudes linked with inner representations of persons from the patient's past, most often parents, siblings or close caregivers, are activated. These attitudes are displaced onto the patient's inner image of the therapist and the therapeutic relationship. A mixing of representations from the past and the present thereby arises. On this basis the patient perceives and acts in the therapeutic relationship as if a past relationship still existed.
>
> *(p. 37)*

The understanding of transference holds great significance for the psychodynamic therapist. This is due to the fact that these *unconscious* expectations serve as a key to comprehending how the patient navigates their relational difficulties, including the *internal conflicts* that have developed within significant relationships early in the patient's life. If patients expect others to let them down or become angry, they might prefer to keep their distance and not trust those around them. This inclination to maintain distance may have been adaptive if they were raised by a rejecting and aggressive parent—it effectively reduced the risk of conflict and of experiences of being let down. However, assuming that people will betray us can hinder our ability to form secure and intimate relationships in the present. And if a patient thinks that their therapist will let them down or get angry, it will be hard for them to trust and talk openly in therapy. The patient thus *transfers* their old expectations onto the therapist, resulting in a mixing of representations from the past and the present, as Gullestad and Killingmo explain in the definition cited above.

Reactions like these may pose a challenge for therapists. When patients believe that you will betray them, they may struggle to open up to you. However, this also presents an opportunity. As the phenomenon unfolds in the therapist-patient relationship, there is a chance to explore and understand the dynamics behind it and to use the therapeutic relationship as a platform for discovering new ways of relating. This lies at the heart of psychodynamic therapy:

> In psychoanalytic psychotherapy, our patients' perceptions of us are not incidental to treatment and they are not interferences or distractions from the work. They are at the heart of therapy.
>
> *(Shedler, 2006, p. 23)*

The psychodynamic project also involves recognizing when one attributes characteristics of people from the past to those in the present: "That was then, this is now." I might have been surrounded by people who let me down in the past, but that is no longer the case. I no longer have to assume that I will be let down, even if that has been my experience in the past.

Malan's Triangle of Person

In short-term dynamic therapy there is a tradition of schematizing the transference process using the triangle of person. David Malan (1979)[1] was an early adopter of this model to describe transference. The triangle of person is illustrated in Figure 3.1.

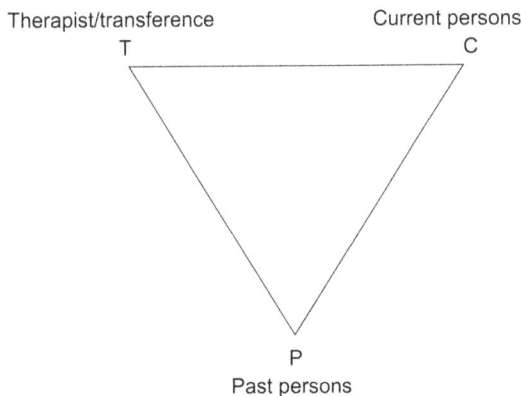

Therapist/transference
T

Current persons
C

P
Past persons

Figure 3.1 The Triangle of Person

The experiences that patients carry with them from their past, particularly from important individuals in their early life (referred to as P for past persons), manifest in their interactions with current individuals in their life (C for current persons). These past experiences (P) are also transferred to the therapist in the transference (T). The triangle of person will be further elaborated upon later in the book in conjunction with the triangle of conflict (Malan, 1979).

The Sweet Child

The conversation with the Sweet Child clearly exemplifies the manifestation of transference in therapy. The following excerpt takes place one hour into the first session, a *trial therapy*, as per tradition in ISTDP, which typically spans a couple of hours (Coughlin Della Selva, 2004). The session has thus far delved into the Sweet Child's feelings of numbness and exhaustion in the face of her challenges, how she experiences diminished joy, a sense of obligation toward her family, and ambivalence toward discussing her struggles. She intricately details how opening up about her personal experiences contradicts her perceived role within the family, where she feels compelled to ensure the well-being of others. An essential aspect of caring for others has involved shielding them from her own problems, leading her to conceal her true feelings.

Hiding from the Therapist

As the session transpires she notices a sense of relief as she opens up about her difficulties, and relatively quickly she reveals how she views me and the therapy relationship through the lenses of her early important relationships (Shedler, 2006).

P: I have always been like .... As soon as I start talking about things, it just feels very liberating, you release tension just by putting things into words.
T: Right?! So right now you feel good feelings for yourself. That is quite important because that's some of what you're saying is difficult for you. Just to be allowed to feel good.
P: *TEARS UP*
T: And there's something happening behind your eyes as well .... So now you have the opportunity to let it through, if you want to. You don't have to be alone with it anymore ....
P: No .... *CRYING*
T: You've been holding it in for so long, you can let it through ....
P: *CRYING*
T: All these painful feelings. You don't have to pull yourself together anymore.
P: That's what I've always done!
T: That's what you've always done! And now you're doing it here with me as well.
P: I only cry in private.

T: You're crying …. Okay …. So in that sense, we can understand why you're looking away and your legs are crossed, and your body ends up in a closed position.

P: Yes.

T: Because this is something you have to do alone. But how is it for you to always cry in private? You've been alone. Alone with all these feelings! Do you want to do the same here with me?

P: Not really. I don't want to be alone with them, but that's …. That's the only way I really know.

The Sweet Child is a highly intelligent young woman who has willingly sought therapy in order to strike a better balance between caring for others and caring for herself. She has expressed a genuine desire to learn new ways of managing her feelings effectively. Nevertheless, she suppresses her feelings when they arise by pulling herself together, *as she has always done.* Her previous experiences of expressing feelings to others are having a significantly impact on her relationship with me as her therapist: She pulls herself together as we interact, only revealing her feelings in private, since *that is the only way she knows.* Her past experiences with expressing feelings have had a profound impact on how she interacts with me when they arise. This is *transference.*

Consequences of Hiding from the Therapist

T: So what exactly happened just now, because it was there. You felt these feelings coming, didn't you?

P: Yes.

T: Then there was something that …. Because now they're gone, do you notice that?

P: Yes.

T: If we rewind a bit, what did you notice happening? What happened on the inside that first made something emerge …. And then there's something that tells you that you shouldn't do this, and now you've ended up here.

P: I feel very vulnerable if I'm going to really cry ….

T: Right. So you could have started really crying here ….

P: Yes, but somehow my body tells me that this is too vulnerable and too open, so please save this for another time. *LAUGHS*

T: *LAUGHS* Yes, let's save this for another time.

P: Yes. And it was like that at the assessment interview as well. I started crying when I talked to the other guy. At least a little. Then I pull myself together and then I go home and then …. Ueehhh. Like, a lot.

T: And again, you ought not to share this with anyone. You have to keep it to yourself. How do you end up feeling? And how would this affect your project here with me? If you're going to use that same mechanism here?

P: It might be a bit destructive … for this project!

T: Yes, it would, wouldn't it?

The Sweet Child realizes that it would be destructive for her progress in therapy, *for this project*, if she continues to pull herself together and only express feelings in private. At best, therapy will offer her intellectual understanding of her issues. However, she will not have the opportunity for new *corrective emotional experiences* (Alexander & French, 1946) in therapy. In the given example, the transformative experience would be *experiencing* that there *actually is a difference* between the past and the present. She *experiences* that her therapist accepts and validates her inner world, which ultimately makes her feel better. It is actually good news that she interacts with her therapist exactly the same way she does with everyone else. This signifies that the underlying mechanisms contributing to her problems are right in front of us, and the Sweet Child and I can work on changing these processes directly within the therapeutic relationship.

New Insight

An important initial step is becoming aware that transference is occurring and that one's perception of the present may be influenced by past experiences. This understanding is exemplified by the Sweet Child, as evident in the following excerpt. She has realized the detrimental nature of relating to me as she has to others. Comprehension of this phenomenon is crucial, not only for the Sweet Child, but for all patients.

P: After I'd been at the assessment interview, and came home crying, and in a way could cry openly on my own, and do that for a little while …. Then, afterward, I felt a bit like …. Hah! It was nice!

T: But you have to do that alone!

P: Yes, that's what I'm used to!

T: Right, that's what you're used to. That's the rule. When it comes to your feelings, they're not for sharing with others.

P: So … I feel that it may have something to do with the fact that many of those I have tried to talk to in the past—that is, friends—they ask in good faith and would like to hear how things are going …. But to be honest, it's too much for them! And then you distance yourself, right? It can be difficult to meet people in grief … in crises and stuff like that.

T: So you are you thinking right now that that applies to me too? Am I able to deal with this?

P: I know that it doesn't actually apply to you, because … it's your job! Well, yes, I think the fact that I closed down earlier when I was about to open up is a kind of behavioral pattern that I've become used to! Because I'm afraid that I'll open up, and then I'll scare the crap out of someone I love.

T: Right, so you …. And these ways of handling yourself, which you have learned … we realize where you learned them, don't we? We understand where it's coming from. So, in a way, it transferred onto me—and suddenly I'm one of those who can't handle this. If you look at me …. I don't know who's sitting here now, for you, who can't handle it. Does it look like I'll be able to handle it?

P: Yes .... It does.

T: How is that for you? If you actually take a look at the person who's sitting here. How is it for you to think—I believe he can handle it.

P: Actually very nice ....

T: Mmm.

P: But also very new ....

T: But it's something new. Yes, it is.

Protecting Others (Including the Therapist ...)

It is vitally important that the patient understands the phenomenon of transferring her old expectations onto the therapist. Only by recognizing that past experiences are distorting her perception of the therapist will it make sense for her to challenge herself to approach the situation differently. In the previous excerpt it was evident that the Sweet Child had grasped this concept, which then allowed us to delve into further exploration:

P: Ugh, yes .... It's a kind of physical barrier. *POINTS TO HER CHEST*

T: Right, sitting here *POINTS TO HER CHEST*. What would you call that? These feelings that tighten up and stop things there?

P: I remember when I was younger, I thought I had a kind of shield.

T: Oh right, like that ....

P: So that people wouldn't, in a way, see how I really felt. So I had like ....

T: So there you have your protection. You protect yourself from ....

P: No, it's not me who protects myself, I protect others!

T: Yes, you protect others! Yes, okay, it's an inner shield, to stop things from getting out! So you're protecting me!

P: Yeah! Yes! Right now, not because I want to, but because it's the only thing I know how to do.

T: Who are you protecting? Who am I right now? Who am I to you? Do you understand the question?

P: Yes .... Or yes and no. I've always protected everyone around me. Family. Friends.

T: Mm .... Right. And are you going to protect me?

P: I realize it's actually really stupid, but .... Yes.

T: You realize that actually .... On the one hand you want to, but on the other, you have quite a few reservations! So I wonder what the two of us can do together, if you want to ... to get past those reservations, to get through this shield, which isn't meant to protect you, but meant to protect others from your feelings! All these mixed feelings. All that grief and love. And all that makes this feel bloody unfair. So there are quite a lot of feelings. So, what can you do right now?

P: Try not to shut down when I notice those feelings coming.

Again, she vividly illustrates her commitment to safeguarding others—even her therapist—from her feelings. At both conscious and unconscious levels, it is as if she has a deep-rooted belief that her feelings would prove excessively burdensome, difficult, and draining for those around her. From childhood she distinctly recalls envisioning a shield protecting those in her proximity. It is noteworthy that she employs the term "shield" itself. Shields are used protect oneself from arrows, swords, spears, and other harmful weapons. Hence, she strives to shield those dear to her from her inner world, ensuring their protection and averting any harm she might cause.

P: When I talk to others while feeling something, be they my boyfriend or friends, when I have to put something difficult into words, or something that has happened, I start to cry when I say it. Because it's so hard to even begin to talk. And as soon as I get going, I can switch it off.
T: So we're up against many, many years of habits here?
P: *NODS*
T: Right
P: So don't take it personally!
T: Do you notice what happened there?
P: Yes, I tried to protect you too!
T: Yes, you did!
P: That's what I do best!

One-Person or Two-Person Psychology?

So far, so good. The therapist and the Sweet Child have reached an agreement that she has a tendency to protect others by concealing her true feelings. She realizes that by protecting the therapist, she could sabotage the whole therapeutic process—something she does not want to do. This mutual understanding is crucial in ISTDP and empowers patient and therapist to collaborate efficiently. For the Sweet Child, this is essential: How can she use therapy to discover a healthier balance between caring for herself and for others if she is prioritizing the therapist's well-being over her own?

But how can one know that she actually means what she is saying? She has a tendency to hide her true feelings! Maybe she realizes that the therapist appreciates it when she *says* she isn't protecting him, unlike how she protects everyone else. Or maybe she has noticed one of the therapist's own difficulties, such as feeling anxious when handling other people's feelings. How can you tell if what happens in therapy is *transference*, meaning how the patient is treating the therapist based on past experiences? There is a possibility that she has accurately perceived something in the therapist!

The fact is that it's impossible to know for certain. Psychotherapy involves testing hypotheses and gathering evidence in collaboration with the patient to either strengthen or weaken the hypotheses that have been developed. In the case of the Sweet Child, several indicators suggest that she encounters difficulties when she constantly puts others' needs before her own: She recounts that her problems began when she had to take care of her mother, she struggles to open up emotionally to others, and she describes how throughout her life she has always had the role of taking care of others. All of these aspects are interconnected, and her statements are consistent. She establishes strong rapport during sessions and comes across as credible.

The therapist must also assess whether they acknowledge their own fear of feelings. If several patients consistently avoid expressing their emotions during therapy sessions, the therapist should reflect on their own role in this dynamic. They should consider seeking supervision and, if necessary, undergo therapy themselves to cultivate a greater sense of safety when confronted with others' feelings. By conducting these kinds of assessments, the therapist can strengthen or weaken the hypothesis regarding whether the observed phenomenon is indeed at the core of the patient's problem or not.

In a compelling series of articles published in the *Journal of the Norwegian Psychological Association*, Flåten (2021) and Gjerde (2021) raise valid concerns about ISTDP and its potential to foster inflexible therapists who fail to genuinely consider a patient's possible concerns or disagreements. These critical observations shed light on a crucial issue that arises when therapists overlook the importance of humility in recognizing that the phenomena they observe are not absolute truths, but rather hypotheses that can be strengthened or weakened. It is evident that adopting a dismissive stance toward patients' concerns is neither desirable nor appropriate in ISTDP or indeed in any other therapeutic approach.

Relational Criticism

Lewis Aron was an early and systematic critic of the classical psychoanalysis view of the therapist's role, a view that has also strongly influenced ISTDP. This perspective highlights that the therapist can actually understand the patient's essential truth and should convey it to the patient.

Aron (1990) was a pioneer in *relational psychoanalysis*, challenging the conventional view of transference as a process solely driven by the patient, unaffected by the therapist. Traditionally, therapists were seen as blank screens for patients to project their unconscious onto (Greenberg, 1986). Aron advocated for a shift away from this one-person psychology framework, explaining phenomena occurring in therapy as only influenced by the patient, that is, from one—1—person. He argued for the adoption of a two-person psychology approach that recognizes the active contribution of two persons, both therapist and patient, to the transference phenomena, emphasizing the need to consider both perspectives in order to truly grasp what is occurring.

Paul L. Wachtel (1981) makes a significant theoretical contribution to this discussion by connecting Piaget's (1952) concept of schema to the phenomenon of transference. According to Wachtel, transference is rooted in our childhood experiences and interactions with those closest to us, molding schemas that shape our perceptions and expectations of others. When encountering new people, such as a therapist, they can be *assimilated* into this pre-existing mental schema, meaning that the patient adapts their schema only to a limited degree when engaging with the therapist. The patient's perception of the therapist is thus mainly influenced by their existing schema. The therapist becomes *assimilated*, or integrated, into the existing schema. Alternatively, the patient could *accommodate*, or adapt, their schema when interacting with the therapist. By doing so, the patient rejects the constraints of their existing schema and embraces characteristics of the therapist that do not neatly fit in. This allows for a more accurate and realistic representation of the therapist.

One of the benefits of this approach is that it introduces the idea that a patient's perception of their therapist does not have to be based solely on their personal history or solely on an accurate understanding of the therapist. The patient brings with them a pre-existing understanding of relationships in the form of a schema. When interacting with the therapist, the patient will assimilate (integrate) the therapist into this existing schema to a certain extent. Some aspects of the therapist will engender accommodations to the schema, and it is through this accommodation that meaningful change can take place in psychotherapy.

This perspective on transference makes clinical sense. The perception that the patient has of the therapist is inevitably influenced by a blend of the patient's personal expectations and the therapist's true attributes, a blend that may vary. When the perception of the therapist is mostly assimilated into pre-existing schemas, it would resemble the traditional concept of transference. Thus, if this perception of the therapist also causes problems for the patient, addressing and working through it becomes a vital component of psychodynamic therapy.

Countertransference

This brings us to another key concept in psychodynamic therapy: countertransference. Early psychoanalytic theory suggested that emotional reactions from therapists toward their patients—especially those that are challenging or uncomfortable—were undesirable (Gullestad & Killingmo, 2019). Such reactions were seen as signs that the therapist had not undergone sufficient analysis, pointing to the need for further psychoanalytic treatment. However, in modern psychodynamic therapy, this view has shifted. As previously mentioned, it is now widely accepted that therapists, being human, inevitably influence the therapeutic relationship. Emotional reactions to patients are not only expected but are considered a natural part of any relationship, including therapy.

This means that both the patient and the therapist will experience transference reactions. Just as the patient transfers expectations from past experiences onto the therapist, the therapist will do the same toward the patient. For example, a therapist who was bullied or excluded as a child might carry an expectation that others dislike them. As a result, they could mistakenly interpret the patient's negative feelings as personal dislike, when in fact, these feelings are a crucial part of the patient's therapeutic process and are unrelated to the therapist personally.

Definition

Gullestad and Killingmo (2019) distinguish between the therapist's transference reactions and countertransference reactions, presenting an updated definition:

> As we define the concept of countertransference today, it refers to the therapist's reactions to unconscious communication by the patient.
>
> *(p. 127)*

The authors make it clear that not all of the therapist's emotional responses are classified as countertransference; only those tied to the patient's unconscious ways of relating to the therapist fall under this term. While the therapist's transference reactions reveal more about the therapist themselves, countertransference reactions offer insight into the patient. According to Gullestad and Killingmo (2019), countertransference is "the royal road to the subtext of human communication" (p. 127). By examining their countertransference, the therapist can gain knowledge that go beyond the patient's explicit communication. For instance, while the patient's words may seem friendly and pleasant, the therapist might notice a feeling of irritation rising within themselves. This reaction, which doesn't align with the patient's outwardly friendly demeanor, could be valuable information, suggesting that there may be hidden aggression beneath the patient's seemingly gentle exterior.

As discussed earlier, it is impossible to be certain whether the therapist's emotional reaction is countertransference or their own personal transference. The therapist, too, has an unconscious mental life that influences the therapeutic relationship, making it difficult to separate the responses rooted in their own conflicts from reactions to the patient's unconscious communication. However, it remains essential—perhaps even crucial for effective therapy—that the therapist maintains a kind and curious inward gaze. This may not only help prevent the therapist's own transference reactions from hindering the patient's growth, but also allow access to insights about the patient that cannot be gained through explicit communication.

Summary

In this exploration of important concepts and foundations of psychodynamic therapy, I have so far detailed the existence of unconscious mental phenomena (Chapter 1). It is often these unconscious phenomena that hinder the patient from resolving their issues on their own, leading them to seek therapy. These phenomena are characterized by internal conflicts (Chapter 2) that, for various reasons, prove too complicated and painful for the patient to effectively manage alone. The patient's ways of coping with these internal conflicts often manifest in the transference (Chapter 3) with the therapist. This gives the therapist an opportunity to directly address the patient's challenges within the therapeutic relationship while gaining insight into the patient's unconscious processes by examining their own countertransference reactions. Profound comprehension of unconscious processes, internal conflicts, and transference is crucial for the therapist to establish a strong working alliance with the patient in ISTDP. Exploring the systematic use of this understanding to construct a therapeutic framework is the focus of Part II.

Note

1 Menninger (1958) was the first to describe the triangle of person; Malan (1979) integrated it with the triangle of conflict.

Chapter 4

Defense Mechanisms

The next psychodynamic phenomenon that is crucial to understand in order to become a skilled ISTDP therapist is *defense mechanisms*. This phenomenon is thoroughly described in the psychoanalytic literature,[1] with Anna Freud (1937) being one of the pioneers. Defense mechanisms are the psychological mechanisms human beings use to avoid anxiety-provoking internal states, such as unacceptable thoughts, feelings, impulses, and desires.[2] The defense mechanisms of significance for the psychodynamic therapist are those that are unconscious, automatic, and create difficulties for the patient. Focusing on the patient's avoidance of difficult internal phenomena is crucial in this type of therapy (Blagys & Hilsenroth, 2000).

Shedler (2006) establishes a parallel between the human psyche, systems theory, and biological processes, as these processes all seek to achieve equilibrium or homeostasis. For instance, when exposed to high temperatures, our bodies instinctively strive to maintain a constant internal temperature by sweating. Sweating serves as a natural defense mechanism against overheating and is crucial for maintaining good health. However, this defense mechanism can also present challenges. If a person remains in a hot environment without hydrating, dehydration can occur, leading to severe consequences, even death. What was initially an adaptive response to a difficult situation has now become a grave concern. The workings of the psyche mirror this pattern. Our psychological defense mechanisms aim to establish a psychological equilibrium, but sometimes, in the pursuit of balance, new problems emerge.

Defense Mechanisms in Everyday Life

The utilization of defense mechanisms is a common and familiar phenomenon. We continuously defend against unwanted inner states, both consciously and unconsciously, in our daily lives. Encountering individuals behaving in ways that we find objectionable is also a regular occurrence. When faced with such situations, we may choose not to directly challenge the person's actions. Instead, we may *knowingly* opt to employ defense mechanisms. For example, we might rationalize the individual's behavior by considering underlying reasons, such as his difficult relationship with his alcoholic father, which helps to mitigate our feelings

DOI: 10.4324/9781003516217-6

of anger. This process of rationalization—understanding and identifying underlying causes—serves as a defense mechanism, effectively tempering our emotional responses.

A group of young men in their twenties gathers together to watch a film. As they are engrossed in the story, one of them suddenly feels a wave of sadness washing over him. Although tears gather behind his eyes, he hesitates to show his vulnerability in front of the other guys. Instead of allowing his feelings to come through, he opts for an alternative route. He consciously shifts his focus to something entirely unrelated, such as the impressive size of their new TV. This deliberate act serves as a defense mechanism, shielding him from impending tears. By redirecting his attention, he creates a necessary distance from his emotional reaction, safeguarding his composure.

In the example above, a defense mechanism is intentionally used to maintain psychological balance and avoid discomfort. Instead of confronting complex situations and unpleasant inner states, the individual in question chooses to avoid them. In this example, the defense mechanism causes minimal or no problems. On the contrary, it may even enhance smooth and successful social interactions. Imagine if everyone openly shared their emotions and thoughts in social situations without any form of self-censorship. It would create chaos and be incredibly wearisome.

Unconscious Defense Mechanisms That Cause Problems

Most of the time our defense mechanisms operate unconsciously, beyond our control. They kick in automatically when we are faced with internal and painful conflicts. Unbeknown to us, we detach from our emotions in an attempt to avoid experiencing the pain.

A child grows up alone with a mother who is depressed. The mother's response to the child's curiosity, laughter, and nagging is often negative. When the child acts independently, helps with household chores, or acts caringly toward the mother, her reaction is usually positive. The child quickly understands what the mother likes, and behaves well to make her happy—for example, by not being too loud or playful. This results in further positive interaction with the mother, on whom the child is completely dependent.

The child comes to the realization that inviting friends over from school or being late home from school isn't worth it. Gradually, looking after the mother becomes a deeply ingrained habit; it becomes second nature, woven into the fabric of daily life. Both positive and negative feelings become tied to the mother's negative reactions, and the child avoids experiencing and expressing them. In this given situation, with a mother who is feeling depressed, this becomes the child's best opportunity to forge a positive bond with their mother. The child's best solution becomes disregarding their own needs and feelings in favor of their mother's well-being.

The problem, of course, is that the child carries the lesson of self-neglect with them into later stages of life. The once effective coping mechanism from childhood no longer proves effective. Once the child has grown into an adult seeking egalitarian relationships, ignoring their own needs will cause problems. Simultaneously, this strategy, or defense mechanism if you prefer, has become automated and is no longer a conscious decision. It's just how they treat themselves, even with people who will tolerate their feelings. The defense mechanism has become part of whom the person is; a part of their personality or *character*. Therefore, in psychodynamic theory such integrated and unconscious defense mechanisms are referred to as *character defenses* (Gullestad & Killingmo, 2019; Kuhn, 2014).

As children we acquire a multitude of skills that become second nature to us as adults, becoming unconscious knowledge. In Chapter 1, I provided the example of tying shoelaces, a seemingly effortless task that still requires conscious effort to alter. This very concept applies to defense mechanisms as well. The defense mechanisms we lean on and incorporate into our daily lives as children persist into adulthood, regardless of the changes in our environment. What may have been an effective strategy to navigate tough situations in our younger years no longer serves us as adults.

The forthcoming extract from the dialogue with the Sweet Child exemplifies this and demonstrates how her unconscious use of defense mechanisms in response to her internal struggle leads to complications.[3]

The Sweet Child

In Chapter 2, I described how the Sweet Child struggled to find a balance between taking care of her parents and taking care of herself. Both her mother and father are seriously ill. At the same time, she has a life she appreciates and wants to live to the full. How can she solve this dilemma?

The upcoming therapy segment begins fifteen minutes into the first session, roughly where the excerpt in Chapter 1 left off. My starting point in this conversation is a psychodynamic understanding of psychological difficulties, which suggests that the way one attempts to resolve internal conflicts can actually create new problems. I am trying to figure out how she handles her conflicts, and how well or poorly her approach works. I wonder what defense mechanisms she uses, and whether these create new problems for her. To find out, I ask her how she copes with her conflicts.

T: It sounds like things are terribly complicated inside you. Could you say a little about how you're coping with this conflict? When you're living with all these conflicting feelings and the role of being the sunbeam. Having your mother as a non-optimal role model, whom you are so fond of, and who has been a home carer herself. Your father, who has been ill for so long. Your mom who is getting sick now—you might spend the next thirty years as their carer. Your life with lots of possibilities; very exciting! It's a massive conflict isn't it?

P: Mmm. *NODS*.

I remind her of what we have talked about. She was born into a family where she was given the role of being the sunbeam. Her father was sick, and her mother had been selflessly taking care of her own parents for a long time. Despite these challenges, she still has a chance of a good life. My assumption is that this is complicated to live with and may contribute to her psychological problems. It will be my job to find out if this assumption is correct.

T: How do manage this? What are the consequences of all this for your daily life? How is it for you on the inside?

P: There are a lot of ups and down. Some days I somehow manage to ... keep it at bay and get quite a lot done. But other days I notice that I become completely ... apathetic. I just can't get started. I can't ... sit down. I'm writing a master's thesis, and then I have a job on the side. I thought about it .... The guy I talked to when I was here last time, he asked me about productivity and stuff like that. If it had affected it. I said that it hadn't. But I've thought about it a lot in the last week, and yes! Actually!

T: So you become apathetic. What else do you notice?

P: Sometimes I notice that I'm becoming a little numb. That it's better not to feel anything than to feel it all the time.

T: Okay. So this is a way of turning off feelings?

P: *WHISPERS* Yes.

T: Of turning off this conflict that we just had a look at?

P: Guess so.

Sometimes, by making a conscious effort, the Sweet Child manages to keep the difficulties at bay. However, there are moments when she fails to do so, rendering herself apathetic and numb in the face of her internal conflicts.

So what is the connection to *defense mechanisms*? Defense mechanisms come into play when our internal conflicts become too anxiety-provoking. The Sweet Child says, "it is better not to feel anything, than to feel it all the time." She notices that making herself passive and numb also makes things easier because then she doesn't have to feel! This is not a conscious strategy but rather an automatic and unconscious response. But despite her lack of conscious awareness, it is still something she does. It is an unconscious defense mechanism that serves to shield her from confronting distressing feelings.

The defense mechanisms she employs serve to disconnect and distance herself from her feelings and internal conflict, helping her to avoid facing them directly. The issue is that when you switch off your emotional life, you become apathetic, devoid of vitality, devoid of energy. And without energy, you become ineffective and have problems with productivity. The way the Sweet Child tries—more or less unconsciously—to resolve her conflict leads to new problems.

The Sweet Child also sees other ways in which she has avoided her internal conflict. She has actually used a number of defense mechanisms:

P: I have also ... ehh .... Last August I quit my job, the one I've had for the last three years, because I was about to hit the wall. I was burning the candle at both ends. I was working very much. I think that was probably my survival tactic. Working A LOT.

T: Okay.

P: And I've always been like that, when I'm at work with colleagues, I manage to leave the difficult stuff at home and that gives me a little break.

The Sweet Child describes how she has tried to distract herself. Instead of taking time to connect with herself, pay attention to her feelings, and reflect on the situation, she has worked to an excessive degree. She has *distracted* herself from her internal conflict, again semi-aware of what she is doing. I summarize what I've comprehended so far to check if we both have the same understanding of how she deals with things.

T: So you have some strategies that make you not have to fully connect to what is inside you.

P: I think so, yes.

T: Working a lot, numbing yourself out, becoming apathetic. Or distracting yourself.

P: Somehow it has …. That apathy came after I quit my job. When I did that, I was sort of forced to actually pay some attention to myself.

She continues to discuss her job and how she attempted to cope with her challenges by working intensely, which ended up having a negative effect on her. Again we see that the defense mechanism she uses causes new problems:

P: That's where I've been working for the last three years, and it's been great fun. But as things got more difficult back home, I kind of …. I just took on all the work I could get! So when something came along, I just, yes, yes, I can take it!

T: It's good that you see that! When there was more to deal with at home, you took on more work. So that's been your way of dealing with it, then.

P: Mmm. Then I realized that it wasn't working, because I got so exhausted! And somehow I wasn't myself anymore. I noticed that I didn't have the energy to be socially active. I actually enjoy working out. And suddenly I didn't. I kind of felt like I had lost myself. So I quit that job to actually force myself to pay some attention to myself. It was a month and a half after I did that, that I realized maybe I should speak to someone, and reached out to you.

T: Okay, so that's when you reached out. So what was happening was that you used work as a strategy to keep difficult feelings regarding …. Did your mom get sick at that time too?

P: Well, Mom has been sick for … uh … actually a year and a half. It progressed very slowly in the beginning and then lately it has progressed awfully quickly.

T: So you quit your job, which had been your strategy to distract yourself, because you saw that it wasn't healthy for you. But what happens then is that when you start to pay attention to yourself, rather than dealing with these complex feelings, you turn off and become apathetic?

P: Yes.

Initially, she uses one defense mechanism—namely, to distract herself by working. She realizes that this strategy is making her so exhausted that she no longer feels like herself. Saying yes to everything to distract herself from what is difficult on the inside does not solve her problem. Hence, when she stops distracting herself, the conflict is still there. Then another defense mechanism kicks in, one that is unconscious, which is about detaching from herself. She observes the outcome of this mechanism as apathy, numbness, and emptiness, yet she is unaware of the unconscious actions leading to these symptoms. That is why she is asking for help.

Malan's Triangle of Conflict

The Sweet Child has employed defense mechanisms to distance herself from her internal, unconscious conflicts. These conflicts revolve around the dilemma of how to confront her parents' ailing health and their need for assistance. Instead of embracing this new reality, she has consciously distracted herself with work and unconsciously numbed out her feelings. She has evaded facing the conflict, neglecting to seek a constructive resolution. This begs the question: What other options exist? If she were to confront this conflict head-on, what are the psychological implications?

David Malan, a British psychoanalyst, is a valuable resource when it comes to comprehending alternatives to using defense mechanisms. Malan played an instrumental role in the early development of short-term dynamic therapy (Malan, 1979), pioneered his very own Brief Psychotherapy (Malan, 1963), and served as the ghostwriter for the renowned ISTDP classic, *Unlocking the Unconscious* (Davanloo, 1990).[4]

One of Malan's (1979) key arguments is that psychological conflicts manifest themselves through complex feelings. These feelings come to the surface when the patient is confronted with a situation that triggers their conflicts. In order to evade the conflict, the patient uses defense mechanisms. Drawing upon Ezriel (1952), Malan developed a triangle to visualize the connection between feelings that have become anxiety-provoking due to being associated with a conflict, and the defense mechanisms employed. This conceptual tool, known as the triangle of conflict (see Figure 4.1), serves to elucidate the interplay between these elements.

Impulse/Feeling

At the bottom of the triangle of conflict is impulse/feeling, marked I/F (see Figure 4.1). These are the primary feelings that are connected to the conflict, each accompanied by specific impulses (Normann-Eide, 2020). Feelings in this context are defined as the internal, physiological activations we experience when we are

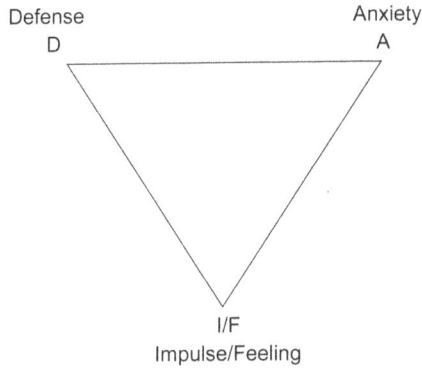

Figure 4.1 The Triangle of Conflict

emotionally triggered. The impulse is the action tendency triggered when we are physiologically activated by the feeling. The easiest way to understand this is through an example:

The Sweet Child explains the challenge of taking in the positives in her life while struggling with feelings of guilt. It is difficult for her to prioritize her own well-being and live a fulfilling life filled with joy. *Joy*, as described by Normann-Eide (2020), is a powerful feeling that is experienced physiologically as energy, vitality, spontaneity, and a zest for life. It ignites a natural impulse to smile, laugh, and cultivate even more joy. However, experiencing happiness and wanting to laugh becomes complex when a loved one is facing serious illness and needs our support. In such situations, we often find ourselves grappling with grief. *Grief* is experienced in an intensely physical way, causing a heavy sensation in the stomach and throat. It triggers an impulse to cry and seek solace from someone close, as Normann-Eide (2020) explains. When someone is emotionally close to us, we naturally feel *love* for them. Love manifests physiologically as a sense of calmness, well-being, and often warmth and relaxation. It brings up an impulse to do something good for our loved ones. To further understand the physiology of emotions, their associated impulses, and their original adaptive function, refer to Table 10.1. Further insights on ISTDP's perspective on feelings can be found in Chapters 10 and 15.

Wanting to prioritize self-care and simultaneously feeling the need to mourn and take care of loved ones can be a complex and paradoxical situation. Prioritizing oneself above those who are ill often leads to feelings of guilt. *Guilt* manifests as restlessness, pressure on the chest, and stomach pain, causing immense distress and prompting a strong desire to maintain one's sense of community and connection with others (Normann-Eide, 2020). Conversely, prioritizing others before oneself can compromise personal well-being and subdue positive feelings. The Sweet Child carries within her an internal conflict that gives rise to a web of intricate and conflicting emotions.

Anxiety

What happens when we have internal conflicts that arouse conflicting emotions? It causes an unpleasant feeling with physical symptoms such as muscle tension, increased heart rate, upset stomach, and trouble concentrating. These uncomfortable bodily sensations are symptoms of anxiety and are marked *A* for *Anxiety* on the triangle of conflict (see Figure 4.1).

The human body reacts physiologically to what is perceived as a threat. In the Sweet Child's case, the threat is to her psychological balance, which triggers an alarm signal to restore equilibrium, as in other biological systems (Shedler, 2006). Freud (1936) referred to these signals that announce impending danger as *signal anxiety*. Anxiety is a *signal* that we are psychologically engaged with something that is both threatening and filled with conflict.

If the therapist observes that the patient is becoming anxious, it would be a signal that they are nearing the core of the unresolved internal conflict. In psychodynamic therapy, the goal is to assist the patient in resolving their internal conflicts, as explained in Chapter 2. At the same time, the patient is presented with a dilemma: Should they allow themselves to shine their spotlight on the conflict, to become familiar with it, even if it provokes anxiety and unease? For the patient to be willing to do this, a good working alliance is required (Bordin, 1979). When the patient chooses to confront their anxiety and delve into the conflict, it becomes an imperative aspect of the therapeutic endeavor to ensure that the anxiety does not escalate to an overwhelming level.[5]

In everyday speech, anxiety is commonly described as both thoughts and as bodily sensations. In ISTDP, anxiety is defined as the physiological response that arises within us when we confront a perceived threat (Coughlin Della Selva, 2004). The activation of the somatic and autonomic nervous systems controls these bodily responses, which typically include tension, heavy sighing respirations, restlessness, palpitations, flushing, sweating, nausea, blurred vision, and dizziness.[6] Human beings dislike feeling anxious and try to avoid anxiety-inducing situations.

Defense Mechanisms

The Sweet Child's mixed feelings (I/F) make her uncomfortable and anxious (A). To avoid this discomfort, she employs *defense mechanisms (D)*. *Defense mechanisms* are marked with *D* for defense (see Figure 4.1) in Malan's (1979) triangle of conflict.

The defense mechanisms used by the Sweet Child, and also the situations in which she employs them, are becoming clear. Figure 4.2 illustrates what has been discovered so far in the conversation.

The Sweet Child does good things for herself even if her parents are ill. This is *the situation* (see Figure 4.2) that sparks mixed feelings in her, such as joy, grief, love, and guilt (*impulse/feeling—I/F*). Experiencing these conflicting feelings is

Symptoms: Numb, tired, indifferent, unproductive

Distraction	*Defense*		← Anxiety	*Anxiety*	Tense muscles

Distraction
Overworking   *Defense*   ← ———————— *Anxiety*   Tense muscles
Detachment   D   A   Rapid pulse
                                                                            Restlessness

Situation: ——————————→   I/F
Do good things for herself   *Impulse/Feeling*
even if her parents are ill   Joy, grief, love, and guilt

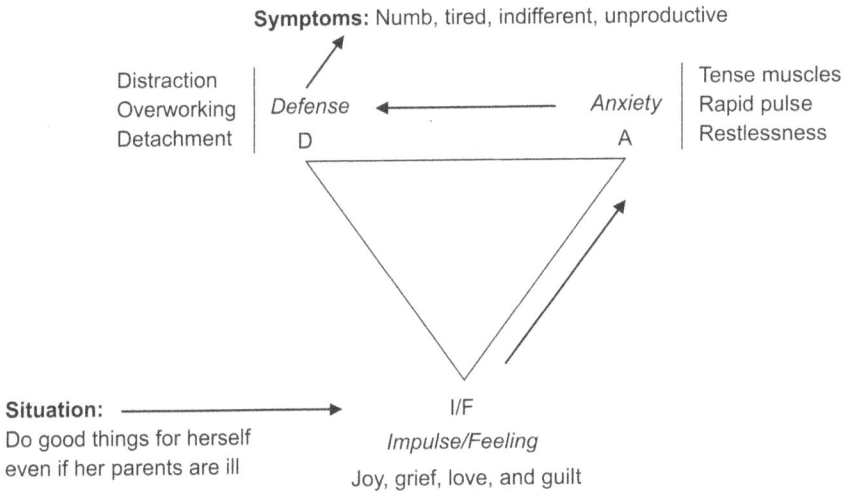

Figure 4.2 The Triangle of Conflict applied to the case of the Sweet Child

causing her considerable discomfort and anxiety *(anxiety—A)*, which manifests as tension, rapid pulse, and restlessness. To cope, she resorts to defense mechanisms like distraction, overwork, and detachment *(defense—D)*. However, relying on these mechanisms gives rise to her symptoms, leaving her feeling drained, numb, indifferent, and unproductive. In her pursuit of psychological balance, she inadvertently creates additional challenges for herself.

The Sweet Child

The Sweet Child is seeking therapy because she feels numb, indifferent, lacks energy, and is being unproductive in her studies. These symptoms are a consequence of defense mechanisms such as distraction and detachment. In ISTDP, the therapist aims to help the patient experience conflicting feelings while not being overwhelmed by anxiety, in order to resolve internal psychological conflicts. If this is achieved, the patient will no longer need defense mechanisms and the symptoms should go away.

In Chapter 3, I discussed the unique opportunity that arises when the psychological phenomena that cause problems are present in the therapy room. This gives the therapist and patient a chance to process these issues while they are actually taking place. In the upcoming pages I will demonstrate how the Sweet Child uses defense mechanisms during the therapy session. The Sweet Child reacts when I stay quiet and don't say anything. She becomes frustrated and starts to lose faith in my ability to help her. I remind her of her boyfriend, who also goes silent when she tries to express her feelings. As a result, she feels angry with him and with several others who are unable to accept her the way she would like.

Laughter as a Defense Mechanism Against Anger

Anger is a feeling that plays a crucial role in providing us with the energy needed for healthy self-assertion and self-care behaviors (Normann-Eide, 2020). Central to the Sweet Child's struggles are difficulties in asserting herself and expressing her needs; consequently, when she feels angry, I see it as a positive. I curiously inquire into whether she relates to this feeling and the energy it provides, in a constructive way.

T: Who is making you angry by not helping you?
P: I can think of several people. *FIDDLES WITH HER FINGERS*
T: Does anyone in particular come to mind?
P: *SIGHS* My sister.
T: OKAY. Please tell me more ….
P: She's a trained medical doctor, for better or worse. And sometimes, when I try to talk to her about all these things, it feels like my sister disappears. She brings out Dr. Lise, as I call her, who is sort of the professional version of her.
T: What do you feel toward her then?
P: I get angry, because it …. *SIGHS* It feels condescending!
T: So she's condescending toward you. How are you experiencing that anger right now? When you imagine her being condescending by becoming Dr. Lise?
P: I tense up here! *POINTS TO HER SHOULDERS*. Ahhh! Sitting up in the chair completely differently! *STRAIGHTENS UP*. I notice that when I thought of her, I became like—argh!

The Sweet Child says that she gets angry and tenses up in her shoulders. She straightens up in her chair and raises her voice. This is a sign that she allows herself to feel the self-assertive energy that we call anger. Many find this feeling difficult to experience, partly because they confuse the *feeling* of anger with aggressive *behavior*. I therefore wonder if she allows herself to feel and experience this feeling. The alternative is that it will give her anxiety, which would motivate her to use defense mechanisms (see Figure 4.1).

T: Mmm. What do you notice then? If you're really going to allow yourself to experience these feelings, so that you can get to know them?!
P: *SIGHS* *LAUGHS* Oh, I'm so not used to this!

I ask her what she experiences when she gets angry and the Sweet Child laughs and says she is not used to this. When she laughs, her anger seems to subside. Thus, the Sweet Child defends against her anger by laughing it away. Rather than facing her anger in the session, she relies on laughter as a defense mechanism. She also mentions that anger is an experience she is not used to, and her anxiety about the feeling becomes evident in her heavy sighs and fidgeting. This interplay of feelings, anxiety, and defense can be shown through Malan's triangle of conflict as depicted in Figure 4.3.

Laughs | *Defense* ⟵——————— *Anxiety* | Tense chest (*SIGHS*)
D   A | Fiddling (restlessness)

Situation: ——————————⟶   I/F
Perceiving her sister   *Impulse/Feeling*
as condescending   Anger

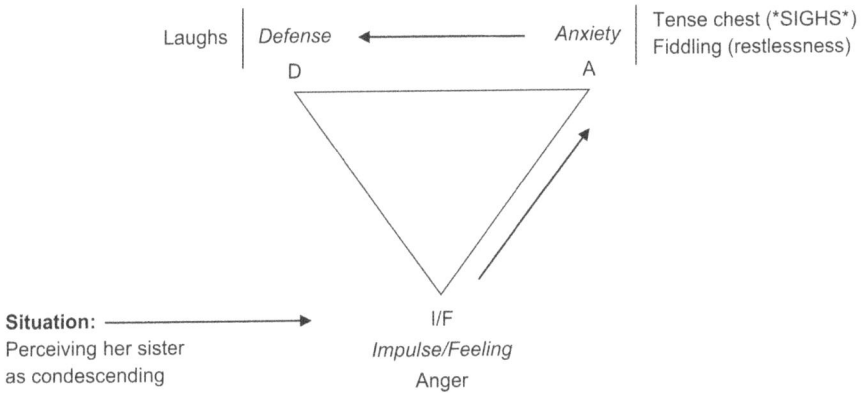

Figure 4.3 The Triangle of Conflict applied to the case of the Sweet Child

Weeping as a Defense Mechanism Against Anger

Even though she laughs it off, her body posture tells me that anger and irritation are not far away. I invite and challenge her again to let her feelings through, even if it feels unfamiliar to her.

T: Sure. And if you let yourself experience this anger toward your sister—Dr. Lise?!

P: Ah! She's so annoying! Really annoying! Her jargon changes completely and she starts using medical terminology. And suddenly, it feels like my sister disappears. *SIGHS*

P: *TEARS UP*

T: So that's what she does. But now tears are coming to your eyes. What happens to your anger as the tears come?

P: Eh …. My anger …. If I get really angry, I start to cry.

T: How is that for you?

P: I've never really been able to clearly express anger.

T: How is it for you when you start crying? Is it okay for you? Do people take you seriously?

P: *SIGHS* Not at all!

Sometimes it can be challenging to determine whether tears are an expression of the emotion of grief, a necessary feeling for humans to navigate through loss, or if they are weepy tears that function as a defense against anger and cause complications. The key to unraveling this is through asking the patient. In the present case, the Sweet Child explicitly states that her tears are troublesome. As she begins to cry and becomes weepy, her anger becomes subdued, making it arduous

Symptom: Not taken seriously

Weeping | *Defense* ⟵———————— *Anxiety* | Tense chest (*SIGHS*)
         D   A   Fiddling

Situation: ————————⟶   I/F
Perceiving her sister   *Impulse/Feeling*
as condescending   Anger

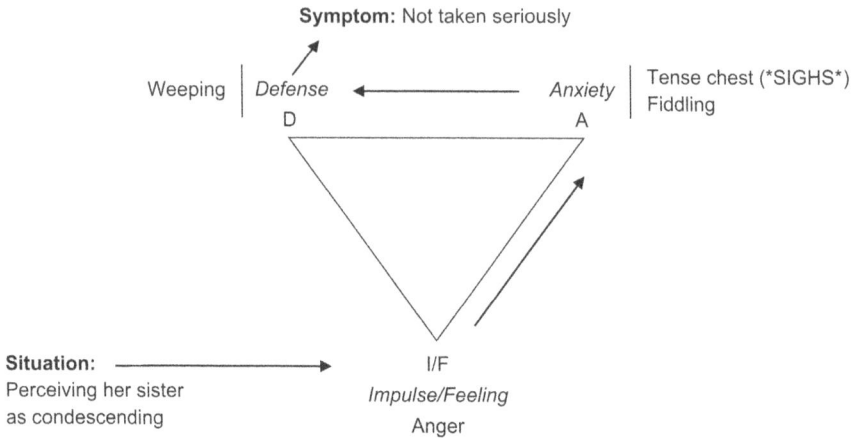

Figure 4.4 The Triangle of Conflict applied to the case of the Sweet Child

for her to effectively express this feeling. As a consequence she does not feel taken seriously in the manner she desires (refer to Figure 4.4).

Self-Attack as a Defense Mechanism Against Anger

Weeping in the face of anger is a familiar response in her daily life, and it also becomes evident during the therapy session. However, this response leaves her without the energy that anger would give her to assert herself properly. When this happens in therapy, it presents an opportunity for us to address and work with this mechanism in real time. I am fully aware that the Sweet Child has plenty of internal resources. Is it within her ability to halt the tears through sheer willpower? Once again, I challenge her to experience and explore her anger in our session together.

T: Okay. So let's see if we can do something about that. How do you notice this anger, if you don't wash it away with your tears? This anger toward your sister?

P: *SIGHS* I'm angry because she bring out Dr. Lise to handle this whole situation so much better than I can.

T: Okay, so there's a bit of envy too?

P: Mmm.

T: How do you feel this anger toward her … for her … using Dr. Lise, both to distance herself from you and to deal with it … One more person who is better off than you. How do you experience this anger toward Lise?

P: *HOLDS HER HANDS AROUND HER NECK AS IF TO STRANGLE HER-SELF* It's like this … here.

T: Right. But that's your anger turned back on yourself, it's you strangling your-self, do you agree?

P: *NODS* Mmm.

A common defense mechanism when feeling anger toward loved ones is to redi-rect it toward oneself. In order to avoid feeling anger toward someone you deeply care for, you convince yourself that it must be your fault. You start blaming your-self, thinking that it was something you said or did that caused the trouble. By doing so, you take the blame away from the person who is actually the target of your anger, and this helps to diminish the intensity of the anger. This is what the Sweet Child is doing here. Instead of allowing herself to experience anger toward her sister, Lise, she takes a stranglehold on herself. She literally strangles her feel-ings and words.

The Consequence of the Defense Mechanisms

As the therapy session progresses the Sweet Child begins to realize how she avoids her anger, and that it is having negative consequences on her life.

P: I'd like to be able to tell and show her that I'm angry! I can't show that feeling! *TEARS UP*

T: So if we keep reality out of here for a little while. Let's see in your imagination what it is you want to show her. What's inside you?

P: *FIDDLES RESTLESSLY*

T: If you allow yourself to take your feelings seriously? This isn't about what you're going to say to Lise in reality, but about what's inside of you. Because that's why we're here; to get to the bottom of all your complicated feelings. And we hear that you're quite angry with your sister.

P: *SIGHS*

T: And we see that rather than …. First you strangle yourself when feeling anger toward your boyfriend, then you strangle yourself when you're angry at your sister. We see your hands go like this *I MIMIC A STRANGLEHOLD ON MY-SELF*. So who makes you angry? It's Lise, isn't it?

P: *NODS*

T: And who ends up suffering?

P: *WHISPERS* Me ….

In this segment, the Sweet Child comes to realize something significant. Laughing off her anger, weeping it away, and turning the anger on herself only leads to her suffering in the end. Instead of experiencing her *feelings* toward her sister (referring to experiencing anger on a physical level, not resorting to ag-gressive behavior), she engages in self-destructive actions that bring her nothing but distress.

Detachment as a Defense Against Anger

T: So what can you do with that pattern right now? What can the two of us do—me and you?

P: Dig into it .... *SIGHS*

T: So if you were to let this out .... If you allow yourself to really let it out right now .... How do you experience it in your body? If you're not going to take it out on your throat?

P: Now I'm getting numb. I don't feel anything.

T: Isn't that interesting?

P: Yes.

T: The numbness arrived. The reason you came here.

P: When you asked, it was a bit like .... I don't feel anything! Nothing in my body! I think I'm very good at thinking, not so good at feeling!

For a little while the Sweet Child doesn't laugh in response to her feelings, and neither does she weep. She makes a conscious effort to stop herself from choking her experience of anger and to overcome the defense mechanisms which during the session she has now become aware of. Then suddenly one of the symptoms she came to therapy for appears: she becomes numb. She realizes that when confronted with her anger, she unconsciously suppresses the physical sensation of energy and empowerment that accompanies such a feeling. Automatically, she turns to the defense mechanism *detachment*, with the consequence that she becomes numb. The task at hand is to help her become more consciously aware of all of this and then take action to address the automaticity of these defense mechanisms. Figure 4.5 shows this schematically using the triangle of conflict.

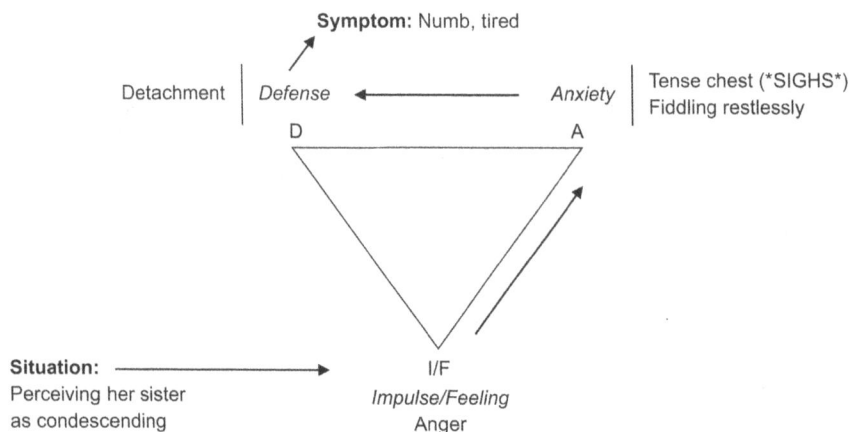

Figure 4.5 The Triangle of Conflict applied to the case of the Sweet Child

In this chapter, I have discussed defense mechanisms and emphasized their role in avoiding unconscious conflicts. The purpose of defense mechanisms is to maintain inner balance; however, they can often lead to trouble. This sets the stage for the next chapter, which delves into the ways psychodynamic theory and therapy comprehend psychological symptoms and suffering.

Notes

1 See also Blackman (2004) and Vaillant (1992) for thorough reviews of the psychodynamic understanding of defense mechanisms.
2 This definition of defense mechanisms is based on Freud (1962), Coughlin Della Selva (2004), and Frederickson (2013).
3 Read Chapter 4 of the book *Co-Creating Change* by Frederickson (2013) for a detailed explanation of how defense mechanisms are understood in ISTDP.
4 At the 2022 IEDTA conference in Venice, both Ferruccio Ossimo (2022) and Patricia Coughlin (2022a) described the close collaboration between David Malan and Habib Davanloo. Malan wrote *Unlocking the Unconscious* (Davanloo, 1990), which presents Davanloo's ideas, but did not claim credit for his contribution to the book.
5 Please refer to Chapter 14 for further insights on regulating anxiety. Much has also been written in the ISTDP literature about the regulation of anxiety. For instance, notable works include Frederickson (2013, 2020) and Abbass (2015).
6 In Chapter 2 of *Co-Creating Change*, Jon Frederickson (2013) provides a comprehensive review of the relationship between the different nervous systems and symptoms of anxiety.

Chapter 5

Symptoms

It is common to see reports in the media that the number of people with mental health problems is increasing (Bazaz et al., 2021). According to the Norwegian Psychological Association (2022) website, half of Norway's population will experience mental illness at some point in their lives. The association defines mental disorder as mental distress of such an intensity that it can be diagnosed according to the guidelines of ICD-10 (WHO, 1992). All the sources above describe mental disorders as something a person has, gets, or suffers from, and that they can be diagnosed like other types of illness.

The ICD-10 is the World Health Organization's manual for classification of diseases, mental disorders included. The manual describes mental disorders similarly to physical illnesses, and categorizes diagnoses on the basis of observable symptoms in the patient. This way of understanding illness is often called *the medical model* (Huda, 2019). The medical model has some advantages. It makes communication, research, and teaching about mental disorders easier. It can be stated that the patient has been diagnosed with depression, that research has been conducted on methods for treating depression, and that it is possible to both teach and learn these techniques. ICD-10 serves as a reference guide that provides detailed descriptions of depression and outlines the symptoms associated with this diagnosis. This approach to understanding mental disorders is effective when using methods such as cognitive therapy, with specific treatment manuals for diagnoses like depression, social phobia, and panic disorder (Wenzel, 2021). The symptoms and diagnoses are seen as diseases to be treated and eliminated.

Psychodynamic Understanding of Symptoms

Psychodynamic theory offers a unique approach to understanding mental illness. According to this perspective, depression and anxiety are not *illnesses* that require treatment. The symptoms, however, are directly correlated to the way in which the patient engages with their inner self and their psychological conflicts (Gabbard, 2017; Gullestad & Killingmo, 2019). When helping the patient with their suffering, the therapist seeks to understand the *underlying psychological processes that lead to symptoms*. Symptoms occur when the patient's internal conflict is

DOI: 10.4324/9781003516217-7

managed in a way that causes complications; as a consequence, emotional symptoms and ailments make psychological and phenomenological sense and are not at all random—on the contrary, they are directly related to whom the patient is, their available internal resources, and the coping strategies to which they resort.

This does not mean that the psychodynamic therapist is unable to help the patient to alleviate their symptoms. An increasing body of research demonstrates the effectiveness of psychodynamic therapy in addressing common symptoms of mental illness. In his classic article "The Efficacy of Psychodynamic Psychotherapy," Jonathan Shedler (2010) presents a range of scientific studies demonstrating the positive impact of psychodynamic therapy. Several studies published more recently, such as Steinert et al. (2017) and Leichsenring et al. (2015), also support this form of therapy's positive effects on psychological symptoms. The path to relief from symptoms does not, however, involve addressing the symptoms directly. Instead, it entails assisting the patient in managing their underlying unconscious conflicts in constructive ways.

As described in Chapter 4, Malan's (1979) triangle of conflict (see Figure 5.1) illustrates how psychodynamic therapy explains symptoms. When symptoms occur, they arise because a specific *situation* triggers *feelings and impulses* that are interconnected with an internal, unconscious conflict. These feelings are complicated and thus cause *anxiety* and discomfort. Sometimes, this very anxiety will be the problem the patient seeks to solve in therapy. In such instances, symptoms may manifest as bodily pain, tense muscles, palpitations, nausea, perspiration, dizziness, and more. The patient's symptoms are physiological symptoms of anxiety that are triggered by complex emotions.

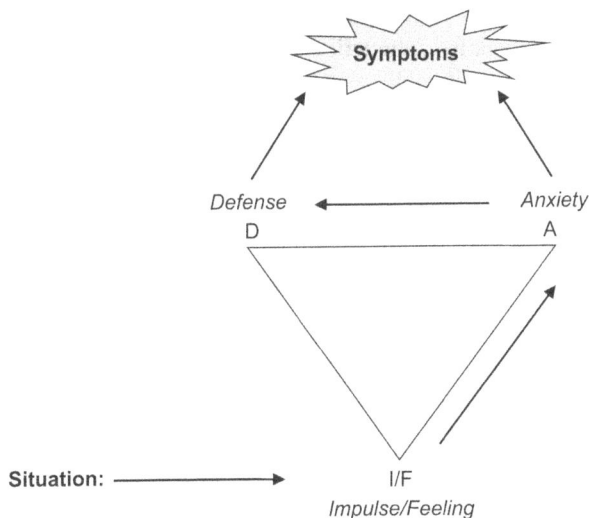

Figure 5.1 The Triangle of Conflict and its Relationship to the Symptom-Generating Situation and Resulting Symptoms

The patient may also try to avoid the anxiety that their feelings trigger by resorting to defense mechanisms. However, some defense mechanisms can engender new problems and lead to additional symptoms. This concept is illustrated in Figure 5.1.

To understand what is meant by the phrase "symptoms make psychological and phenomenological sense," let's consider a few examples.

The Depressed Alcoholic

The Depressed Alcoholic was a 43-year-old man who sought help due to his battles with depression and an emerging alcohol issue. He expressed sensations of weakness, guilt, and worthlessness, alongside a lack both of motivation and momentum to act, all of which are common symptoms associated with depression. Activities that previously brought him joy were now failing to bring him any pleasure, and this had persisted for the past three months. Additionally, he had difficulty falling asleep and often woke up early. To cope with his sleep troubles, he resorted to consuming a bottle of wine before going to bed, a result of gradually increasing his alcohol intake over the past six months. He confessed that this routine was an attempt to find solace and achieve some sleep, a pattern he had experienced a couple of times in the past.

Based on this description of symptoms, the patient met the criteria for the following diagnoses according to ICD-10: F33.1 Recurrent depressive disorder, current episode moderate and F10.1 Harmful use of alcohol (WHO, 1992). Taking into consideration the medical model (Huda, 2019), it would be appropriate to initiate treatment for depression. This may involve the administration of antidepressant medication (Cipriani et al., 2018) and cognitive therapy for depression, with a focus on challenging negative automatic thoughts and promoting behavioral activation (Wenzel, 2021). Additionally, due to the alcohol abuse, a gradual withdrawal from alcohol would also be recommended. According to the diagnoses and current research, the patient would likely benefit from this treatment approach. However, it is important to acknowledge that the effectiveness of antidepressant medication is moderate at best when compared to talk therapy (Shedler, 2010).

Psychodynamic Understanding of Symptoms

When conducting psychodynamic therapy, I begin with an alternative approach. My belief is not that he suffers from the illnesses of depression and alcoholism but rather that he is grappling with an internal conflict that he is struggling to address. Therefore, I need to gather more details than those described above. As a psychodynamic therapist I am not focused on identifying his symptoms alone—I aim to develop hypotheses about the unconscious internal conflicts that are at the root of his symptoms so that I can help him address the underlying causes of his suffering. Such hypotheses are essential to developing a collaborative, psychodynamic project between therapist and patient.

He had already given me several indications of where we could initiate the investigation of his issues. He began drinking six months prior to commencing treatment. What had occurred half a year ago? Why did he start drinking like this? Three months before seeking treatment, he began experiencing symptoms of depression. What had taken place three months prior that triggered them?

Six months before he began therapy, his wife of fifteen years made the decision to file for divorce. When questioned about his feelings, he nonchalantly responded, "It's okay, I suppose I wasn't surprised." He furthermore revealed that his ex-wife had moved in with a new man three months ago. Once again, he expressed that it was okay, stating, "She must be allowed to do as she likes." So, here is a man who was abandoned by his wife for another man. Although he claimed to be fine, he began drinking and became depressed around the same time that this happened. Although it cannot be definitively confirmed that these events and symptoms are related, as a psychodynamic therapist I incorporated this information into the ongoing formation of my hypothesis.

He also disclosed crucial information when I inquired about his symptoms. He mentioned that he had experienced depression several times before, which led to the diagnosis of *recurrent* depression. A medical perspective on recurrent depression would describe it as a condition characterized by episodes that come and go, possibly due to its chronic nature or the patient's enduring biological susceptibility to the illness. In psychodynamic therapy it is crucial to explore what may have preceded these depressive episodes. Is it possible that something similar had occurred on these occasions, triggering an internal, unconscious conflict that he had struggled to confront?

In the session with the Depressed Alcoholic it became apparent that his first episode of depression occurred during his second year of high school. Coincidentally, his parents divorced during the same period, and his father entered into a new relationship. The second episode of depression surfaced in his mid-twenties after a significant breakup. It was evident that he had experienced turmoil in close relationships prior to his depressive episodes. While the correlation could be coincidental, I collaborated with the patient to develop a hypothesis to explore this connection further through investigation.

The Precipitating Trigger to Symptoms

After his wife left him, things seemed to go well for the most part, and he managed to function effectively at work. Their relationship had not been particularly close, he realized. However, as evening fell, he was overcome by feelings of loneliness and sadness. He found this experience quite distressing, as it would cause palpitations, make him tense, and lead him to wander around restlessly. The thoughts that kept recurring were that he should regain his composure and continue living as he did before the breakup. He became aware that he felt better whenever he consumed alcohol. Put into Malan's triangle of conflict, it would look like Figure 5.2.

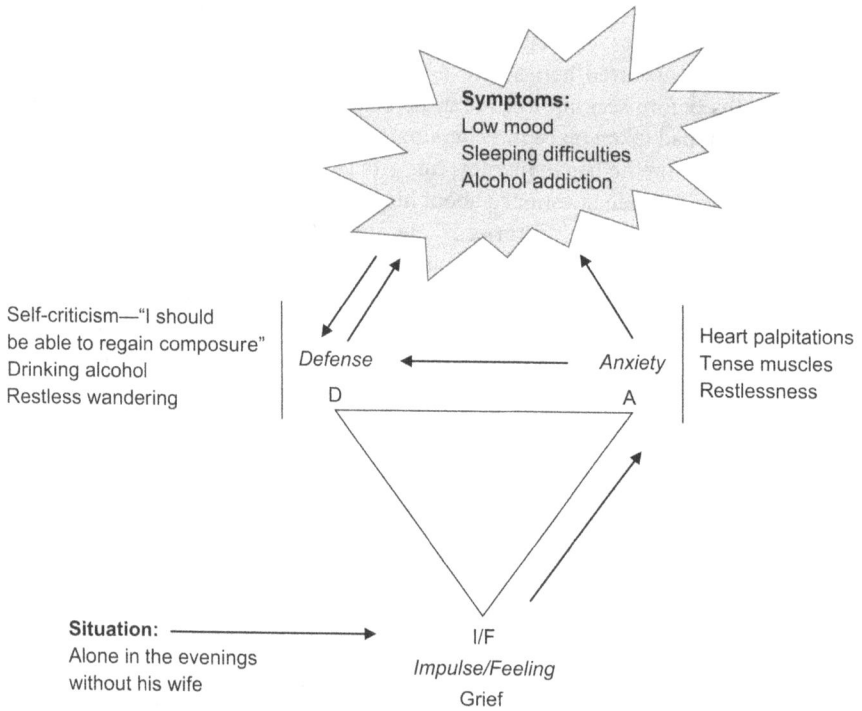

Figure 5.2 The Triangle of Conflict applied to the case of the Depressed Alcholoic

When his wife started dating the new man, he once again became restless, tense, and sensed his pulse increasing. He ruminated on his inferiority compared to the new man and fixated on the guilt he felt about the breakup, as he had devoted himself to his work over the years, often prioritizing it over his wife. Confronted with these thoughts, he felt miserable and dwelled extensively on the poor choices he had made. The corners of the triangle of conflict are becoming increasingly apparent. However, the feelings elicited by his ex-wife finding a new partner remain unclear. This is a crucial aspect to explore in the psychodynamic project; refer to Figure 5.3.

What He Had Learned from His Father

The patient dwelled on his perceived inferiority, as he scolded himself for experiencing sadness and indecisiveness, thinking that this was not how a man should behave! This brought to mind his father's desire for him to be strong. As a young child, the patient often felt uneasy at school. Despite his father's enthusiasm for him to engage in soccer and vigorous play, it was not something he truly enjoyed.

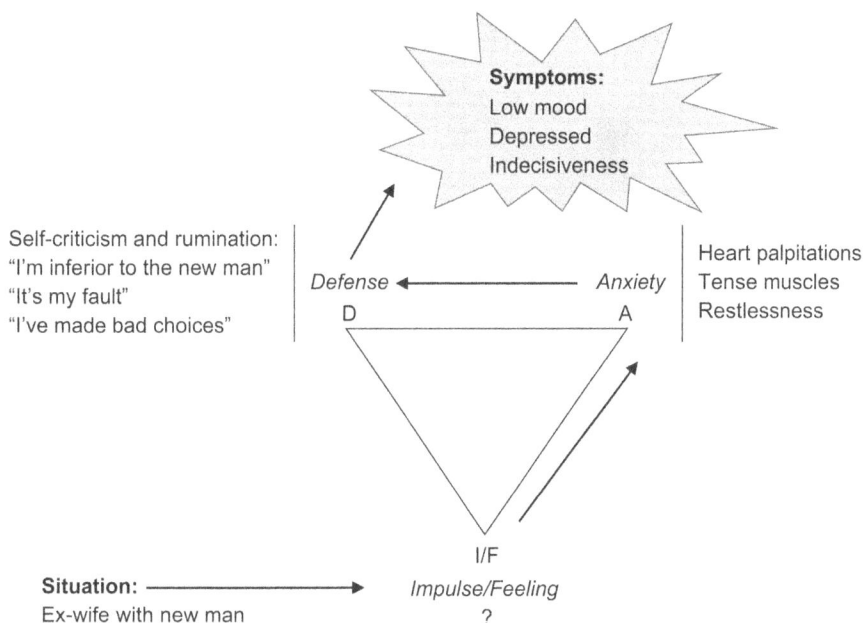

Figure 5.3 The Triangle of Conflict applied to the case of the Depressed Alcholoic

He vividly remembered his father's words, urging him to regain composure and focus on the positives, as real men don't cry or show fear. Figure 5.4 illustrates this correlation, with an arrow tracing back from the symptoms to new defense mechanisms, ultimately reinforcing the symptoms.

He also recalled how much he resented his father leaving his mother, which made him feel a mix of anger and sadness. When he tried to discuss his feelings with his father, he was dismissed with a curt "That's life!" His father was adamant that everything would be fine now that his son was a big boy, and continued, determined to live his own life.

The Therapy

During therapy we focused on the patient's emotional response to the breakup. Gradually, he was able to process his feelings of grief regarding his lost relationships with his father, ex-girlfriend, and ex-wife. Importantly, he achieved this without criticizing himself, like his father had criticized him before. The ability to mourn a loss and still feel like a man was a novel experience for him. Moreover, he was able to take responsibility for his role in the breakup without descending into unproductive self-criticism. He realized that he had become distant from his

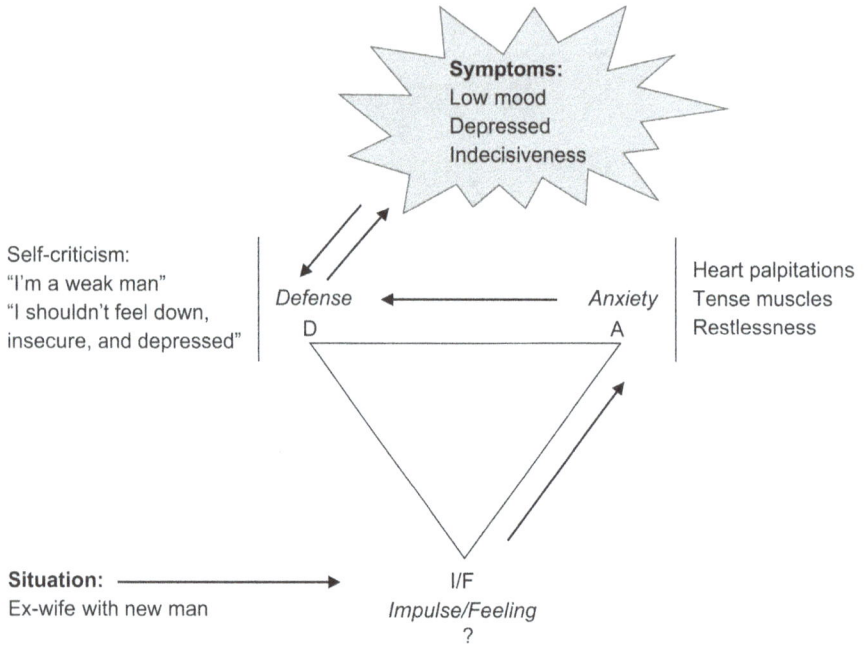

Figure 5.4 The Triangle of Conflict applied to the case of the Depressed Alcholoic

wife and had been spending too much time working. Moreover, he recognized that he had been following in his father's footsteps, who had also neglected his family. He allowed himself to experience his anger toward his ex-wife, who had found a new partner while still in a relationship with him. The anger was the unfamiliar feeling that we needed to understand, indicated with a question mark in Figures 5.3 and 5.4. The anger toward his ex-wife made him realize that he was still harboring anger toward his father, who had abandoned the family. Instead of making an effort to mend the relationship with the family, just like the patient's wife had done, his father had found a new partner.

It became evident that instead of grieving the loss of his wife, he had numbed his pain with alcohol. He had internalized his father's belief that true men do not cry, and whenever the urge to cry arose, he felt anxious. He also realized that instead of getting angry at his wife's and father's infidelity, he had been unjustly blaming himself for being worthless, feeble, and inadequate. In this way, he justified their actions: they had not done anything wrong; rather, it was a consequence of his worthlessness, weakness, and inadequacy. As he gradually embraced his feelings, he observed that his self-criticism faded away. He quit drinking and the depression lifted. During a follow-up interview one year after his treatment ended, he reported feeling great and no longer having issues with drinking. He had also begun

Self-criticism and rumination:
"I'm inferior to the new man"
"It's my fault"
"I have made bad choices"
"I'm worthless"
"I'm inadequate"
Drinking alcohol

Symptoms:
Low mood
Depressed
Indecisiveness

Tense muscles
Heart palpitations
Inner restlessness

Defense ←—————— Anxiety
D   A

Situation: ——————→ I/F ——————→ Alternative:
Ex-wife with new man   *Impulse/Feeling*   No symptoms
Alone without his wife   Anger   Energy and strength
                                        Grief   New relationship

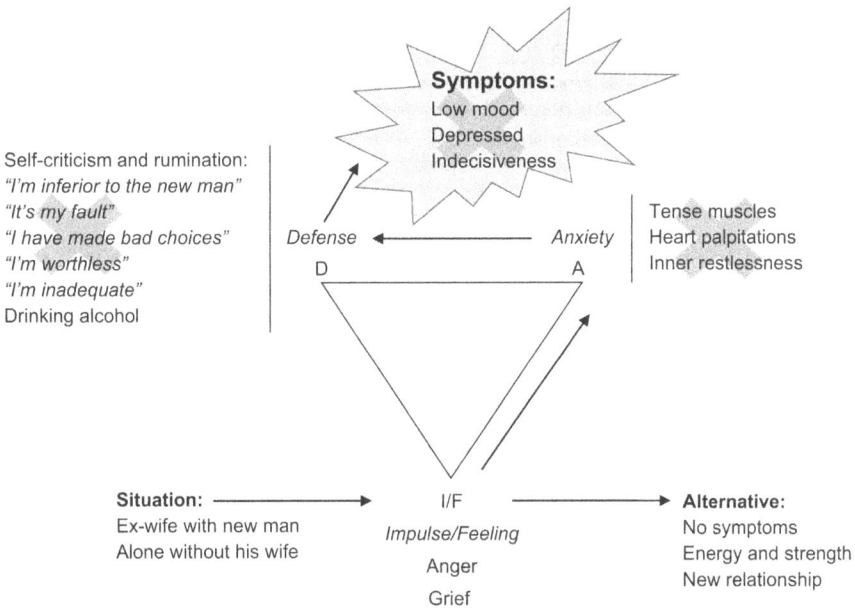

Figure 5.5 The Triangle of Conflict applied to the case of the Depressed Alcholoic

a relationship with a woman and made the decision to reduce his workload in order to truly give her a chance. Figure 5.5 illustrates this. Once he had grown comfortable experiencing grief and anger, these feelings no longer triggered anxiety within him. Consequently, he no longer felt the need to resort to destructive defense mechanisms when confronted with them. As a result, he was able to embark on a new relationship without exhibiting symptoms of mental illness.

The psychodynamic therapist has the ambitious goal of not only reducing the patient's symptoms but also equipping them with the necessary tools to take control of their lives and achieve self-mastery. This approach helps prevent the potential recurrence of symptoms, and for many patients, recovery continues even after treatment concludes (Shedler, 2010). The patient in this particular case experienced a notable abatement in depression and effectively put an end to his drinking habit. Interestingly, this positive outcome was achieved with minimal discussion of the symptoms of depression and alcohol consumption. Instead, our substantial focus was directed toward exploring his emotional reactions to break-ups and infidelity, specifically in regard to grief and anger. We also discussed extensively how he had unconsciously adopted his father's strategies and manner of dealing with his emotions. He had internalized these approaches and repeated to himself the same things his father had said to him. This had a detrimental effect, leaving him feeling distressed and depressed. Alcohol became a means of coping with loneliness and grief, initially proving quite effective but eventually posing problems.

Psychodynamic therapy, in contrast to the perspective of ICD-10, does not view symptoms merely as manifestations of an illness. They are, however, an essential outcome of how the patient manages their internal, unconscious conflicts. Once these internal conflicts are resolved, the patient will no longer need to use symptom-creating defense mechanisms.

The Sweet Child

The Sweet Child sought therapy due to her difficulties in looking after her own needs while her parents were ill. She grappled with feelings of guilt, low mood, emotional numbness, and decreased productivity. Furthermore, she had ceased engaging in exercise, an activity in which she truly took joy. She frequently found herself brought to tears and facing challenges in prioritizing her own self-care. Just like in the case of the Depressed Alcoholic, one could have begun by considering different diagnoses. She described some of the key symptoms of depression, such as guilt, low mood, reduced activity levels, and loss of joy; effective measures might have involved addressing negative thoughts, engaging in behavioral activation, and considering medication for depression. But would this truly be the best course of action for the Sweet Child? Would it genuinely resolve all of her problems, including those concerning the path she should take in life? I highly doubt it. Her challenges were intricately linked to how she had grappled with the dilemma surrounding her parents' illness and her role within the family.

Overworking to Avoid Internal Conflict

The Sweet Child's struggle is partly due to her mother having been a home caregiver for her parents. The way she fulfills that role is to deprioritize her own needs, and the Sweet Child realizes that she might easily fall into the same pattern. She senses that on some level it would be easier if her sick parents passed away, but these thoughts fill her with guilt. And to make matters even more complicated, she was born into a family grieving the loss of her older brother. She was assigned the role of the "sunbeam," responsible for bringing happiness to the rest of the family. It was through her efforts to manage all of this that her symptoms began to surface. The way she deals with internal, unconscious conflicts is what is leading to her problems (see Chapter 4).

P: I have also ... ehh .... Last August I quit my job, the one I've had for the last three years, because I was about to hit the wall. I was burning the candle at both ends. I was working very much. I think that was probably my survival tactic. Working A LOT.

T: Okay.

P: And I've always been like that, when I'm at work with colleagues, I manage to leave the difficult stuff at home and that gives me a little break.

(...)

T: It's good that you see that! When there was more to deal with at home, you took on more work. So that's been your way of dealing with it, then.

P: Mmm. Then I realized that it wasn't working, because I got so exhausted! And somehow I wasn't myself anymore. I noticed that I didn't have the energy to be socially active. I actually enjoy working out. And suddenly I didn't. I kind of felt like I had lost myself. So I quit that job to actually force myself to pay some attention to myself. It was a month and a half after I did that, that I realized maybe I should speak to someone, and reached out to you.

Faced with her mother's illness, the Sweet Child found solace in throwing herself into work. For her, it was a survival tactic, a way to escape from the difficult realities at home. However, she soon realized that this coping mechanism was taking a toll on her, leaving her exhausted and overwhelmed. What had initially brought distraction had now created a whole new set of challenges. This is visually represented in *the triangle of conflict* (see Figure 5.6).

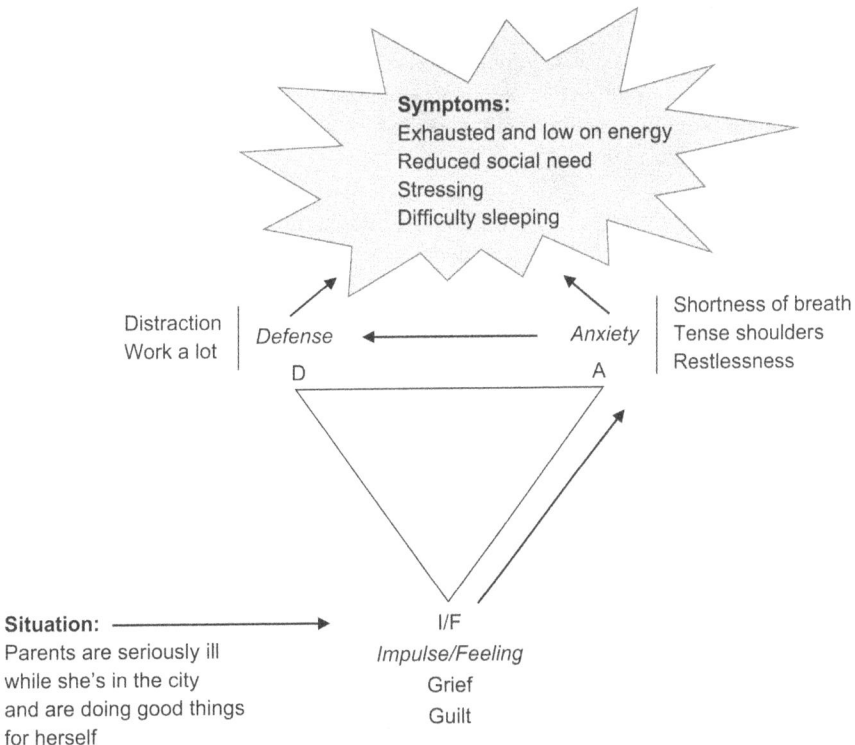

Figure 5.6 The Triangle of Conflict applied to the case of the Sweet Child

If the Sweet Child had sought therapy at this time, her symptoms would have been exhaustion and weariness. She would likely have described herself as highly stressed, experiencing symptoms such as restlessness, shortness of breath, tense shoulders, and difficulty sleeping. These symptoms were a direct result of her excessive workload. The Sweet Child realized this without going to therapy, so she quit her job in order to take better care of herself.

One Defense Mechanism Takes Over from Another

Even if she removes one defense mechanism (*working a lot*) that causes symptoms (*exhaustion*), the underlying conflict and the challenges still persist. The direct mechanism that produces symptoms is gone, but not the underlying cause of the symptoms. The situation is similar to using acetaminophen to cure a fever. Although the fever may be alleviated, the underlying cause of the fever is not being addressed. If you believe that everything is all right again just because the fever is abated by taking acetaminophen, you will not know whether you have truly eliminated the underlying illness that triggered the fever.

When the Sweet Child isn't working as much, she once again has to actively deal with the fact that her parents are ill. This is of course still fraught with conflict for her, and in the face of this, something else happens: She becomes apathetic and numb. Even if a symptom and a defense mechanism are gone, the conflict remains. If she cannot handle the complexity and conflict within her, she will need a new defense mechanism to protect herself.

P: Sometimes I notice that I'm becoming a little numb. That it's better not to feel anything than to feel it all the time.
T: Okay. So this is a way of turning off feelings?
P: *WHISPERS* Yes.
T: Of turning off this conflict that we just had a look at?
P: Guess so.

Figures 5.6 and 5.7 depict the same struggle: coming to terms with her parents' serious illness while also striving to lead a fulfilling life in the city. The only thing that has changed is the defense mechanism used in the face of this: she used to work a lot; now she is shutting down. The cause of the suffering is the same but the symptoms are different.

This argument highlights the fact that simply treating the symptom is not always sufficient. If the underlying problem is not resolved, the patient will either experience heightened anxiety or be forced to make use of new defense mechanisms. As a result, the patient experiences new and different symptoms. Psychodynamic therapy aims to address the root causes of conflicts that drive symptoms. This helps patients avoid the onset of symptoms when faced with challenging life events in the future.

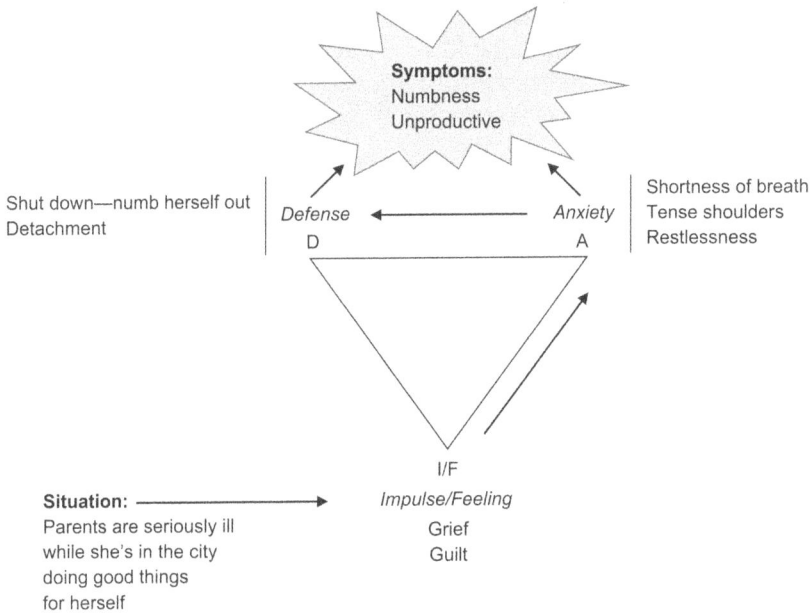

Figure 5.7 The Triangle of Conflict applied to the case of the Sweet Child

When Symptoms Appear During the Therapy Session

As described in Chapter 3, psychodynamic therapy places its focus on the phenomena unfolding within the therapy room. That is because it provides a unique opportunity to work on the difficulties as they play out, as the therapeutic pair has the actual causal mechanisms of the patient's symptoms right in front of their nose. This occurred during the Sweet Child's session when we were discussing her anger toward her sister, who she felt was being condescending. It became evident that she had employed numerous defense mechanisms to cope with her anger, prompting me to question what she—and we—could do about this tendency to evade anger.

T: So what can you do with that pattern right now? What can the two of us do— me and you?

P: Dig into it .... *SIGHS*

T: So if you were to let this out .... If you allow yourself to really let it out right now .... How do you experience it in your body? If you're not going to hold yourself around your throat?

P: Now I'm getting numb. I don't feel anything.

T: Isn't that interesting?

P: Yes.

T: The numbness arrived. The reason you came here.

P: When you asked, it was a bit like …. I don't feel anything! Nothing in my body! I think I'm very good at thinking, not so good at feeling!

T: But when …. Part of the reason you're here is because you're going numb, isn't it?

P: Mmm.

T: And just now you went numb. Do you remember what I asked you?

P: What I noticed in my body when I got angry. *SIGHS*

T: And what happened then?

P: Woooof!! *GESTURES DOWNWARD* Felt nothing! *LAUGHS* *TEARS UP*

T: How do you understand that? That when I ask you how you feel this anger toward Lise, you do this …. *SHOWING A STRANGLEHOLD ON MYSELF*.

P: *SIGHS*

T: You stop it there. And when I say that you attack yourself—is that what you wanted to do? No, you didn't. How do you feel your anger toward Lise? Woooof …. How are we supposed to understand that? This must be very important. Because we triggered your symptom right there.

P: Maybe I'm angrier than I realized *SIGHS*.

In the therapy session, the same pattern unfolds as in the rest of her life. When confronted with unpleasant feelings, she shuts down. It becomes challenging for her to tap into her anger when her sister fails to provide the desired support and comes across as condescending. However, the consequence of shutting down is that she becomes emotionally numb (see Figure 5.8). When this occurs in my presence,

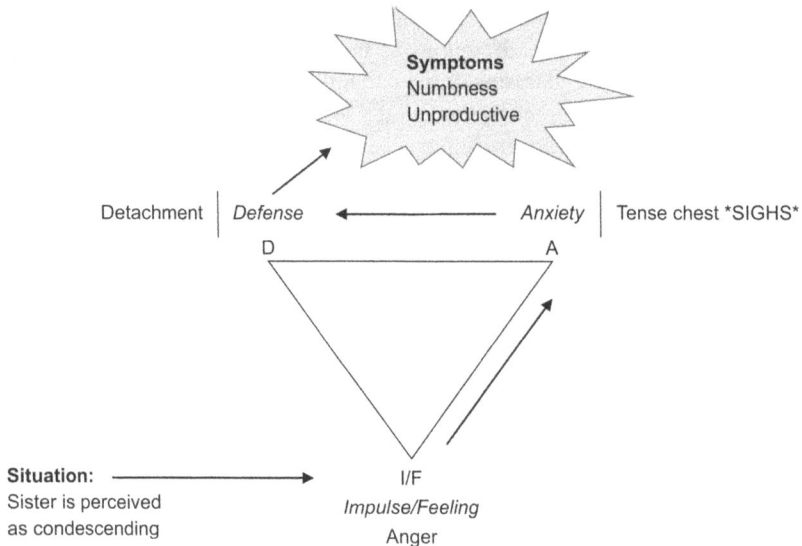

Figure 5.8 The Triangle of Conflict applied to the case of the Sweet Child

it provides us with the opportunity to address this issue together in therapy. By supporting her in processing her anger and helping her gain confidence in embracing this feeling, she will no longer need to depend on defense mechanisms. This emotional response will no longer provoke anxiety, and she can harness the energy that anger provides for healthy self-assertion.[1]

In psychodynamic therapy, psychological problems are not viewed as symptoms of diseases but rather as a result of how individuals relate to their internal, unconscious conflicts. This approach is essential for ISTDP therapists to grasp as it both forms the basis for building strong working relationships with patients and informs almost every intervention in therapy of this type. In the second part of the book, I demonstrate how to use this understanding as the basis for establishing a successful therapeutic collaboration with the patient.

Note

1 Chapter 7 delves deeper into the Sweet Child's story, illustrating our efforts to help her embrace and gain confidence in the feelings she had long kept at bay.

Chapter 6

Developmental Psychology, Genetic and Social Factors

Traditionally, psychodynamic theory has explained mental disorders as the result of internal conflicts that stem from complex relational experiences during childhood. To a large extent, this understanding remains valid: the way we navigate conflict-laden situations with our primary caregivers tends to be generalized and carried over into adulthood. As children, certain coping strategies may have served us well, but as adults these very strategies can present substantial challenges, as discussed in Chapter 5. Since Freud's early works, research in the field of developmental psychology, genetics, and social factors has greatly contributed to our understanding of the causes of mental difficulties. To truly grasp ISTDP and how to establish robust, collaborative projects, it is crucial to comprehend how this knowledge can be integrated into a psychodynamic therapeutic project.

Developmental Psychology

In psychodynamic therapy there is a greater emphasis on early experiences compared to several other types of therapy (Blagys & Hilsenroth, 2000). There is a firm belief that past experiences, from infancy to adulthood, shape the development of personality and psychological challenges (Gabbard, 2017). This fundamental idea lies at the heart of psychodynamic theory: childhood and upbringing exert a profound influence on the adult psyche. During this critical period, individuals acquire vital skills to navigate the complexities of life—be they practical, relational, or psychological.

Freud (1920) introduced this understanding early on in his description of psychoanalysis. He described different psychosexual stages[1] associated with different periods in life. In these stages, the child's energy was directed toward various erogenous zones on the body and involved various psychological developmental challenges that the child had to solve in relation to their caregivers. Depending on how these challenges were resolved, there would be different mental consequences later in life. This was one of the first theories of developmental psychology that aimed to explain children's development through stages. Many psychoanalytic theorists have since written about how childhood experiences, and how they are handled, impact the adult psyche (Erikson, 1950; Klein, 1960; Mahler, 1968;

DOI: 10.4324/9781003516217-8

Winnicott, 1971). These theories regarding the relationship between childhood and adulthood serve as the foundation of all psychodynamic therapies.

Modern empirical research has established a clear correlation between parenting style and positive adjustment in both adolescence and adulthood (Masten, 2015). Additionally, studies have shown that negative childhood experiences have a significant impact on the mental health of adults (Hughes et al., 2017). These findings provide empirical support to the psychoanalytic understanding that childhood experiences play a crucial role in shaping the mental health of adults.

While there are correlations between early life experiences and later mental health problems, it is crucial to understand that this is not a simple relationship of cause and effect. Not everyone who has undergone challenging events in childhood, such as poverty, abuse, or natural disasters, will necessarily develop severe mental difficulties, although there is a significant correlation (Infurna et al., 2016; Masten, 2015). What truly matters is not the experiences themselves but the individual's ability to navigate and process them in a way that does not exacerbate their challenges.

In their book, Gullestad and Killingmo (2019) delve into the concept of trauma. Their main focus lies in how the grave event—the trauma—for example, a sexual assault, is dealt with psychologically. Such an event can be profoundly traumatic for an individual, resulting in severe challenges. For another person, the incident can be dealt with constructively and motivate them to stand up for themselves and fight. For both, the incident is a serious breach of integrity. But the incident is not equally *traumatic* for them. Sometimes, the root of this difference can be traced back to the past. If you carry a burden that suggests the world is generally secure, allowing the abuse to be perceived as an isolated incident, it becomes more manageable to confront and address. If a person has experienced repeated abuse, further instances of abuse can trigger memories of past trauma, further cementing the belief that the world is inherently unsafe, leading to significant psychological consequences. Additionally, this new abuse may awaken memories of previous violations along with associated emotions that need to be addressed. When this type of experience is combined with an innate temperament that makes self-regulation difficult, it becomes evident that different individuals may handle similar situations in markedly distinct ways (Rothbart et al., 2011).

Malan's Triangles

In short-term dynamic therapy, Malan's triangles (1979) are used to describe the relationship between past experiences and current problems, as I explained in Chapters 3 and 4. The triangle of person in Figure 3.1 shows how experiences from people in the past (P), with current people (C), and with the therapist (T) are connected.

The triangle of person and the triangle of conflict (Figure 4.1) are mutually dependent on each other to make sense. Through experiences with significant people in the past, inner conflicts with associated feelings (I/F) are shaped. Since these

Therapist/Transference   **Current People**

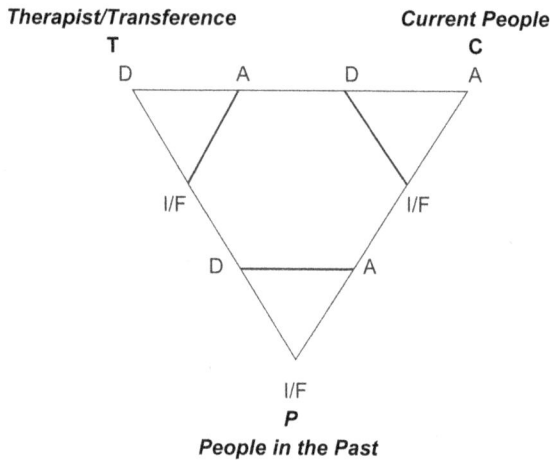

Figure 6.1 The Triangle of Conflict and The Triangle of Person combined

feelings are linked to conflict, they provoke anxiety (A). Due to these anxiety-provoking feelings, one learns to use defense mechanisms (D) to maintain a psychological equilibrium (see Chapter 4).

The triangle of a person illustrates that the lessons learned are carried into adulthood. The feelings are still anxiety-provoking, and the person will automatically use the same defense mechanisms they learned as a child. The triangle of conflict unfolds equally with individuals from the past (P), current individuals (C), and the therapist (T).

To illustrate this concept, the two triangles can be merged as depicted in Figure 6.1 (Molnos, 1986).

There is thus a triangle of conflict in each corner of the triangle of person: The way we navigate our feelings, anxiety, and defenses remains consistent across individuals, be it in the past, the present, or even with our therapist. The triangles (Malan, 1979; Molnos, 1986) provide therapists with a simple tool to diagram the intricate psychoanalytic theory that explains how our childhood coping mechanisms manifest in the present.

The Sweet Child

To understand how developmental psychological factors influence psychotherapy, it is once again useful to examine the case of the Sweet Child.

Formative Life Experiences

The Sweet Child shares experiences from her upbringing that have made it especially challenging for her to cope with her parents falling ill. One is that her mother has been a home carer in a way that has been self-sacrificing, as the Sweet Child explained in Chapter 1. As we grow up, we learn, among other things, through imitation how to handle various situations. The lesson that the Sweet Child has learned about how to be a home carer is not particularly helpful for her. The Sweet Child sees this, but it is still difficult: "I don't want to repeat what I grew up with, but it feels so natural to me to do it!." Her mother made a selfless sacrifice in order to care for her own parents. Isn't she going to receive the same care from her own daughter now that it is she who is ill? This poses a complex emotional dilemma for the Sweet Child. The experiences she has carried with her from the past (P) are making it difficult for her in the present (C).

Another significant experience from the Sweet Child's childhood that profoundly impacted her was being born into a family in mourning. Her brother had died of cancer at the age of twelve, a year and a half before she was born. At a very young age, she took on the role of the family's "sunbeam," striving to bring happiness to everyone, and she succeeded. Of course, this was not a conscious decision, yet by being a source of positivity and joy, she was able to lighten the atmosphere and, in turn, find it easier to be herself. Thus, she continued to pursue her compassionate actions, carrying with her a profound obligation to show concern and care for others into her adult life.

Protecting the Others

The Sweet Child's problem lies in putting herself second, just as she has observed her mother doing. Her altruistic nature has brought positive things into her life: she has many friends, a boyfriend, and has had exciting jobs and responsibilities at a young age. She is highly regarded, and in the session she presents herself equally so. However, this way of living creates problems when her parents fall ill and need help. Should she continue to be their "sunbeam" and make them happy, at the cost of her own plans in life, even though that would run contrary to her own wishes? At the same time, it is unsettling and anxiety-inducing to abandon a coping strategy that has been crucial and, in many ways, beneficial to her.

In Chapter 3, the Sweet Child talked about how she did not reveal to me, nor to those around her, her true feelings. Since she was a child, she had thought that she had an inner shield that protected those around her from her burdensome feelings. By keeping her true feelings to herself, she believed she was being helpful to those around her. This coping mechanism made it even more challenging for her when she encountered difficulties that she struggled to handle on her own. The strategy she learned as a child she applied not only with me but also with those around her.

Internalizing the Family Culture

The Sweet Child also discusses how her family culture has influenced her as she has grown up. She finds it hard when friends seek her help with their problems because she feels jealous and resentful that they have an easier life than her. At the same time, she does not think she should react like this, as she has always been taught that grief and problems are distinct entities:

P: As I have grown up in a family that has dealt with a lot, both illness and death and all kinds of things, Mom and Dad have always been very eager to tell me that I shouldn't compare grief and problems. So we can't expect .... So .... When friends of mine come to me with their problems they experience them as real problems! Because that's what they're struggling with. So I've always learned not to compare it.

T: Okay! Is that really possible? You've been taught not to do that. But at the same time you say that you've experienced a great deal of envy and bitterness.

P: Yes, I wish we could exchange problems. It would be nice to have a break.

T: *SPEAKING IN A LOW VOICE* So now the big question is: Are you going to allow yourself, right now, to let all these feelings through?

P: *WHISPERS* Yes.

T: Or are you going to put this lid on them? Right now, as you sit here?

P: *SIGHS* I came here to feel it, to dig into it. So I realize that it's a good idea! But I think it'll be difficult!

The Sweet Child realizes the difficulty in accepting feelings of envy and bitterness due to the challenges she has faced in life. These are things she has become accustomed to putting a lid on, and her family has valued this "lid" highly.

Moreover, she understands that the way her family has discussed her brother's death, and also emotions in general, has had an impact on her. While she has participated in conversations about grieving for her brother, she has not addressed the complications she—and only she—has faced in being the family's "sunbeam."

P: So my feelings connected to that, and that sadness, I've been able to talk about. But I probably haven't talked about a lot of other things. Because from my point of view, that would result in giving Mom and Dad more worries and more to think about.

Resources

It is important to acknowledge that the Sweet Child carries with her numerous good experiences from her upbringing. She depicts a profoundly intimate bond with her father, as later elucidated in Chapter 7. All the evidence suggests that she has developed a secure attachment (Ainsworth et al., 1978) to her parents, which is likewise associated with positive therapy outcomes (Levy et al., 2011). She has made meaningful friendships and had many successful experiences at school and in her free time. All of this will equip her with effective strategies to navigate life and will serve as valuable assets for her (Masten, 2015).

Genetic Factors

Psychodynamic theory is based on the understanding that psychological difficulties arise from interactions with significant others, usually from a young age. At the same time, twin research has revealed a significant genetic influence on mental disorders. It is not surprising that disorders such as bipolar disorder, schizophrenia, and ADHD have a high degree of heritability, ranging from 70% to 85%. Personality disorders, anorexia, addiction problems, panic disorder, depression, and generalized anxiety are all also significantly influenced by heredity (Bienvenu et al., 2011; Petterson et al., 2019; Torgersen et al., 2012).

How does psychodynamic theory and therapy relate to this? Can psychodynamic psychotherapy be effective in treating disorders with a strong genetic component? Research into its effectiveness suggests that psychodynamic therapy is highly effective in treating personality disorders, anxiety, and depression. Promising findings have also emerged for the treatment of anorexia and drug addiction. This therapeutic approach thus appears to be effective for disorders with a moderate degree of heredity (Abbate-Daga et al., 2016; Fonagy, 2015; Keefe et al., 2014; Shedler, 2010; Warshaw, 2022).

For disorders like bipolar disorder, schizophrenia, and ADHD, which have the highest levels of genetic heritability, the picture becomes more uncertain. Allan Abbass has published case studies demonstrating positive outcomes for patients diagnosed with both bipolar disorder and psychotic disorders (Abbass et al., 2015, 2019). As of the spring of 2022, finding research on psychodynamic therapy for ADHD is a challenging endeavor.

How can we comprehend the intersection of psychodynamic therapy and genetic heredity? Individuals possess varying degrees of genetic susceptibility to various mental disorders. Nonetheless, no research has demonstrated complete heritability, which would imply that all individuals with genetic vulnerability would develop the disorder. Therefore, it is evident that additional factors impact the expression of genetics. Freud (1966) observed early on how internal and external factors can have varying effects on individuals. One of the key factors contributing to this lies in the way one's biological makeup is nurtured, both by oneself and by the surrounding environment. It is fascinating to observe how two children can be born with distinct temperaments: the first may possess a fiery disposition, requiring assistance to find inner tranquility; meanwhile, the second may exhibit a cautious nature, necessitating guidance to develop self-assertion. Consequently, these unique traits call for distinct approaches to upbringing and regulation by their parents, enabling them to thrive and flourish through life (Rothbart et al., 2011). In this manner, siblings may have vastly distinct experiences despite having relatively similar upbringings, ultimately leading to remarkably different life trajectories.

Each human being is born with a unique genetic makeup, granting them diverse opportunities and vulnerabilities. We approach the world with the genetic predisposition we have been given, and have to rely on our surroundings to meet our needs in a *good enough way* (Winnicott, 1990). Only through this help can we discover how to cope with ourselves. If we do not receive the necessary assistance to address our temperament and inherent vulnerabilities, we may develop internal conflicts that can give rise to symptoms under certain circumstances. Psychodynamic therapy is an effective way to help patients manage and navigate these conflicts.

The Man with a Manically Guilty Conscience

The Man with a Manically Guilty Conscience was a gentleman in his forties. For more than twenty years he had been living with a diagnosis of bipolar disorder, type 1 (WHO, 1992), a highly hereditary condition. Stabilization and medication had so far been the recommended treatment approach (Geddes & Miklowitz, 2013). He had experienced multiple episodes of mania throughout his life, leading to numerous admissions to the emergency ward. During periods when he took his medication, he functioned with stability: he sought help from the healthcare system as needed and performed decently in his job. Nevertheless, he had stopped taking his medication several times, which quickly led to new manic episodes. During these periods of reckless behavior, he betrayed and hurt those closest to him, leading several to withdraw from him. Furthermore, he put himself, his family, and his friends in financially difficult situations.

From his early years, The Man with a Manically Guilty Conscience had battled a deep-seated belief that something was inherently wrong with him. His tumultuous behavior led to frequent disruptions at school, and at home he suffered physical punishment from his violent father. Despite brief periods of stability in his adolescence and adulthood—such as obtaining an education, having romantic relationships, and maintaining employment—during therapy, a recurring pattern emerged: he would abruptly cease taking his medication when things seemed to be going well. This destructive decision led to manic episodes just before an important exam, after proposing to his girlfriend, and after taking on more responsibilities at work. Upon closer examination he discovered a recurring pattern in his life: a relentless feeling of anxiety whenever things were going well for him, leading him to sabotage all that was good. Feeling bad somehow felt safer, like a familiar state that alleviated his anxiety. Yet at the same time he was unwittingly sabotaging his own life.

Slowly but surely, through therapy, he became aware that he carried a constant feeling of guilt for everything he had ruined throughout his life. He was deeply enraged by the insufficient assistance he had received, a situation made even more intolerable by the realization that he himself had made it challenging for those trying to help him. This intense anger was thus also tinged with a sense of guilt. At the beginning of the therapy he lacked a clear awareness that he carried a burden of guilt and a troubled conscience. In other words, the guilt was *unconscious*. As long as he was harming himself and feeling unwell, he was disconnected from this feeling. In a way, he gave himself the punishment he thought he deserved, thus shortcutting the experience of guilt. As he gradually improved and began desiring to rebuild relationships and achieve a stable life, all the feelings linked to his past resurfaced.

An important theme in therapy was how he could manage his guilt without resorting to self-punishment, such as discontinuing medication. He also invested significant effort in repairing relationships with individuals he deemed important in his life. He eventually acknowledged his anger for all the punishment he had received growing up, and he mourned all the losses he had suffered. Gradually, he began to feel that he deserved something good in life, despite the forbidden feelings and the earlier episodes of asocial behavior. As a result, he stopped discontinuing his medication during stable periods and began contacting the emergency ward at the first signs of manic phases. By seeking help to prevent the episodes, he was able to avoid harming himself and those close to him.

Psychodynamic therapy could not cure his bipolar disorder, a condition predominantly influenced by genetics. However, it played a pivotal role in helping him confront both his conscious and unconscious guilt. This guilt had surfaced due to the complex interplay of his genetic predispositions and the reactions of those closest to him. By developing a healthier relationship with his guilt, he was able to adhere more effectively to bipolar treatment recommendations. Additionally, he succeeded in repairing his relationships with some of the most important people in his life. This highlights a crucial point: In psychodynamic therapy, therapists strive to assist their patients in addressing conflicts that have emerged from the interplay between their inherent personality and the responses they have encountered from others throughout their lives.

The Man Who Refused to Be Smart

To illustrate the complex interplay of genetics, upbringing, and psychological challenges, let's consider another case where genetic factors play a significant role, specifically ADHD.

A student in his twenties began treatment seeking help for difficulties with concentration and depressive symptoms. He started therapy at the same time as he completed an assessment for ADHD. The assessment, which included a WAIS test,[2] revealed significant challenges with processing speed and short-term memory. At the same time, the tests indicated an intellectual level well above average. In therapy, he discussed the challenges he faced growing up, where he was consistently told that he had the potential to do better than he was demonstrating. He was often placed at the front of the classroom due to his difficulty in keeping up, and he was not permitted to go out and play until he had completed his homework, leading to a significant amount of time spent on schoolwork. During the therapy sessions, he shared his self-perception as lazy, sluggish, and unintelligent—a perception heavily influenced by the criticisms of his teachers and parents. Moreover, he possessed beliefs that discouraged him from engaging in study groups, fearing that he would burden others. This mindset aggravated his depression and reinforced his tendency to withdraw from social interactions.

Accepting the assessment findings, which revealed neurological challenges affecting memory and speed, was difficult for him. It also highlighted that he was indeed highly intelligent. Throughout his entire life, he had constantly been told to gather his strength and resolve, leading him to perceive himself as lazy and unintelligent. The therapy focused on helping him to accept his difficulties, to mourn the reality of his handicaps, to manage his anger toward those who had placed unreasonable expectations on him, and to begin prioritizing self-care. He also had to allow himself to appreciate and showcase his abilities. He eventually applied for extended time for the exam, arranged for a place in the reading room with less disruption, and stopped labeling himself as lazy. He continued to struggle with short-term memory and processing speed, and psychodynamic therapy did not cure his neurological issues. However, it did enable him to cope with his biological limitations in a compassionate and constructive manner. His depressive symptoms diminished and his academic performance showed significant improvement.

The Sweet Child

As I have mentioned several times, the Sweet Child experienced fatigue, numbness, depression, and reduced productivity after her parents became ill. I have no knowledge of the Sweet Child's potential genetic vulnerability to mental health issues; there was not much history of mental illness in the immediate family. Her mother likely experienced fatigue from caregiving and may have faced psychological challenges at some point, but there is no indication that genetics played a significant role in this. Her father was diagnosed with early-onset Alzheimer's, a disease that has a significant genetic component (Bienvenu et al., 2011). At the same time, there is little evidence to suggest that a genetic susceptibility to Alzheimer's disease directly contributes to the challenges faced by the Sweet Child.

What is likely, however, is that she possessed many genetically determined *positive* traits. From an early age she was a gentle, easily regulated, and sociable child who was empathetic and took care of those around her:

P: That's what Mom and Dad say as well: I was a little girl who was really agreeable, never quarreled, and behaved nicely.

These types of personality traits are highly influenced by genetics (Bratko et al., 2017). She excelled in school and was on the verge of completing her master's degree. Academic prowess is closely correlated with high IQ, which also exhibits a significant degree of heritability (Plomin & Deary, 2015). A sociable personality and high IQ are linked to good functioning in adulthood (Masten, 2015). The Sweet Child's agreeable personality and strong cognitive abilities allowed her to become the family's "sunbeam." These attributes also helped her find solace within a mourning family and excel as a student. However, at the same time, this is also part of the problem for the Sweet Child. Her sociable and empathetic nature, coupled with her ability to handle things with little help, have led her to prioritize others over herself.

We are all shaped by our genetic background. Some individuals inherit genes that make them susceptible to certain issues, while others have genetic traits that make adaptation easy. Psychodynamic therapy understands mental disorders as consequences of how individuals manage their genetic heritage and life experiences. Therapy cannot alter the biological and genetic foundation with which one is born; that much is indisputable. Therefore, the objective should be to discover constructive ways to live *with* it.

Mental suffering arises when individuals face internal conflicts that overwhelm them with anxiety or when they utilize defense mechanisms that lead to difficulties. Inner conflicts arise from the interaction between the inherent qualities of individuals and how these qualities are received by their closest caregivers. Achieving a comprehensive understanding of mental disorders via a psychodynamic framework therefore encompasses both genetic and environmental factors.

Social Factors

Social factors can significantly impact psychological well-being, both as protective factors and as risk factors. For example, a strong social network and human support serve as a shield against psychological distress, while a lack of social support stands out as a clear risk factor for such disorders (Masten, 2015; Sehmi et al., 2020).

Several factors can elevate the risk of mental health issues. These include stressful life events such as divorce, unemployment, physical illness, the loss of a loved one, accidents, socioeconomic status, and sexual harassment (Horowitz, 2002; Sheldon et al., 2021). More common occurrences such as falling in love, partying, physical illness/injury and sleep deprivation can also trigger psychological problems, at least in patients diagnosed with bipolar disorder (Proudfoot et al., 2012). These social factors are involved in a complex interplay with genetic and developmental psychological factors, where all can reciprocally impact each other (Brody et al., 2013).

The psychodynamic understanding of psychological difficulties is well supported by the research presented in the preceding section. As discussed in Chapter 5, certain circumstances can trigger inner, unconscious conflicts in patients. For example, the Sweet Child's suffering was related to the illness of her parents, while the Depressed Alcoholic was affected by his divorce. These are common life events that can be hard to cope with and heighten the risk of psychological issues.

It is crucial to remember that not everyone who experiences such incidents will suffer from psychological problems. The determining factor is whether the situation will trigger internal conflicts, along with accompanying feelings that are not properly dealt with. Does the person have a strong social support system with whom they can share their challenges? Or do they withdraw, criticize themselves, and get drunk? A social network can serve as a crucial support system, providing individuals with the necessary tools to effectively navigate challenging situations. Having someone to talk to can significantly reduce emotional overwhelm, leading to a decreased reliance on defense mechanisms and their associated negative consequences.

Psychodynamic therapy does not view the social factors mentioned earlier as direct causes of psychological distress. It is not your *experiences*, such as the mentioned life events, that decide whether you develop mental health issues. While death, illness, and divorce are undoubtedly challenging, it is how you *cope with them* that truly impacts your psychological well-being. A social network does not directly and magically protect you. Instead, it offers support, a listening ear, and a constructive alternative to isolation. Those who have faced tough situations must actively seek out and utilize these resources for the social network to be effective. Otherwise, resorting to harmful defense mechanisms may become the only option.

The Sweet Child

The Sweet Child has a lot of friends. She has a boyfriend, engages in many extracurricular activities, and holds multiple jobs, which allows her to expand her social network. This protects her from mental illness. She explicitly stated that she had utilized her job as a distraction from her parents' illness (see Chapter 4). She exhausted herself by working excessively, leaving little surplus for the activities that could safeguard her from psychological problems, such as socializing and exercising. Her defenses against mental difficulties began to falter as the situation became more complex.

In addition, she has mentioned challenges of maximizing the potential of her social network:

P: So ... I feel that it may have something to do with the fact that many of those I have tried to talk to in the past, i.e., friends, they ask in good faith and would like to hear how things are going .... But to be honest, it's too much for them! And then you distance yourself, right? It can be difficult to meet people in grief ... in crises and stuff like that.

Her experience is that she does not get the support she needs when she opens up. This could, of course, be due to the fact that her environment does not cope with it very well. But it is also possible that she tends to withdraw instead of fully opening up:

P: When I talk to others about feelings, be they my boyfriend or friends, when I have to put something difficult into words, or something that has happened, I start to cry when I say it. Because it's so hard to even begin to talk. And as soon as I get going, I can switch it off.

The Sweet Child is able to open up to those around her, yet when she begins to cry, the situation becomes overwhelming. She hides her tears and works hard to keep her composure, which hinders her from fully engaging with her social network. She has even told me that she believes that concealing her true feelings is a way to protect her loved ones—and the Sweet Child is, after all, a sweet child whose role is to be a sunbeam for everyone around her.

Social factors are also central in triggering the Sweet Child's difficulties. Her father has been ill for a long time, and now that her mother has also fallen ill, it has put her in a difficult situation. Her mother used to be the one who looked after her father, but is now less able to do so. This new social situation is proving to be challenging for the Sweet Child to cope with. Again, it is essential to note that what occurs is not as significant as how it is dealt with. Her parents' illnesses awaken inner conflicts in the Sweet Child. She is someone who ought to be there for others. She ought to embrace the role of the sunbeam. She ought to be the good daughter and do as expected. She ought to protect those around her by not telling them how she really feels. She ought to raise her inner shield so that her feelings do not escape and hurt others. She volunteers to help her parents. The problem is that these strategies will ultimately demand that she sacrifice herself and her own life. The Sweet Child does not want that. The complex social changes within her family are putting her usual coping strategies to a serious test.

In my view, it is crucial for modern psychodynamic theory to incorporate all the aforementioned factors. The interplay between developmental psychology, genetic elements, and social factors will undoubtedly impact the individual patient. Consequently, it becomes imperative to consider and examine all these factors carefully, as they serve as the foundation for developing accurate hypotheses and establishing effective working alliances with each unique patient.

Notes

1 Freud named these, respectively, the oral phase, the anal phase, the phallic phase, the latent phase, and the genital phase.
2 The Wechsler Adult Intelligence Scale (WAIS) (Wechsler, 2008) is a widely utilized assessment of cognitive abilities.

Chapter 7

The Sweet Child

The Sweet Child has been illustrative for this part of the book. She has been a help-ful child who has supported everyone around her; she has also helped to illustrate how core phenomena and concepts in psychodynamic therapy manifest in practice. In this chapter I describe how her therapy proceeded and how we addressed her complex feelings related to her conflicting life themes.

From Insight to Practice

So far, the Sweet Child and I have developed a shared understanding of her prob-lems and how they are impacting her life. She recognizes the origin of her strate-gies and how, by avoiding complex feelings, she triggers her symptoms. We also agree that she protects me, her boyfriend, and her friends in the same way as she has protected her parents: she has a shield that prevents her feelings being ex-pressed, in order to spare those around her from being burdened by them.

P: I think I'm bad at caring for myself, and I'm also pretty bad at receiving care from others.

The Sweet Child sums it up nicely: she recognizes that the consequences of her approach to life are that she neglects self-care.

T: Right. We see that two of your main ways of dealing with things ... one is directed *outward*, taking care of others. Taking care of me, even! Just like your mom did. Then we see the other way, when you bypass the first. Because you come back here and start doing good things for yourself. Then you become numb....

P: Mmm. There are some days where it's just easier not to think than to think.

T: Right.

P: Escape into a book or Netflix or something, to not have to decide what you really feel.

T: So now we are beginning to understand this. We see the pattern. So, what will be our next task? Yours and mine?

DOI: 10.4324/9781003516217-9

P: Well, I don't know!

T: We're beginning to understand this. You can see it, you're a smart young woman. What's the next step after you understand?

P: *LAUGHS* Might have to start practicing, then.

T: Do you want to do that?

P: *NODS*

Once again, the Sweet Child demonstrates her great capacity. She understands that once you have understood and gained insight, the next step is to put it into practice. *Insight*[1] plays a crucial role in short-term dynamic therapy. Without it, therapists and patients are left without information about how to proceed, which could obviously lead to misunderstandings. But insight alone is not enough to bring about change. For short-term dynamic therapy to be truly effective, patients must also have new experiences. To achieve this, as the Sweet Child understands, one must practice—practice new ways of dealing with one's feelings.

T: And so we're up against how many years of experience? Twenty? We're up against something that's your identity.

P: Yes. I think it's pretty solidly built in.

T: I wonder what you can do to start opening up, here with me? To take control and put yourself in the driver's seat. Allow yourself to do good things for yourself. What can you do right now?

The Sweet Child falls silent and gazes at me with a slightly puzzled look in her eyes. I wait without speaking, letting the silence linger for some time.

P: *SIGHS* If you ask me, I'll ask you!

Although changing lifelong patterns is complicated, it is possible—and the Sweet Child has proven to be a resourceful woman. Therefore, I believe she already knows how to do this, even though she may not realize her ability to take control and open up. As it would involve delving into painful feelings, a new unconscious defense mechanism arises. She becomes passive, believing she is incapable of doing something she actually has the capacity for—and it is important to note that believing you cannot do something is entirely different from actually being incapable of doing it.

Honest Conversations About Reality

As therapists, we are quite limited in what we can do for our patients. We can help them recognize their destructive patterns, help them find alternative ways of dealing with them, and support them when they test out new, unfamiliar approaches. Only our patients can *implement* the necessary changes. As psychotherapists, we are not surgeons operating on our patients; rather, we are comparable to personal trainers in a gym who offer comprehensive training plans—ultimately, it is the patients themselves who must actively engage in the training.

It is time for an honest conversation about reality. There can be no doubt that the hard work has to come from the Sweet Child herself. However, it is crucial for me to be warm, empathetic, and emphasize that I am there for her, as a caring attitude is an essential part of any therapy. I see she is in pain, but I cannot walk the painful road *for* her. Instead, I am there to walk *with* her.

T: Right. *SPEAKING SLOWLY AND IN A GENTLE VOICE* And I'm here. And I really want to help you. But at some point, there is a switch you have to flip on your own.
P: Mmm.
T: And I would love to get inside your head and help you and turn things around.
P: *LAUGHS, TEARING UP*
T: *TALKS GENTLY* All I can do is to help you see what it is, but then you have to turn things around on your own.
P: Mmm.
T: That's the harsh reality.
P: *NODS* *TEARING UP*
T: *SPEAKING SOFTLY* But I'd really like to be here with you while you do it. And look at whatever comes from that.
P: *SIGHS*
T: So that you don't have to be there all alone!
P: *WHISPERS* Yes ….
T: *SPEAKING SOFTLY* Because that specific task is yours, but then the success can be yours too. And then freedom can be yours.
P: *WHISPERS* I'd really like to have that!
T: Yes, I understand that.
P: *CRYING INTENSELY*

The Sweet Child has understood my message: she understands that she has to do it alone, and she also knows *what* to do. When I communicate the message in a warm, empathetic, and clear manner, she begins to express the feelings she has been avoiding. The ability to exude both warm affection and unwavering clarity is a crucial aspect of being an effective ISTDP therapist.[2]

Feelings and Insight Hand in Hand

Feelings come in waves, and eventually the Sweet Child stops crying. She has let some of her grief pass through her, and I wonder how that experience was for her. We have talked about practicing letting her feelings come through, and now she has just done so. A goal of ISTDP treatment is to help patients be able to think and feel at the same time and in a balanced way. This is crucial, as the combination of insight and emotional experience is linked to positive outcomes in therapy (Coughlin, 2017). I therefore invite her to reflect on what just happened:

T: Okay .... Mm .... Do you know what happened just now that made you .... Because you actually did it a little more, did you notice? What was it you just did?
P: Yes.
T: This is important! A little more than before? Do you agree, or am just being an optimistic psychologist?
P: No, I think I agree! *LAUGHS* It felt different than before.
T: So, what did you do? Because you just did it! Before you stopped again ....
P: So .... Really, it's overriding the voice that says, "Pull yourself together—straighten up!", sort of.
T: Okay, so there's a voice that says, "Pull yourself together, straighten up?"
P: Well, not straighten up ... don't open up, in a way! Keep it together! *LAUGHS*
T: So, you notice that there's a voice: Keep it together, don't open up!
P: *NODS*
T: Wow! Well heard, or noticed, or however I should put it. What was it like for you to let it through for a couple of seconds?
P: It was actually very nice. At the same time, it was painful, but yes ....

We both acknowledge that she has done an excellent job. I offer praise; she accepts it with a laugh, and then realizes something crucial: her success was not just a coincidence, but the result of her own actions. Earlier in the session, our focus was on bringing her previously automatic and unconscious defense mechanisms into conscious awareness. She has recognized that she has been withholding and detaching from her feelings when they emerged. Now she has the ability to override the voice inside her that urges her to pull herself together and hide her true feelings. Furthermore, she expresses something important: it feels very nice, despite it also being painful.

T: So, it's nice to let these painful feelings through. But then the voice comes.
P: It's kind of been there for so long that it ... yeah, I think it's going to take some time to silence it .... I mean ... I've never cried in front of a stranger before!
T: But now you have the opportunity.
P: It might be the case that the better I get to know you ... a bit of feeling secure, and stuff and ... because ... so ... with my boyfriend, I can ... let it through and cry much longer. And feel that, real ... yes ... redemptive connection, before it stops.
T: And we'll get to know each other better over time. But the question is: Is it about you needing to know me better? Or is it doing it that feels really scary?
P: *WHISPERS* It's very scary! *LAUGHS* It is!
T: It's really scary to open up to me, right now.

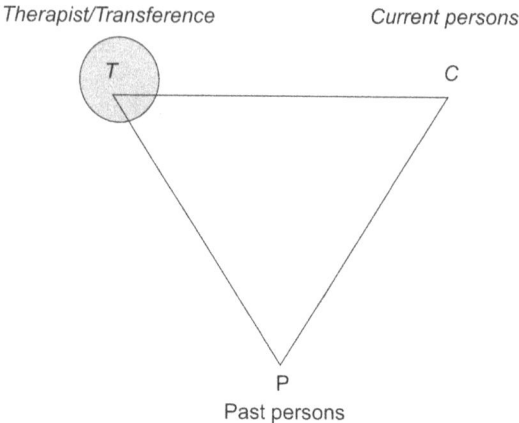

Figure 7.1 The Triangle of Person with Emphasis on the Therapist/Transference Corner

It feels unfamiliar and scary for her to open up to me. Understanding what is going on in the session becomes clearer if it is drawn onto Malan's triangles. The interaction between me (the therapist) and the Sweet Child is placed at the T-corner of the triangle of person (see Figure 7.1).

The illustration in Figure 7.2 depicts the dynamics of the triangle of conflict. Speaking openly to me (*situation*) evokes the *feeling* of sadness in her, with the accompanying *impulse* to cry. But crying in front of me is scary, and it makes her

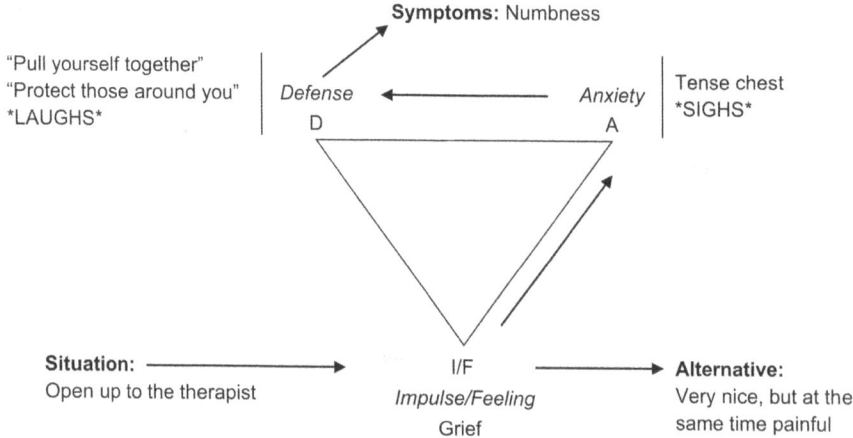

Figure 7.2 The Triangle of Conflict applied to the case of the Sweet Child

anxious. She then tells herself: "Pull yourself together." However, when she does not pull herself together and instead tolerates the discomfort, she notices that it feels very nice, but at the same time painful.

Being Tolerated and Getting Help

At this point in the therapy we are addressing a critical mechanism that is central to the Sweet Child's problems as it manifests in the therapy session: she is protecting me, just as she has protected everyone else. However, we now have the opportunity to transform this protective strategy within the therapy setting. This is precisely what we mean by working in the transference, as discussed in Chapter 3.

T: We have already seen that you think you ought to protect me. You have to make sure I won't get disappointed, if I'm not good enough at my job and can't help you.

P: *LAUGHS*

T: Suddenly, a lot of this is about me!

P: Yes!

T: "So how did that therapy turn out for you? Not so well, but I think the psychologist had a great time!"

P: *LAUGHS* Yes, he had a great time!

T: Yes, made sure he had a great time.

I crack a joke that makes the Sweet Child laugh. The joke highlights the seriousness of the situation, and the Sweet Child seizes the opportunity. She leans forward in the chair and looks me straight in the eye.

P: I feel so vulnerable sitting like this! *CRIES*

T: What comes up when you sit like this?

P: *SIGHS* No one really knows how I feel, like 100%! *CRYING* People only know fractions. My boyfriend is the one who knows the most.

T: So now you have the opportunity to tell me everything.

So far in the session we have focused on her tendency to avoid acknowledging her feelings when she is around other people. With this newfound understanding she boldly leans toward me, locking her gaze with mine while trying to resist protecting me. However, despite her newfound understanding, this behavior makes her anxious, and she sighs. At the same time, it saddens her that no one, not even her boyfriend, truly knows her. She starts crying and, faced with her grief, I sit quietly and offer supportive sounds.

Feelings Toward the Therapist

When I sit quietly for a while, it reminds her of her boyfriend (the C-corner of the triangle of person)—see Figure 7.1. He has done exactly the same thing.

P: But he hasn't ... well ... since he meets me with silence, it makes it difficult for me to continue. Because I'm the kind of person who needs a little something ....

T: Okay. Did I meet you with silence, right now?

P: Yes! A little! The fact that you just look at me ... and are completely silent .... It's the same as in my relationship with my boyfriend—it stops there!

T: So, you react a little toward me, since I don't quite help you through it?

P: Yes .... At least with my boyfriend, I've thought that when he meets me with silence when I .... But you give much more feedback than what he does! *LAUGHS*

T: But still. But still!

P: When he meets me with silence, it feels so vulnerable to keep talking and reveal myself. I need a question or a "mm-hm."

T: So, you need that from me too?

P: Yes, maybe something like that. That's why I struggle when you just sit there looking at me.

When patients start to cry, I naturally become quiet, striving to be fully present in an empathetic manner. This approach has proven effective for many patients. However, the Sweet Child has a unique experience with silence. She has long been alone with her feelings, and when I remain silent without clearly acknowledging her experience, it is as though she is alone once more. This is a great example of how what works for one patient may not necessarily work for another. At this point it is crucial to address the feelings that the Sweet Child experiences in response to my actions. She has rarely shared with anyone directly how she reacts to their actions and what she needs from them. Now she has the opportunity to do precisely that with me.

T: If you would be willing to try to test out being completely honest with your feelings .... What do you feel toward me, in that moment, when I become quiet and don't help you continue? When I kind of go flat, or ... I don't know what's going on. How do you feel toward me? If you're dead honest. If you're not going to protect me. If you can take away parts of the shield that's supposed to protect others. What do you feel toward me at that very moment, when I am not giving you the help you need?

P: That it should be your job to help me go further.

T: Yes, right! So that's your thought, right?

P: A bit like, come on! Ask me a question!

T: Yeah, right. That's your thought again. And your feeling when I don't? When I don't do my job, and don't help you go further by not asking you questions?

P: Frustration.

A Corrective Emotional Experience

The patient notices that she feels frustrated when I stay silent, just like she does when her boyfriend and numerous others stay silent. However, the difference now is that with me challenging her, she is able to express her frustration. This leads to a new experience for her, and there is something about this that evokes a sense of sadness.

P: *TEARS UP*

T: *SPEAKS GENTLY* Okay. Just let it flow through. Just allow this wave to come....

P: *CRYING*

T: Let it last as long as it lasts, you don't have to do anything about it. No need to force it through, no need to take it away.

P: *CRYING, WIPING TEARS*

T: Just let it be as it is. No need to do anything with it, just let it come through. Your body knows how to do it, if you just trust your body.

P: *CRYING* *SOBS*

T: Because, you actually know how to do this. You were really good at it when you were a newborn.

P: *LAUGHS* Yes ... *WIPES TEARS*

T: How was it for you this time?

P: I notice that I feel more each time.

T: Okay.

P: Without necessarily being able to separate it—into what it is! It's just *a lot*!

T: It's just a lot! Right!

P: But it feels like you want good things for me.

T: It feels like I want good things for you. Right. How is that for you? To look me in the eye and feel like I want good things for you?

P: It's very nice. And then it's very strange to show feelings for the first time for someone who doesn't *PULLS BACKWARD DEMONSTRATIVELY* become terrified!

The Sweet Child has just opened up to me about how she feels, exposing her sadness and grief. She has also been open and honest about her frustration with me when I stay quiet. Being honest and open about her feelings toward someone, for the first time ever, is good. It is nice, and it feels like I want good things for her. In addition, this is an important *corrective emotional experience* (Alexander & French, 1946), as I do not withdraw from her and her feelings. She can freely express how she feels without the recipient—me—becoming terrified. This experience is absolutely crucial for her to be open about her feelings toward other people in her life. Facilitating profound emotional experiences like this is a fundamental component of ISTDP (Davanloo, 1990).

Losing a Parent

The Sweet Child expresses her anger and frustration toward me, her boyfriend, and her sister, as we have not been able to provide her with the help and support she needs. Being in touch with this anger brings back memories of her being angry with her father. This is a common phenomenon in ISTDP: when patients allow themselves to fully experience their complex feelings toward people in their daily lives, it often triggers the recall of old memories in which similar feelings were once activated. These memories often reveal the formative experiences that have led to the patients' suffering. The spontaneous sharing of such new memories is a clear sign that *the unconscious therapeutic alliance* is strong (Davanloo, 1990; Kuhn, 2014).

P: Initially, I was very angry when Dad got sick. That was my first reaction *CRYING*. And then I have had a very guilty conscience for being angry with him.

T: Aha, so there's the guilty conscience, too.

P: It may be that there has been anger for quite a long time that has not been let out. I became very frustrated and angry when Dad changed.

T: Of course.

P: He wasn't Dad anymore, and he's not now, either.

The Sweet Child remembers how her father changed from being a socially competent man into making a spectacle of himself in social situations. She has been struggling with a feeling of shame, been burdened by a sense of responsibility for helping him, while simultaneously criticizing herself for not being able to do so. She realizes that she is sick of this, but finds it difficult to voice it out loud.

P: I … I'm just really sick of his illness shaping so many parts of our lives—for those of us that are around him—and imposing so many limitations.

T: So what do you feel, in your body right now, when you say you're sick of it—what's happening now? There are some tears coming, threatening to tear down this "sick of it." What do you notice—what do you feel toward him? Do you feel anything, or are you going numb again?

P: I'm going numb.

Expressing all that she is sick of in relation to her father brings up her anger toward him, as she is speaking of it. This is really complicated for her: she quickly disconnects from herself and becomes numb. But this time she does not *stay* numb, but instead starts crying when she *realizes* that she is going numb. She recognizes her defense mechanism of detachment, understands the harm it causes, and this insight is deeply painful for her. In ISTDP, grief that comes with realizing the negative impact of one's defense mechanisms is considered an important step in the therapy process.

P: *CRYING AND SOBBING*
T: This hurts ... It's okay to let it go through ... It's fine, just take this wave as well .... Grief and guilty conscience and everything. And instead of feeling these complicated, angry feelings toward your father that give you such a guilty conscience, because you love him so much, he was such a lovely person until you were 15 ... you rather go numb....
P: *CRYING*
T: Mmm. It's okay, just let it through.
P: *CRYING*
T: Mmm. Let the wave come through.
P: *THE TEARS GRADUALLY COME TO A HALT* I think a lot relates to this.
T: It has become pretty obvious to us, hasn't it, as to when you go numb?
P: Mmm. I've lost my dad! But he's still there, just not as himself! And that is so frustrating!
T: Of course it is!
P: I want everyone to know him as he was!
T: Of course!
P: Not like a grumpy old man who is really cranky and rude.
T: You don't like that father, do you? There's a whole bunch of complicated stuff here, do you see that? You want everyone to see him as ... because he was so nice! You had fifteen years with him. And now he's not himself anymore. You have lost him. In a way, he is dead.
P: His body is still there, but Dad as he was is gone.
T: Oh, so you've lost your dad. Your dad is gone.
P: And now Mom has changed too.
T: Okay, so now you're losing your mom, too.
P: That's what I'm afraid of.
T: Have you lost your mom, or is she still there somehow?
P: She's there, but she's in so much pain. She has really changed as a result of being on so much pain.

The Sweet Child shares how she feels angry toward her father, who has repeatedly embarrassed both himself and her. Her grief becomes evident as well. She has lost the father she once had; he is actually gone. Furthermore, her mother has also changed, and she fears losing her too. The Sweet Child has lost one parent and now faces the potential loss of another.

First Anger, Then Good Memories, Then Sadness Again

Together, we continue our work to help the Sweet Child experience her anger toward her father. She is explaining how in recent years he has become an irritable and grumpy man, even with his grandchildren. At first she feels strong and energized when she allows herself to feel angry, but then she starts to cry. On the one hand, she knows that crying defensively means that others will not realize that she is actually angry. At the same time, she has a sense of regaining control when crying compared to feeling angry.

P: It's easier to regain control than to … especially when what I really want to do is scream!

T: And then your hands came up …. Scream!

P: I don't feel like screaming in here!

T: Okay, but what would you have screamed? In your imagination, you don't need to scream in here. Let's work on *feeling* it rather than *acting* it out. In your imagination. Allow yourself to feel it in your body, and picture in your imagination what this is all about. So that you can practice feeling it, not avoiding it. Screaming is kind of a way to avoid feeling it by acting it out. But the impulse to scream is important. What does it look like? Where do you picture it? Where are you screaming?

P: In the woods. That was Dad's sanctuary …. *CRYING*

T: That was Dad's sanctuary.

P: He was a keen outdoorsman. So I grew up in the woods. *CRIES AND SOBS*

T: Okay, just let it come through …. So there they are, the good memories!

P: *NODS*

T: What did the two of you do in the woods? Please tell me!

P: *LAUGHS AND CRIES* He taught me about different kinds of trees and moss and rock. Flora and fauna. He had studied forestry. So….

T: This is very important. Because these are the good memories that are starting to surface.

P: Yes. We were always out in the woods. We were always hiking on Sundays. When I was three years old, I could name all different species of trees and types of lichen and … the whole works. It was, in a way, our special shared thing.

T: So that's what you did. Nice job, teaching a three-year-old girl all of that!

P: We have a video of me walking around, naming all the tree species in the forest.

T: That he taught you.

P: That he taught me.

The Sweet Child remembers how angry she became at her father after he fell ill. He made a spectacle of himself in social situations, and he changed. Being angry at someone who has dementia and thus cannot do anything about the change that is occurring, is a complicated feeling. She has therefore more or less consciously tried to suppress her anger. The problem is that when you suppress one feeling, other feelings tend to follow. Thus, it is only *after* she allows herself to feel angry toward her father that the good memories resurface. This is a common occurrence in therapy: in order to access the good memories, one often first needs to process feelings of anger. The emergence of new memories is also a strong indicator of a solid *unconscious therapeutic alliance* (Davanloo, 1990; Kuhn, 2014). Still, pleasant memories of her father are also mixed with complex emotions, inevitably evoking feelings of grief over her loss.

P: But now he can't .... He's mostly cognitively affected, but also a little physically too. So he can't go hiking in the mountains anymore, or in the forest. We used to hike in the mountains a lot. And we had the woods right outside our door, so that was what we did the most. Holidays and weekends we always spent in the mountains. But he isn't able to go there anymore.

T: So that's one more thing you've lost.

P: I still go there, but that's when I feel like screaming. Because I can't bring him with me! *CRIES*

T: Just let that one through, too. He can't be with you anymore.

P: *CRIES*

T: But you still know all the species of trees ...

P: *LAUGHS AND CRIES* Yes ....

T: It's terribly sad ...

Angry Impulses and Guilt

Anger led to good feelings. Good feelings led to sadness. And grief brings up fresh memories and another round of anger:

P: Yes ... *CRYING* He can't join me ... and that .... He can't join me and that .... He wants to intensely, but whenever he has tried to go hiking, he has become confused and helpless. Totally weird and different. So that's where I want to scream. Sometimes I do scream, even.

T: So all these feelings come up. And the woods become quite important. Because it's somehow the room where all these good feelings toward your dad, all the good memories, all this rage ....

P: Yes, and also ... Dad has ... I think in a way Dad's way of grieving my brother's death was exercise and being out in the woods. It has been his sanctuary.

T: So you have copied his ways of handling things as well.

P: Yes.

T: Go out into the woods and scream. Working out to get rid of things.

P: Throw some rocks *LAUGHS*. That's even better than screaming.

T: So there is the power in your hands.

P: Yes, it's so good to throw stones.

T: Who are you angry at? In the woods?

P: Dad's dementia. Because that's where I'm able to be angry at the disease and not at him.

T: Right. But that's your rationality, isn't it?

P: *WHISPERS* Yes ....

T: That ... that's your adult brain explaining how it's all connected. So here is a ... in that way you can be allowed to feel the rage. Stone-throwing and shouting and .... But when we talked about feeling it toward your boyfriend, this comes *TAKING A STRANGLEHOLD ON MYSELF*, when we talk about your sister, this comes *TAKING A STRANGLEHOLD ON MYSELF*. It's back at you. Speaking of this rage toward your dad, you numb yourself out. If you call it dementia, you can feel it. But actually, it's all about him. If we put away your rational brain.

P: I know it is.

T: So how do you feel that rage toward him? The stone-throwing ... the screaming rage.

P: Mmm. Well ... I've thought several times, when I've been out in the woods and felt angry ... for him, and for everyone around him, it would have been better if he took a walk in the woods and fell down a mountainside. It's what he wants the most, to keep hiking in the woods, but he can't ....

T: So here is a rage that could very well end in death.

We are beginning to grasp why the Sweet Child has found it difficult to experience her true feelings. When she refrains from using her defense mechanisms, the internal conflict within her becomes unmistakably apparent. She cherishes her many good memories of her father, who was close to her and played an important and present role in her life. The Sweet Child has an abundance of love for her father, but now that he has changed, she feels so angry that she sometimes wishes he had died. This internal struggle is deeply painful, and instead of facing these conflicting feelings, she has been avoiding them.

P: *SIGHS* Yes .... Yes, actually. But it's horrific to say that!

T: So how do you notice this rage that could almost kill him? We've already seen strangulation. But that's directed back at you.

P: *NODDING* *WHISPERS* Yes ... *SIGHS * Yes .... Sometimes I wish I just, well, ohhh ....

T: Yes, let it come ....

P: *SOBS* I want to scream at him too!

T: Right, so what are you screaming? In your imagination, if you were to let this out completely unfiltered? Leave your brain to one side. You have more than enough brains to understand. If you're to be allowed to let this out freely, what do you want to scream, what does your body want to do? If everything is allowed to come out?

P: It's like, I don't dare to say it out loud! *LOOKS AWAY*

Internally, she is aware of what she wants to shout at her father—but saying it out loud and sharing it with someone is very difficult for her. She doesn't want to say it out loud, and she distances herself from me by looking away. At this point, our mutual understanding that our task in therapy is to assist her in not facing difficult feelings alone, is incredibly valuable.

T: Right. So let's look at it together, so that you don't have to be alone with it.
P: No ....
T: What are you screaming? What are you doing?
P: *LOOKS AWAY AND STARTS TO CRY*
T: Right ... okay, just let it come. It's the guilt, isn't it?
P: *CRYING* *NODDING*
T: Mmm. It's okay. Just let yourself feel this guilt, rather than punish yourself for it.
P: *CRYING*
T: Okay....

Without having said it out loud yet, the guilt stemming from what she wants to scream at her father emerges. The vivid image in her imagination stirs up strong feelings. Guilt, a common feeling when one is angry with a loved one, is one of the most painful feelings we experience. One way to sidestep guilt over anger is to avoid it by criticizing or punishing oneself. Instead of feeling guilty, one resorts to self-punishment and gives oneself a hard time. This form of self-punishment becomes a defense mechanism against guilt. However, this strategy leads to suffering and psychological distress. To live with inner conflict, as described in Chapter 2, one must also learn to tolerate a guilty conscience without self-punishment.

P: *SOBS* I could actually scream, "I hate you!"
T: You want to scream that you hate him. What more? If everything is allowed to come out? If you don't hold back? Those things that you don't feel you can say out loud? Just allow it through, this thing that gives you such a guilty conscience.
P: *CRIES AND SOBS*
P: That it would be easier for all of us if he wasn't here anymore.
T: Yes ....
P: Because my mother and my sister and I cannot relate to each other as we would like to, because everything has to be on his terms. Always.
T: Okay, so he's ruining it for all of you. He's ruining it for you, your sister and your mother. How do you notice this rage? Is it inside you?
P: *LOOKS CALM AND SAD* No, now it went away again.
T: Okay, where did that go?
P: Don't know ....
T: How do you feel right now?
P: Right now I feel relieved! *LAUGHS*
T: You feel relieved. That's a good feeling, isn't it?
P: Yes! It's not like I've told anyone before that I would like to say, "I hate you!" to Dad!

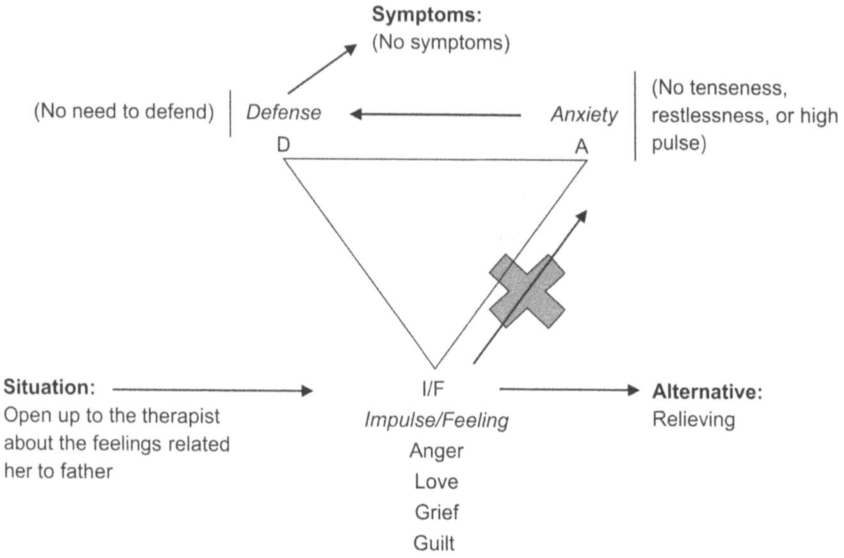

Figure 7.3 The Triangle of Conflict applied to the case of the Sweet Child

This is why, in psychodynamic therapy, the therapist focuses on unconscious conflicts and the associated feelings. When you become aware of and *experience* your feelings, like the Sweet Child does, it brings a sense of relief. She has *experienced and been consciously aware* of anger, love, grief and guilt. She has openly discussed her feelings with someone she truly trusts. As a result, the feelings no longer evoke as much anxiety (as shown in Figure 7.3), and she feels much better.

The Sweet Child expresses an important message: the difference between the *wish* to say something and *actually* saying it is significant. This distinction is challenging for many of us. When we feel something strongly, we get the sense of having *done* something wrong even though we obviously have not. We have just *experienced feelings*. There is a big difference between craving chocolate and eating chocolate. There is a big difference between not wanting to get out of bed, and actually not getting up. There is a big difference between wanting to shout, "I hate you!" and actually shouting it. This distinction is essential to understand when working with feelings and their impulses.

P: I would never say that, though!

T: No, you wouldn't. And that's what's important. It is incredibly important. Because you're treating that feeling as if you're *actually going to say it*. You feel as guilty as if you had actually said that. Do you see that?

P: Yes, yes! *NODS*

T: And as you just said … you will never say that!

P: *LAUGHS*
T: So these are your feelings.
P: Mmm.
T: Such a guilty conscience … because we know what lovely moments you've had with your dad. But then you didn't go numb—you felt relief?
P: Mm *NODS*.
T: Can you let yourself feel that?
P: *NODS* It's so lovely!
T: Right. So just feel …. Let it be there as long as it's there. It's an important feeling. Because this is a bit of that freedom. Allowing yourself to feel what you feel.
P: *WHISPERS* Yes … Mm. It's really lovely.

They Could Have Asked!

The Sweet Child continues to describe how her father has repeatedly ruined family dinners with his inappropriate behavior. What were once pleasant gatherings have now turned into dreaded occasions. In her imagination, she portrays taking the dinner plates into the woods and smashing them. She smashes them in anger, just like her dreams have been shattered. It is a painful and sorrowful image, and she sees herself sitting in the woods amid the broken plates, crying. And she cries alone.

T: What is it like for you to picture yourself crying in the woods? Lonely?
P: Somehow, that's what I feel regarding this whole situation. Even though I have a lot of great people around me, I feel lonely when it comes to how I feel. So far I haven't had anyone to talk to about it. I have a lot of nice people in my life, but only a very few of them know how I truly feel.
T: So … this girl sitting in the woods with the broken plates … is that you *now*, or is it back then? How old is the girl who is sitting there?
P: No, it's me ten years ago.
T: Ten years ago. What does that girl need? She who's sitting out there in the woods after smashing those plates?
P: To be seen.
T: By whom? Who are you going to bring in? Who does she need?
P: Mom. And my sister.
T: What can you do to bring them into this fantasy?
P: I wish they would …. *SIGHS* They were so determined that we should … handle it on our own. I really think I needed a bit more help to deal with Dad's diagnosis.
T: So how do they come and help you? In your imagination? When you're sitting there alone in the woods with broken plates. Sitting there alone, crying.
P: They could ask me how I was actually doing.

T: What else? What happens then?

P: Then I could tell them ….

T: What are you telling them? Out in the woods with the broken plates? Your father's woods?

P: That I'm afraid! *CRIES*

T: So, what do you need then?

P: I think I just needed us to talk more about it. But we didn't do that back then, so … it's kind of hard to start doing it now. And then I felt like I was the one who handled it worst … the relationship with my father. Because I was so annoyed with him. So we went from me and Dad having a very good relationship to …. Actually, we were also the ones who would blow up at each other. Because we were quite similar, we could get at loggerheads. But there were never any major conflicts. But after Dad got sick … I got so annoyed at everything he did …. All the signs of illness he showed were a reminder of the kind of future that was waiting for us.

This part highlights one of the reasons why things have become difficult for the Sweet Child. She has always sensed that she ought to protect her loved ones from her feelings. And when her sister and mother have focused on handling their struggles on their own, it has become increasingly difficult. To get out of her role of helping and supporting others, she would have needed them to ask her and take the initiative to talk about it. They didn't, and the Sweet Child has kept her feelings to herself. The section also showcases the usefulness of *portraying feelings* (Davanloo, 1990): picturing in the imagination how the feeling motivates one to act. It is no coincidence that the Sweet Child's fantasy takes place in the woods. The *unconscious therapeutic alliance*[3] contributes to the images taking place in an important location—the special place that they shared—and the fact that she is sitting there alone, looking like she did ten years ago, brings up important themes of loneliness and lack of help.

Envy

The Sweet Child continues to express her complex feelings. She confesses to feeling envious of her sister, Lise:

P: *SIGHS* I think it's unfair that she got … ten more good years with Mom and Dad than I did. After all, I've gotten less years with everyone. Grandparents. And I didn't even get to meet my brother. And I probably wouldn't have been born if he hadn't died!

T: That's quite intense, isn't it?!

P: They had no plans to have another child. It was the two of them, but then … they decided to have me.

T: That one is actually pretty damn intense. Without his death you wouldn't have existed.

P: No.

T: Better be grateful.

P: *NODS* They had no plans to have another child. But they reckoned it was the only right thing to do after he died, since there was only Lise left. She was only ten.

T: So you were somehow born for Lise's sake. And for your mom and dad's.

P: Mmm.

T: Mmm. How does that feel?

P: It's exhausting to have to be there for everyone else.

She is envious and angry—feelings that are difficult for a lot of people to handle. Yet at the same time she ought to feel grateful since she was never meant to exist in the first place. The Sweet Child has confronted numerous emotional challenges, and it has been exhausting to provide support for everyone else.

Summing Up

The session is coming to an end, and we have achieved a lot in this trial therapy. The Sweet Child is a resourceful young woman, possessing a remarkable talent for articulating her thoughts with precision. She has demonstrated considerable courage in confronting challenging feelings with a person she has just recently met. She has also helped to illustrate the first part of this book, making it easier to understand key phenomena in psychodynamic therapy.

The overarching goal of a trial therapy is to form a foundation for further therapy. The therapist and the patient have the opportunity to establish a strong alliance (Bordin, 1979) through mutual understanding and shared experiences. Hence, I am curious as to what she is left with following the session.

T: What have you understood? If you share what you take away from this, I will fill in what I have in mind.

P: So … I think the way I deal with what I'm struggling with now—the fact that my father is sick and my mother is sick—comes from the upbringing I had. That I …. Mom and Dad could have bad days. And I was very good at paying attention to that, even back then. So don't …. The shield we talked about probably comes from the fact that I didn't want to inflict more worries on them. Or more things to be sad about.

T: This inverted shield.

P: Yes. Keeping what's mine on the inside. And that has probably meant that I'm not very good at feeling …. So, for me to talk about feelings as physical sensations is like speaking a foreign language!

T: And then we see that you're quite good at it when we focus in on it.

P: Yes, it comes down to practice. But I think it's pretty healthy! I don't usually pay attention to my experience. I tend to *think* I'm sad, I'm angry. I don't experience it!

Psychodynamic theory recognizes that multiple factors can contribute to the patient's problems.[4] In the Sweet Child's therapy we have worked on a number of phenomena that created difficulties for her, among other aspects, how unconscious conflicts regarding taking care of herself have led her to use defense mechanisms that have given rise to new problems. She has struggled to find effective alternatives to defense mechanisms; hence she is seeking help. Accepting help has been a complex task for her, not only from friends and family, but also from me. She employs the same strategies with me that she learned when growing up: she protects me. We then worked systematically to explore and comprehend the feelings and conflicts she had with her father, sister, brother, and mother. She found this a relief. But how does she feel when she returns one week later?

Sweet Child O' Mine

One week later, the Sweet Child returns with good news. She said she was tired after the session, but also felt she had acknowledged and effectively processed her feelings. She didn't become numb; instead, it felt good.

Later on, on the same day as the trial therapy, something occurred that illustrates what happens when we stop using defense mechanisms to distance ourselves from our inner world: that which lies in the unconscious begins to surface, presenting us with an opportunity to process it. Once you have toppled the first domino in a rally, and do not stop the next one from tumbling, a lot can come up. The Sweet Child's unconscious, associative network reveals new information that illuminates what has been happening within her. In ISTDP, the type of phenomenon described in the following section is understood as an indicator that *the unconscious therapeutic alliance* (Davanloo, 1990) is good.

P: Later that day, I don't know where it came from, but suddenly I started humming *CRYING* the song "Sweet Child O' Mine."

T: By Guns N' Roses?

P: It's in a movie. Have you seen *Captain Fantastic*?

T: *SHAKING MY HEAD*

P: It's about a family …. If you haven't seen it, you should. A fantastic family, coming-of-age film, about a slightly unconventional family that lives on the edge of society out in the woods. And they play that song in the movie when they bury their mom. *SOBS* *LAUGHS*. That scene has always stuck with me, without me really understanding why. *CRYING* And suddenly last Thursday I was at home and I was humming that song. Where was it coming from? I hadn't specifically been thinking about it. Just started singing the song. Eh … so exactly what it was, I don't know.

T: So, the scene where they buried their mother ….

P: Yes. So I …. You asked me to pay attention and be a aware of what was going through my feelings. And it was so strange that it came right then.

T: A parent's funeral.

P: Well, yes *CRYING*

T: Who did you bury?

P: In my case, it's probably ... *WIPES HER TEARS* ... the old version of Dad. *CRIES* It's so weird. Because I've seen that movie so many times. And every time .... Then that scene hits me in the gut. But also ... they're a bit alternative. They kidnap the mother's coffin from a conventional funeral and take her out in the woods, by the sea ... and do their own thing.

T: Out in the woods?

P: Or out in nature.

T: But you said out in the woods.

P: Maybe there's something there that I haven't thought of. I've never understood why that singular scene has been ... hit me hard. There might be something ... in that you have to say ... or come to terms with the fact that ... the father I would like to get back, I won't get him back.

The Sweet Child is humming "Sweet Child O' Mine." She learned this song from a scene in a movie where a beloved parent is buried in the woods, and the scene has always deeply moved her. And we understand why: she has lost the old version of her father and has to come to terms with the fact that she will never get that father back. Human beings often rely on rituals, such as funerals, to help cope with the pain of losing loved ones. Unfortunately, the Sweet Child will never get the chance to hold a funeral for the old version of her dad. But grieving in the session with me has helped her move on.

P: But I've also noticed this week ... there hasn't been much to put a lid on. I don't know. It feels like, by putting things into words with you last week, things I haven't really said out loud to anyone before, has helped a lot. It was a bit like that—ahhh! Now it's said out loud, and then you can be a little less ashamed. I could say it to you without being met with the kind of disgust and horror that you fear you'll be met with if you say that out loud.

T: As you may have met yourself?

P: Yes, that too. It has been a bit like, there are less repressed feelings. Yes.

T: So you've already gotten a lot of results out of the job you did last time? It was quite a job you did!

P: Yes, that night I was completely worn out. My boyfriend was almost worried about me. Because I was completely kaput. And it feels different.

T: What do you notice?

P: I've felt a bit like ... lighter, somehow. *LAUGHS AND MOVES HER BODY* When I walk, and yes, a bit more relaxed in my body.

T: When you walk ....

P: Yes, not quite so .... Sometimes it feels like it affects the way I walk .... On bad days my way of walking becomes a bit like ... argh. But now there's a strength in my steps. It has been very nice.

In addition to the trial therapy, the Sweet Child had three sessions with me. She also participated in a mindfulness group at the clinic where I work. At termination, she was happy and relieved. She felt liberated, able to express herself more openly with those around her, and she was no longer feeling depressed.

Therapy rarely progresses as quickly and smoothly as it did with the Sweet Child. She was a wise and sweet child, and so she is invaluable when it comes to explaining these psychodynamic processes. For those of you who are new to psychodynamic therapy: do not expect things to progress this quickly or for everything to become this clear right away. Take all the time you need, and one day you might meet a sweet child who can change so quickly too.

Notes

1 Insight is the psychodynamic term for understanding oneself, and is associated with improvement in psychodynamic therapy (Kallestad et al., 2010).
2 David Malan (1979) called this way of communicating being *an iron hand in a velvet glove*.
3 Kuhn (2014) describes the unconscious therapeutic alliance (UTA) as the unconscious and constructive side of the patient's inner self that strives for recovery and good health.
4 In psychodynamic therapy, this is called *multiple causation* (Coughlin, 2022b).

Part II

Dynamic Inquiry and Alliance

T: We're beginning to understand this. You can see it, you're a smart young woman. What's the next step after you understand?

P: **LAUGHS** Might have to start practicing, then.

After reading the first part of this book, it has hopefully become easier to understand psychodynamic theory. However, theoretical comprehension alone is not enough to bring about change. It must be put into practice. Now is the time to delve into how this is accomplished in practical terms—might have to start practicing, then.

DOI: 10.4324/9781003516217-10

Chapter 8

Case Formulation and Alliance

Little has been written about the process of establishing effective and practical psycho-dynamic collaborations or *conscious alliances* (Kuhn, 2014) in Intensive Short-Term Dynamic Psychotherapy (ISTDP), and this is having a significant impact on the field. New ISTDP therapists have often grasped the concept of helping the patient "imagine that they are taking someone's life," which stems from the technique of portraying feelings in one's imagination (Davanloo, 1990). However, they may lack understanding of why and when this technique is relevant to the therapeutic process. They may also have little knowledge of how to create effective psychodynamic healing projects.

In ISTDP literature, as I see it, there is an underlying assumption that this—as well as a fundamental understanding of psychodynamics—is a skill that new therapists possess. Previous generations of psychotherapists may have acquired this knowledge through their basic education. However, in my experience, it is evident that many of today's emerging therapists lack this essential competence.

One complicating aspect is that some ISTDP literature places significant emphasis on therapeutic techniques, mirroring other short-term therapies like cognitive-behavioral therapy (Wenzel, 2021). Habib Davanloo and Aaron Beck, who developed these respective methods, received their training in classical psychoanalytic therapy, which provided them with a profound and comprehensive understanding of their patients. Both were frustrated that progress was slow with this method, and therefore developed efficient techniques to accelerate their patients' recovery. However, they brought with them a fundamental understanding of psychoanalytic theory, which was also ingrained in the first generations of therapists who learned these technical methods.

When today's therapists are taught these effective techniques, there is a risk that what was originally meant to enhance the effectiveness of therapy based on analytic understanding is now being taught as the entire therapy itself. One then runs the risk of having therapists who are only trained in technique, without possessing a comprehensive and profound understanding of theory. If you want to build a house in marshy terrain, being a technically skilled carpenter is not enough: it is crucial to understand that the building site is a bog and to be able to effectively drain the area, dig a proper cellar, and cast a solid foundation wall that remains dry. All of these steps must be completed before beginning the carpentry work.

DOI: 10.4324/9781003516217-11

This concept translates directly to psychotherapy. You must comprehend the terrain, establish a solid and enduring foundation, and determine the type of structure to construct. Before beginning specialized carpentry work, it is crucial to ensure that all of these elements are in place.

At the beginning of a short-term dynamic therapy, there are two main objectives to be pursued. The first is to establish hypotheses regarding the causes of the patient's challenges. This can be referred to as a psychodynamic case formulation, which is co-created through collaboration with the patient. The second objective is to establish a robust working alliance (Bordin, 1979). A case formulation, together with a strong working alliance, offers a comprehensive grasp of the terrain, creates a sturdy foundation, and lays out a blueprint for constructing the house.

Psychodynamic Case Formulation

In short-term dynamic therapy and ISTDP, creating a case formulation hinges on a few key principles. First, the therapist must understand the patient's problems and goals. Together, the therapist and patient need to develop hypotheses on the mechanisms causing the patient's problems, as discussed in Chapters 4 and 5. Furthermore, they need to formulate theories about the psychological processes that perpetuate these mechanisms, even when they cease to be advantageous, as outlined in Chapters 1 and 2. Together, they should explore the specific situations and individuals involved when the problems surface, and when they first appeared. These problems often show up in the patient's interaction with their therapist, as mentioned in Chapter 3. By scrutinizing these situations, they can gain insights into what transpires when the difficulties emerge.

Another way to describe this is using Malan's (1979) two triangles, which were discussed in Chapters 3, 4, and 6.

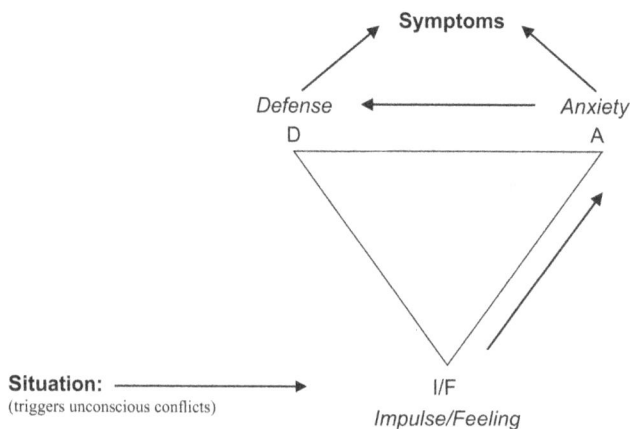

Figure 8.1 The Triangle of Conflict and its Relationship to the Symptom-Generating Situation and Resulting Symptoms

Therapist/transference   Current people
T   C

P
Past persons

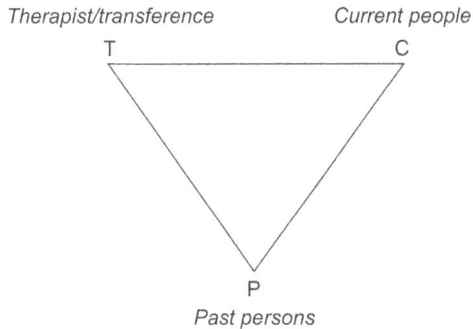

Figure 8.2 The Triangle of Person

These two triangles visually depict the components previously explained as the elements of a short-term dynamic case formulation. Symptom-generating situations with people in the current (C), with people in the past (P), and with the therapist (T) should be inquired into, where C, P, and T represent the three corners of the triangle of person (Figure 8.2). In psychodynamic theory, it is assumed that the unconscious psychological conflicts and the ways they are managed are shaped through interactions with significant figures from the past. These conflicts, and the patient's ways of dealing with them, will resurface both with people in the patient's current life and with the therapist. This forms the foundation of psychodynamic thinking. You can gather information about the patient's conflicts on all three corners of the triangle of person based on the theoretical assumption that they are interconnected.

At each corner of the triangle of person, it is beneficial to reveal the way the triangle of conflict (Figure 8.1) unfolds. The therapist looks for examples of *symptom-generating situations*. This is not a search for feelings *in general*, which is a common misconception among ISTDP therapists. The situations of interest are those that arouse *feelings and impulses (I/F)* toward *people (C, T, and P)*, and that are causing *anxiety (A)*. To avoid these feelings, the patient uses *defense mechanisms (D)* which cause further symptoms. These are the situations and relationships that, for some reason, are linked to the patient's unconscious conflicts, and are the focus of the ISTDP therapist's exploration. If the situation were not connected to unconscious conflicts, the feelings would not have caused anxiety, but would have been merely *experienced*. Situations with people in the current life trigger inner unconscious conflicts and cause the patient to use old strategies to avoid having to deal with the conflict and its associated feelings. These mechanisms are responsible for producing the *symptoms* that lead patients to seek help (Chapter 5).

Here is an imaginary example: For many people, joy is a straightforward feeling. Situations that bring about joy are positive and provide an experience of the feeling of joy in the form of energy, vitality, and vigor. The feeling is simply experienced in its purest form and contributes to an increased quality of life. However, some individuals have a problematic relationship to their feeling of joy. They may have grown up with a parent who was depressed or struggled with substance abuse, causing their expressions of joy to be perceived as burdensome or distressing for their caregiver. Thus, it was not uncomplicated to just *feel* and *experience* joy, as the feeling was associated with pain and difficulties, and possibly criticism and punishment. In current life, in a scenario where the patient is returning home to his girlfriend after experiencing something positive at work, the patient finds himself in a complicated situation: The patient feels anxiety in the face of his feeling of joy and anticipates a lack of interest from his partner *(C)*, reminiscent of the disinterest shown by his parent in the past *(P)*. He will then use a defense *(D)*, such as diverting the conversation to something completely unrelated to what brought him joy. This patient will need help to be able to experience joy without anxiety. Effective emotional management involves allowing oneself to experience and acknowledge one's feelings. It is that simple, yet so challenging. *The alternative to avoiding feelings is to experience them.*

When initiating the process of creating a psychodynamic case formulation, you start by examining the patient's problems and symptoms, while trying to understand what is happening at each of the three corners of the triangle of conflict, in the specific situation the difficulties arise. It is not a structured inquiry that has a right and wrong order; it is, on the other hand, a dynamic process (Davanloo, 1990). While in the dialogue with the patient, the therapist tries to mentally place the information in the correct corners of the triangles as it emerges. The therapist must understand which defense mechanisms produce symptoms. They need to comprehend which feelings cause anxiety, and the specific situations and individuals that trigger these feelings. The therapist must cultivate a genuine curiosity about the patient and their mechanisms. Above all, they must facilitate the patient's own curiosity about themselves.

If this examination is done systematically with symptom-inducing situations in the present (the C-corner of the triangle of person), as well as when symptoms occur in the therapist–client relationship (the T-corner of the triangle of person), and in situations where the difficulties first arose in life (the P-corner of the triangle of person), you will often see patterns emerge. As an ISTDP therapist, it is crucial to be transparent and open about your hypotheses concerning these patterns and the interconnectedness of things. This transparent review of symptom-inducing situations will provide a solid foundation for therapists and patients to develop hypotheses about the underlying causes of the patient's difficulties. With these hypotheses in place, it becomes easier to identify the necessary steps that need to be taken in therapy to effectively help the patient. The comprehension of what happens at each corner of the triangles, and how this correlates to the patients presenting problems, is an important part of a short-term dynamic case formulation, as is the hypothesis about the reasons *why* the patient handles situations in a way that creates problems. I will soon provide an example of how this is put into practice. But before I do that, I want to discuss the other main component of psychodynamic house building— namely, the working alliance.

Bordin's Working Alliance

The therapeutic alliance is often misunderstood as only being about the emotional connection between therapist and patient. Edward Bordin (1979) established a widely accepted definition of the working alliance. His definition is utilized in extensive research on this type of alliance and is commonly measured using the Working Alliance Inventory (WAI) (Horvath & Greenberg, 1986). This definition of the working alliance can be applied to most psychotherapy approaches, including short-term dynamic therapy. Bordin described the working alliance as encompassing three components[1]:

1 Agreement on goals.
2 Agreement on the therapeutic tasks.
3 A solid therapeutic bond.

People seek psychotherapy for specific reasons. They are experiencing psychological problems and believe that a psychotherapist can offer the help they need to resolve these challenges. Patients often struggle to articulate their issues effectively. This may be due to difficulty in finding the right words to describe their challenges, or feeling that the problem is more of a vague discomfort. Perhaps it is also uncomfortable for them to discuss their difficulties in a clear and unambiguous manner. Instead, they alleviate this discomfort by referring to their difficulties in a general and non-specific manner. In order to establish a strong working alliance, it is vital to have a clear, mutual understanding and agreement about the patient's goals. While it may be challenging and uncomfortable, one of the initial steps for both the patient and the therapist is to come to a mutual agreement on the issue to be addressed. This agreement is fundamental in formulating a goal. Once this agreement is achieved, it is crucial to establish a shared understanding of the goal, which encapsulates what the patient aims to accomplish once the problem is resolved.

The next important element in establishing a strong working alliance is agreement between the therapist and patient on the therapeutic tasks. This alignment signifies a shared understanding of the collaborative efforts required in therapy to achieve the goal. Consider exposure therapy for arachnophobia. If there is no mutual agreement on the therapeutic task of gradually confronting spiders, it would be considered both absurd and frightening if the therapist were to unexpectedly place a spider directly in front of the patient. Similarly, in short-term dynamic therapy, it is crucial for the therapist and the patient to reach an agreement regarding the exploration of the painful feelings that the patient has previously avoided. Without this mutual understanding and the shared belief that addressing these feelings will lead toward a resolution of the patient's problems, it becomes perplexing why the therapist would inquire into such feelings. After all, why would a patient willingly confront something that induces pain and is perceived as creating problems?

The final aspect of Bordin's definition of the working alliance is the establishment of a strong therapeutic bond. This involves the establishment of a trusting relationship between the therapist and the patient, characterized by empathy and mutual respect. There seems to be a belief among certain groups that the ISTDP therapist should adopt a distant and cold approach, at least according to Camilla Flåten (2021). This goes against everything I believe in and how I have been taught to practice psychodynamic therapy by all of my supervisors, including Patricia Coughlin, the author of several influential ISTDP books (Coughlin, 2017, 2022b; Coughlin Della Selva, 2004; Malan & Coughlin Della Selva, 2007). It also contradicts research on effective therapy, which clearly specifies that a strong bond is related to a positive effect in therapy (Wampold, 2017). It is important to note that this bond encompasses more than just warmth, empathy, and mutual respect. Anderson and colleagues (2009) developed a measure of therapist characteristics called facilitative interpersonal skills (FIS) that are associated with positive therapy outcomes. In addition to warmth and empathy, this measure includes the therapist's verbal fluency, the ability to manage their own emotions, ability to persuade the patient of the therapeutic project, and the ability to provide hope and to maintain a problem focus. A therapist skilled in these elements will establish a strong bond and alliance with their clients, ultimately leading to favorable outcomes in therapy (Wampold, 2017).

When all three factors proposed by Bordin are incorporated into therapy, the chances of it being effective increase significantly (Laska et al., 2014). However, if the ISTDP therapist neglects to effectively address these three essential factors, patients may quickly have a negative experience with this approach. This understanding is based on my experience from years of supervising psychologists and students of clinical psychology as well as insights gained from being a practicing ISTDP therapist. The therapist and the patient must explicitly agree on the issues to be addressed and what they are trying to achieve—that is, what the *goal* is. In addition, there must be a mutual understanding of the steps needed to take in order to achieve the agreed-upon goal, or the *therapeutic task*. This shared understanding must exist within a relationship characterized by a strong *therapeutic bond*. If these factors are not in place, therapy often involves therapists attempting to persuade their patients to follow the method without the patients understanding the reasons behind the therapist's actions. The patient perceives the therapist as rigid, unempathic, and unresponsive, while at the same time the therapist perceives himself as stressed, worn out, and as the one doing all the work in the therapy. As I understand it, these are the crucial elements in Flåten's (2021) and Gjerde's (2021) unpleasant experiences with ISTDP. By focusing on building strong *conscious alliances*, one can often prevent the occurrence of these negative effects in therapy (Kuhn, 2014). It then becomes much easier to utilize all the powerful and effective techniques outlined in the ISTDP literature (Abbass, 2015; Coughlin, 2022b; Coughlin Della Selva, 2004; Davanloo, 1990; Frederickson, 2013) without confusion or misinterpretations.

Note

1 Some might argue that this definition should consist of four components, with agreement on the problems being the first. However, in Bordin's definition and in this text, this agreement is an integral and essential part of the first component, the agreement on the goal.

Chapter 9

Agreement on Goals

"What kind of problems do you need my help with?" is the initial question I ask all of my patients. I ask this question for several reasons. First, gaining an overview of the patient's problems and symptoms is the initial step in developing a psychodynamic case formulation. I begin by exploring the symptoms and working closely with the patient to gain insight into the defense mechanisms at play, as well as the root causes behind their use. Second, agreeing on which problems and symptoms to solve in therapy is the initial and crucial step toward building a strong therapeutic alliance with a shared goal (Bordin, 1979). The ambition of the Intensive Short-Term Dynamic Psychotherapy (ISTDP) therapist is to effectively address symptoms as those described in ICD-10 (WHO, 1992), but also to contribute to resolution of various life challenges such as relationship difficulties, self-destructive patterns, decision-making struggles, and more. When conducting a dynamic inquiry, as described in this chapter, these types of complaints are handled in the same manner as traditional symptomatic complaints. One could argue that *symptoms* fall under the broader umbrella of *problems*. Specifically, symptoms are problems that impact the patient internally, like feelings of anxiety and depression. However, in this book, the terms problems and symptoms are used somewhat interchangeably.

There are also indications that an early agreement on the problem can positively impact the therapeutic bond. Few things are as empowering to the therapeutic process as the therapist demonstrating a clear understanding of why the patient sought therapy and vividly illustrating the connection between the symptom and the underlying conflict. This happened in the Sweet Child's therapy, discussed in Part I of the book:

P: Now I'm getting numb. I don't feel anything.
T: Isn't that interesting?
P: Yes.
T: The numbness arrived. The reason you came here.
P: When you asked, it was a bit like …. I don't feel anything! Nothing in my body! I think I'm very good at thinking, not so good at feeling!
T: But when …. Part of the reason you're here is because you're going numb, isn't it?

DOI: 10.4324/9781003516217-12

P: Mmm.
T: And just now you went numb. Do you remember what I asked you?
P: What I noticed in my body when I got angry. *SIGHS*
T: And what happened then?
P: Woooof!! *GESTURES DOWNWARD* Felt nothing!

In the midst of our session, the symptom that initially brought her to therapy surfaced: she started to feel numb. This occurred as we were trying to assist her in *experiencing* her anger. As a result, our therapeutic endeavor to support her in managing her feelings gained momentum, boosting her confidence in our project.

Therapists often start by asking about the patient's past before understanding the problem they need help with (Frederickson, 2013). There are several reasons why this presents a problem. One issue is that the therapist does not adequately address the patient's primary concern, which is getting help with their current struggles. Having a clear understanding of the patient's perceived problem is crucial for effective therapy (Anderson et al., 2009).

Another issue is that therapists often analyze the past in a general manner, rather than focusing on understanding how specific events in the past have shaped the current problem. Discussing the past should not be an end in itself. The past should be examined when it is required to comprehend internal, unconscious conflicts that impact the present. In order to accomplish this, it is crucial to first grasp the nature of the problems at hand.

Inquiry

To develop a solid case formulation and establish a strong alliance, it is crucial to obtain a clear overview of the nature of the symptoms, including their severity and history. If you don't agree on which problems to address, you cannot agree on the goal, which is crucial for the therapeutic alliance (Bordin, 1979). Patricia Coughlin (2017) highlights this process, and her approach can be summarized into five questions:

A What are the patient's presenting symptoms, and how do they manifest?
B How severe are the symptoms?
C What are the precipitating event(s) triggering symptoms in the patient's *present life*?
D When did the symptoms first occur, and what were the precipitating triggers *back then*?
E How has the patient managed the symptoms up until now?

These questions are not asked directly to the patient, and the answers do not have to appear in the order given. Instead, the therapist aims to engage in a dialogue with the patient in which these questions are addressed. They serve as structuring and guiding topics for the conversation, rather than as direct questions to the patient.

Table 9.1 Key questions for inquiry

	Example
A. What are the patient's presenting symptoms, and how do they manifest?	
B. How severe are the symptoms?	
C. What are the precipitating event(s) triggering symptoms in the patient's *present life*?	
D. When did the symptoms first occur, and what were the precipitating trigger(s) *back then*?	
E. How has the patient managed the symptoms up until now?	

The questions are inserted in Table 9.1, which will serve as a reference through-out this chapter, providing an overview of the challenges faced by the presented patient.

These five questions will provide crucial information for shaping a psychody-namic project. They serve as the foundation for developing hypotheses about the underlying mechanisms that are causing the patient's difficulties. Once these five questions have been addressed, everything is in place to ask: "Is this the problem you would like me to help you with?"

From Problems to Goals

Once you agree on the nature of the problem, you can work toward reaching an agreement on the *goal* of the therapy. Identifying what will replace the problem is essential, as it paves the way for finding a positive alternative that can replace the symptoms. Sometimes a patient's aim is simply to alleviate symptoms, but more often than not, it goes beyond that: Once you eliminate the negative thoughts about yourself, what would you aspire to do instead? Would you like to dive into your passion for writing without mercilessly nitpicking every single step of the process? And if you refuse to shoulder all the blame for any mishaps in your marriage, what would you do then? Is the objective then to address disagreements and conflicts with your partner in a constructive manner, enabling you to feel like an equal and valued companion? It is important to agree on a *positive* goal. In this context, the term positive refers to the inclusion of something additional or the implementation of certain tasks, such as engaging in constructive writing or addressing disagree-ments productively. In other words, removing the symptom is not enough; there should also be something to take its place once the problems are resolved.

The Girl Who Wasn't a Princess

Learning from the patient (Casement, 1985) is crucial, also when understanding how this kind of inquiry should be implemented. In this part, a patient I have named the Girl Who Wasn't a Princess, a female Australian student in her thirties, will help me illustrate this process. The therapy with this woman was conducted in English and has not been translated from Norwegian, unlike the other transcripts in this book.

"What Kinds of Problems Would You Like Me to Help You With?"

She reached out for help in early spring and had been on the waiting list for a few months when she started therapy:

T: So …. What kinds of problems would you like me to help you with?

P: So, at the time that I reached out and set up the first meeting, I was … I had been living with a classmate who was also kind of a romantic interest, and was also a roommate, and it went really, really poorly …. And I don't really need to get into the details of it, because at the time I was … very fixated on every single thing that had happened …. But at this point it's been a couple months ….

T: At the time of the registration, you mean?

P: At the time of the registration it was …. That was the thing that got me into therapy …. Um, right now I would say my …. The reason I wanted to keep doing this and wanted to keep the appointment even though it's been a while, is because I was really … very suicidal at the time.

T: Okay.

P: And I think that has gone away now ….

T: You think? Or has it?

P: Like, it got so bad …. And it was not just that I was living with this person, but also the winter was really hard …. Obviously not everybody responds to that kind of stress by becoming, like, that self-destructive. And so I wanted to … um … I guess deal with it or talk about it now in the summer when things are generally fine, because I'm anticipating that the next winter is going to be hard.

T: So somehow you reckon that winter has got something to do about it? Like living here in the winter?

P: I think so, and I think it's also … um … There are still parts of that … um … because I lived with him for two months, and there are still parts of it that really bother me and he's still my classmate, and we still can't interact normally. At all!

The Girl Who Wasn't a Princess shares that she felt "very suicidal" while living with a classmate she had a romantic interest in. Within her first few sentences, I quickly grasp her reasons for seeking therapy and the circumstances that led to the onset of her problems. She says that the suicidal thoughts have gone away, but she is worried she will relapse, as she is still struggling with her relationship with this person. She is also working on formulating a positive goal for herself—namely, to address the issue (goal) rather than succumb to suicidal thoughts (symptoms).

Early Sharing of Hypotheses

She also understands that not everyone responds to this type of situation the way she did, and that it makes her vulnerable. In Chapter 1, the focus was on unconscious conflicts and their impact on individual reactions, emphasizing that not everyone responds uniformly in identical situations. In just a matter of minutes into the first session, there is data pointing toward a hypothesis that the Girl Who Wasn't a Princess has an unconscious conflict that has been triggered, leading to her recent state of suicidal thoughts. Neither of us clearly knows what this conflict is about. Part of the psychodynamic approach involves fostering curiosity in collaboration with the patient and formulating hypotheses about the underlying causes of their difficulties.

T: What kind of feelings do you experience right now, as you talk about this?
P: I guess … *HESITATES AND LOOKS AWAY* … regret that I got into it in the first place … um … because now it's like I wish I could move on from it, and I find it really, really hard to move on from um … because it was just, it was an incredibly … personal … *SIGHS* …. When things got bad between us, there were a lot of very personal judgments from him coming toward me and … um … He sort of ….
T: Like, he evaluated or judged you ….
P: Yeah, yeah … *SIGHS* ….
T: You must have some reactions to that?
P: Well, I just took everything he said as the truth and I think that was the thing … um ….
T: Mm. That was a part of the problem?
P: Yeah, well I really liked this person and I think, um, when you sort of idealize someone … then they say something about you and you just accept it. And the things he said about me and then continues to say about me … um … when we talk with each other are just … They're not … accurate?! To myself?! *LAUGHS* Um … But I still … I take it seriously, and always take it really personally and so it's just ….

The Girl Who Wasn't a Princess explains that there were a lot of very personal judgments coming from the person she lived with. And she accepted these judgments as the truth, even though she did not see them as accurate. Already at this point, I have a theory about why she gets into trouble with herself: even though she thinks his judgments are not accurate, she takes them personally and seriously. Why is she doing this? What lies in her unconscious mind that drives her to accept things she sees as wrong? I'm inquiring about this, even though I do not anticipate a definitive answer at this point. My main focus at this juncture is to pique curiosity about the underlying causes of her difficulties and to propose my hypothesis that it revolves around some kind of internal conflict.

T: Can I ask you why? You say that he has these personal judgments, you idealize and take it as the truth even though you say that it's not accurate.
P: Um .... *SIGHS*
T: That's sort of like ... uh ... what's the word ... contradictory ....
P: Yeah.
T: It's conflicting ....
P: Yeah.
T: "It's not accurate, but I take it as a truth."
P: Well, I guess ... with him ... I don't really know how things could have gotten so bad ....

In a brief span of time, significant information has been unveiled and I, as an ISTDP therapist, am eager to share my hypotheses and comprehension with the patient. The goal is not to gather patient information like a researcher, analyze it alone in the office, and then publish the results; it is to establish a mutual comprehension of the problem at hand and, ultimately, an agreement on how it should be resolved. Hence, I am cautious about sharing my thoughts:

P: (...) Because we lived together for about two months .... Within the first ten days I was already very suicidal. You know like, it was bad ....
T: So, something about his presence triggered something in you and instead of, like, dealing with that, you go to, like, you have to die ....
P: Um ... I think I was ... yes ... I think ....
T: So something about his presence .... You and him together trigger something in you. And somehow your "solution" ... and I put that in ... what do you call it? This .... *MIMICS AIR QUOTES*
P: Quotes ...
T: Yeah, quotes, right, quotes ... um ... You have to kill yourself. That's your solution.
P: Um, well, what was happening in the first ten days was really hard. And it continued to be bad. Um ... because this was ... I think I've now learned that this is somebody who is actually quite insecure, but sort of puts on this performance of being very confident .... But one of the ways that his insecurity kind of manifests is that he ... compares people (...). And he moved in .... And then was .... He would flirt with me, and then also talk about another classmate, as if he wanted to date our other classmate within the same sentence. So, for example, he would like, ask to watch a movie with me and be like touching me or touching my hand ... and then afterward would text me and say, like,

"Lisbeth is also interested in this movie, we should watch it again." And I'm like .... It was extremely mixed signals the entire time. And so I took him into the forest. And I was .... That was when it really got bad. Because I think what was happening was .... He was reinforcing me liking him. And then also just sort of making it .... I was just really confused. And the entire time I was really confused. And I just didn't know what to do.

I visualize the triangle of conflict in my mind, filling in relevant details in each of its corners. Already at this stage, I am ready to share my understanding with her, based on the triangle of conflict depicted in Figure 9.1.

T: So, what happened here, if we try to sum up .... On, like, a little bit of a higher level .... He sends out mixed signals. He flirts with you, and at the same time, talks about this other girl.

P: Yeah.

T: And obviously you have some reactions to that. And it confuses you. And somehow, again, the solution becomes suicide. Is that correct?

P: Yeah.

T: That your way of avoiding these mixed feelings that ... these feelings ... that his mixed signals are triggering in you ... is going to thoughts about suicide? Is that a way to see it?

P: I think it was that it was always there in my house. So, I was being assessed in this romantic way. And it was confusing. And I didn't know what was going on. And there was no escape from it. And nobody else saw it happening, that was the other thing!

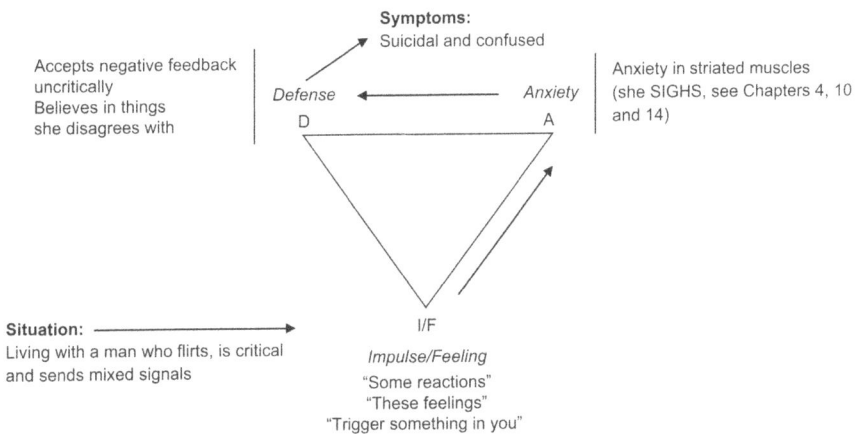

Figure 9.1 The Triangle of Conflict Applied to the Case of The Girl Who Wasn't a Princess

Although I may not fully understand her exact feelings or experience of anxiety, I have a hypothesis that *something* is affecting her at an emotional level. I also suspect she is angry with him and is directing this feeling inward to avoid confronting her rage. However, I want to test this hypothesis without being leading. Therefore, I express this notion as "some reactions," "these feelings," and "trigger something in you." I want to convey that while I may not know exactly what she is feeling, there is definitely *something* impacting her, piquing her curiosity about her inner world. When confronted with this *something*, she unquestioningly accepts the criticism, even though she disagrees with it. Believing in something you disagree with can be confusing. It is also destructive for her, and she ends up feeling suicidal.

While attempting to gain an understanding of the five questions listed in Table 9.1, I am also striving to grasp the dynamics at play on the triangle of conflict. This sets the stage for the subject of Chapter 10, which is what our task together will be: to resolve her problems.

In the conversation so far, several phenomena have been clarified. Her presenting symptoms (suicidality), the triggering situation (a critical and judgmental person who is her roommate, and who sends very mixed signals), and how she has managed her symptoms (accepted the criticism despite not agreeing, thus confusing herself and becoming unsure of herself), have all been revealed. Let me summarize what has been discovered so far on the nature of the Girl Who Wasn't a Princess's symptoms (see Table 9.2).

Table 9.2 Key questions for inquiry applied to the case of The Girl Who Wasn't a Princess

	Example
A. What are the patient's presenting symptoms, and how do they manifest?	"Very suicidal." Difficulty managing the relationship with the person.
B. How severe are the symptoms?	???
C. What are the precipitating event(s) triggering symptoms in the patient's *present life*?	Being romantically involved with her roommate, who is critical and judgmental, and who sends mixed romantic signals. Winter.
D. When did the symptoms first occur, and what were the precipitating trigger(s) *back then*?	???
E. How has the patient managed the symptoms up until now?	Accepts criticism uncritically. Confused/uncertain of herself (i.e., does not trust her own judgment and feelings).

Turning Vagueness into Specifics

Two questions in Table 9.2 remain unanswered: What is the severity of her suicidality, and have similar symptoms occurred before? Furthermore, the Girl Who
Wasn't a Princess has expressed being "very suicidal," although the exact meaning
behind this statement remains unclear. "Very suicidal" can refer to anything from
having thoughts about death to recurring attempts to take one's own life. It is crucial to clarify this, for the patient's safety (I need her to stay alive to help her) and
to understand her symptoms.

To uncover this kind of information, the therapist needs to ask specific and
detailed questions. This level of specificity is crucial in ISTDP and should
guide all therapeutic interventions. Many new therapists struggle with inquiring about their patients' most sensitive and personal experiences, fearing they
might cause offense. Paradoxically, the opposite is often true. Therapists who
courageously ask detailed and specific questions, while of course also showing
empathy, end up creating *corrective emotional experiences* for their patients
(Alexander & French, 1946): Finally, there is someone willing to ask, someone
who truly seeks to understand, and who can endure the challenging truths the
patient expresses.

T: How bad did it get? You said that you were very suicidal. What does that
    mean?
P: Um…. In the worst times … I would wake up … and then spend like two hours
    just sort of lying in bed fantasizing about it. And then you would eventually
    have to get up …. And it was very hard to get … out of that. And I remember
    the feeling … of that … the energy … or the thought of me thinking of killing
    myself had sort of seeped into the walls of the room, that I couldn't be in the
    room anymore without thinking about it.

The statement from the Girl Who Wasn't a Princess about being "very suicidal"
gains more depth. She had suicidal *fantasies*, she stayed in bed for hours, and she
struggled to get out of this painful state. However, "fantasies" is still a vague term,
so I am trying to find out the specific content of these fantasies. The specific content
is crucial for assessing suicidality (Practice Guideline for the Assessment & Treatment of Patients with Suicidal Behaviors, 2003) as well as for gaining a profound
understanding of her symptoms. What are the types of fantasies she entertains
about ending her own life? Can these fantasies help us understand the root of these
problems in any way? Are her fantasies important when it comes to agreeing on the
goal? You will never know unless you ask.

T: So, what kind of fantasies did you have? What did you fantasize about?
P: Um … *LOOKS DOWN* *SIGHS HEAVILY* I guess I would …. It was um
    I remember we … *LOOKS AWAY*. Well, at some point I had gotten a new
    knife from Ikea. And I remember the first time I used it I had this impression

of like—wow—this is really sharp and for some reason that was the thing I always thought I would use .... Because it was so sharp the first time I used it and I thought this would be .... This would work.

She has a knife, she has considered *using* it, and has thought that *this would work*. However, this is still vague. I do not know the nature of her thoughts, whether she actually used it, how close she was to using it, and how she considered using it. Clarity is crucial in order to accurately assess the severity of her symptoms and also to truly understand the difficulties she experiences when she becomes suicidal. The two of us—me and my patient—need to achieve clarity on this matter.

T: How were your fantasies about using it? In what way were you going to use it on yourself?

P: I don't know, I would have had to think about it .... Because a lot of ....

T: So you didn't fantasize about it that time—how you were going to use it?

P: Oh, no ... I would have ... um ... stabbed myself or ... um ....

T: Where?

P: Here *POINTS TO THE HEART*. In the ribs, in the heart, I guess ... *LAUGHS*

T: Uh huh, well, you guess? What was the fantasy at that time? When ....

P: It was more .... It was less the way that I was specifically going to kill myself and more that I knew the location I wanted to do it.

T: Uh huh. Where was that?

P: At my study desk at the university .... Because people were rarely there, but I would have been found within 24 hours ... um .... But then the way that I talked myself out of it most of the time was on logistical things .... You might attempt to kill yourself, but you might not succeed. And then you would have scars and you don't want that .... Or, like my parents live in Australia, and I wouldn't know how to arrange the transport for the body, and so I would have to do that ahead of time and then it.... Right. Yeah. *LAUGHS*

T: So, you didn't do .... Did you make any attempts or did you make plans, or bring the knife up to your study desk .... Or make any preparations?

P: No, I didn't, and I would have bought a new knife to do it .... Because the one that I had had been used for food and I didn't .... I wanted it to be clean, um ....

T: Why?

P: *LOOKS THOUGHTFUL*

T: You were going to die anyway, somehow?

P: I ... it ... well, it was only really sharp the first time I used it, so I needed to get a new one.

The Girl Who Wasn't a Princess had fantasies about stabbing herself in the heart, and perhaps it is no coincidence that it is precisely the heart that is at stake. After all, she has just had her heart broken by a man she was very fond of.

She had numerous arguments against committing suicide. She described ruminating about the circumstances, and she never made any specific plans or preparations. Hence, when the Girl Who Wasn't a Princess said she was "very suicidal," she wasn't talking about actual suicidal attempts nor that she had any specific plan to do so. She was talking about suicidal *thoughts* and *fantasies*. Faced with mistreatment by this man, she responds with thoughts of suicide instead of standing up for herself and taking protective measures.

Inquiry into the History of the Symptoms

At this stage, I have gained a deeper understanding of the manifestation of her suicidal thoughts, as well as a more profound insight into their severity (items 1 and 2, Table 9.3). But I do not know if she has made any suicide attempts earlier in life, which is crucial information when assessing the severity of the symptoms. The ISTDP therapist must also have knowledge of the history of the symptoms, including when they first appeared in life.

T: Uh huh. Have you ever tried, like, uh … committing suicide before? Have you ever made any … like … actual attempts?

P: Um …. *SIGHS AND LOOKS AWAY* No, I have not tried and failed … um …. The closest I got was that I sort of set up myself … um … to … I, like, filled a bathtub with water and was going to drop a radio in it. And so I got in

Table 9.3 Key questions for inquiry applied to the case of The Girl Who Wasn't a Princess

	Example
A. What are the patient's presenting symptoms, and how do they manifest?	• Suicidality: thoughts and fantasies about stabbing herself at her study desk. Difficulty managing the relationship with the ex-roommate.
B. How severe are the symptoms?	• Extensive suicidal thoughts and fantasies, and difficulties getting out of bed. No specific plan or any suicidal attempts.
C. What are the precipitating event(s) triggering symptoms in the patient's *present life?*	Being romantically involved with her roommate, who is critical and judgmental, and who sends mixed romantic signals. Winter.
D. When did the symptoms first occur, and what were the precipitating trigger(s) *back then?*	???
E. How has the patient managed the symptoms up until now?	Accepts criticism uncritically. Confused/uncertain of herself (i.e., does not trust her own judgment and feelings).

with clothes on and was, like, holding the thing .... And I decided not to and I, like, put it out and I climbed back out and I didn't ...

T: When was that?

P: Um, I was around 14.

T: Wow, that sounds painful.

P: Yeah. That time was actually kind of similar, where there was a guy who didn't like me ... um .... But I was .... I had such a crush on this person. I was absolutely obsessed with him and he didn't like me and ... I just kind of was like, well, this person who I like so much, who is so great, um ... isn't interested in me and doesn't like me and it's because I'm ... there's ... I'm insufficient for him to like me.

T: Uh huh. So that's so the same thing again....

P: Yeah.

T: You have some reactions toward him ... but then it's *you* who are insufficient and then *you* are going to die.

When she was fourteen years old, something similar occurred. She prepared for a suicide attempt but ultimately did not go through with it. Once again, it revolves around someone she likes, who does not like her back. Faced with this, she starts ruminating on the idea that she must die. Spontaneously, she recognizes the similarity between recent events and those that occurred when she was 14, and it is no coincidence that she does so. Through our interview, I have outlined my understanding of her situation: when confronted with this man who mistreats her, she experiences negative feelings, and that she avoids those feelings by thinking suicidal thoughts. Without my assistance, she identifies the same pattern when recounting the first time she felt suicidal (see Table 9.4).

The Same Problem Occurs in Various Situations

Our memory system works like dominoes lined up in a row. One specific memory triggers another similar memory, just like one domino chip toppling another.[1] When she recognizes her pattern, a new memory associated with this pattern emerges. While the primary objective at this stage is to obtain an overview of the symptoms and their history, the Girl Who Wasn't a Princess also starts to contribute to the psychodynamic case formulation. She becomes aware of a recurring pattern, and senses that there is an underlying unconscious force that affects her in various areas of her life:

P: Yeah .... And it's that way sometimes in a smaller way with friendships where I'll be ... um ... like, I'll get into a sense of ... not having enough friends or not being friends with the right people or .... Like, everybody else has more friends than me. And then I'll sort of think toward the future and be like, what's the point? *LAUGHS* You know, because ... um ... it ... I'm not doing it right now, so the logic of it kind of .... Obviously, it's a lot more .... It's hard to

Table 9.4 Key questions for inquiry applied to the case of The Girl Who Wasn't
a Princess

	Example
A. What are the patient's presenting symptoms, and how do they manifest?	• Suicidality: thoughts and fantasies about stabbing herself at her study desk. Difficulty managing the relationship with the ex-roommate.
B. How severe are the symptoms?	• Extensive suicidal thoughts and fantasies, and difficulties getting out of bed. No specific plan or any suicidal attempts.
C. What are the precipitating event(s) triggering symptoms in the patient's *present life*?	Being romantically involved with her roommate, who is critical and judgmental, and who sends mixed romantic signals. Winter.
D. When did the symptoms first occur, and what were the precipitating trigger(s) *back then*?	At the age of fourteen, the boy she liked didn't like her back, leading her to prepare for a suicide attempt.
E. How has the patient managed the symptoms up until now?	Accepts criticism uncritically. Confused/uncertain of herself (i.e., does not trust her own judgment and feelings).

understand when I'm not thinking that way, why I do it … um …. But it is …
I … I guess when I feel that way, I sort of look toward the future and I'm like
… if I can't even make friends… or if I can't even find a partner that I really
like … um …. You know, like …. Why keep going, I guess? I don't …. It's so
odd because I've never really had to think through this when I'm not feeling
that way … um ….

T: So why keep going? Why keep on living?

P: Well, I guess it's kind of like … um … It gets to be that way when people have
good … um … internships also and when people have really good professional
networks … um … where people will get jobs through friends or something
like that. Or their friends are working for a politician or something prestigious,
and then they get a job … um …. I guess when I look at … you know … my …
I don't have an internship right now and then I have a lot of really nice friends
actually but, um …. Sometimes I don't see them very often and I kind of ….
Yeah, I guess I look to the future and I'm like … how could I possibly have the
career or the life that I want … um ….

T: So facing this … that your friends have something that you don't have, or that
you're not as close to your friends as you would like to …. That obviously triggers a lot of emotions … it's again, like … why should I live? It's like, back onto
you, like in a destructive way.

Thinking: What's the point?
Thinking: I can't find a partner.
Thinking: How could I have
the life that I want?

Symptoms: Suicidality

Defense
D

Anxiety
A

Striated muscles
(see Chapters 4, 10, and 14)

Situation:
Friends have something she
doesn't have

I/F
Impulse/Feeling
Negative feelings

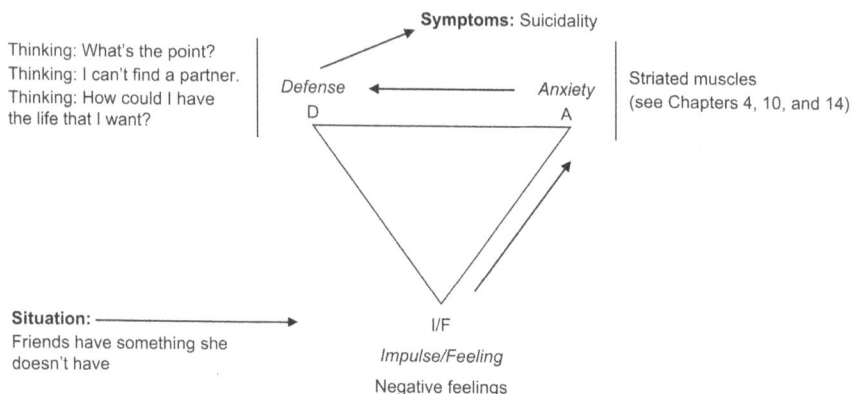

Figure 9.2 The Triangle of Conflict applied to the case of The Girl Who Wasn't a Princess

P: Yeah.
T: And even the most … the ultimate destructive way … suicide, sometimes ….
P: Yeah.
T: So, there's a pattern here, isn't there?
P: Mm … *NODS AND LOOKS AWAY*
T: That somehow you avoid these complicated, painful feelings … negative feelings … in self-destructive ways

Again, we see the same pattern: when she has negative feelings, she starts thinking she is worthless, that life is hopeless, and that she should die. The triangle of conflict describing her emotional struggle with her friends (Figure 9.2) is identical to the triangle of conflict describing her emotional conflict with the critical man (Figure 9.1). She avoids challenging and negative feelings by thinking self-destructive thoughts.

Memories from Childhood

By involving the Girl Who Wasn't a Princess in the dynamic inquiry process, she begins to actively engage herself. She sees connections, and she shares them. Without actively thinking it through, that is, unconsciously, the patient sees relevant connections. This is a characteristic of what Habib Davanloo (1990) referred to as the unconscious therapeutic alliance. If I had interviewed her by asking only direct questions, this would not have happened.

P: Now I feel more like … I didn't have that good of a relationship with my mom. Um …. And I think I didn't … really realize that it was not a normal mother relationship until I went to college and started talking with my brother about it … um …. But I think I didn't …. I could sense that there was this sort of absence of … love in my life …. And … she … is … well, we can get into it … um … but ….

T: Yeah, I think this is an important … uh … theme…. We'll come back to it…. Something about ….

P: Yeah, we could go back to it, but to finish what I was saying … um … I think that I did sort of sense … going into my early teenage years that there was sort of an absence of something that I needed …. And I assumed for a really long time …. Because I had sort of grown up watching … um … you know, like, princess stories where, like, the end … result is that like people find true love and they live happily ever after …. And I guess I had sort of assumed, like … I don't … I didn't feel good and I knew I didn't feel good …. But I just needed to find the perfect partner for me, and then that would be everything, and then I would be fine …. And I think when the person I liked didn't like me back … um … there wasn't any … like, I didn't … I thought that was going to be everything. You know, I thought that was going to fix … or provide … this thing that I didn't have.

A boyfriend might have had the ability to sort things out and make life good, just like the prince can in princess stories. The only problem is that the Girl Who Wasn't a Princess isn't a princess. Instead, she must come to terms with the reality that her relationship with her mother has not been normal and has lacked love. Failed relationships with men have become more than just unsuccessful romantic relationships; they represent a missed opportunity to find genuine love, a love that ideally should have been provided by her mother. Later in the therapy she revealed that she had leukemia as a child. She felt that no one really understood how it had been, making it a very lonely experience. The man she met had relatively recently recovered from bowel cancer. She vividly describes the experience of finally meeting the prince of her dreams, who could truly understand her as they had both survived serious illnesses. And, in the beginning, he was equally eager and dedicated to her. It is not surprising that things became complicated when he abruptly changed.

Psychodynamic Case Formulation and Agreement on Goals

I could have chosen to ask the Girl Who Wasn't a Princess the five questions from Table 9.1. What is your problem? How serious is it? What triggers it? When and how did you experience it for the first time? And how have you handled it so far? It would be a semi-structured interview, during which I would gain some insight into her symptoms.

This is not the way to conduct an inquiry in ISTDP. Instead, the therapist aims to cultivate a flexible and dynamic dialogue. In addition to gaining a comprehensive understanding of the symptoms, their severity, and their history, a collaborative foundation is established by developing a psychodynamic case formulation.

Several times throughout our conversation I say things like "something about being in his presence triggered something in you, and instead of dealing with it, you end up thinking you have to die," and "that is your way of dealing with these feelings regarding his mixed signals. This triggers you, and you end up thinking suicidal thoughts. Is this a way of understanding it?"

From the beginning, I aim to foster a mutual understanding with the patient and gather her perspectives. It is not me—*the therapist*—who alone must do the inquiry and create an understanding of the patient's problems; it is a collaborative effort. I keep the five questions in mind when I do the inquiry, and make a mental remark when I find relevant information. If I notice that pertinent information is missing, I will inquire further into it. The goal is to create a dynamic dialogue where we collaboratively seek clarity. When we achieve this goal, as I and the Girl Who Wasn't a Princess do, the patient actively engages in the therapeutic process by contributing insights and making connections. She understands that her conflict is more fundamental than just suicidal thoughts: it revolves around being rejected, which is particularly complicated for the Girl Who Wasn't a Princess. She has hoped that getting a partner would compensate for the love she has been lacking in her relationship with her mother.

A psychodynamic case formulation, which was one goal of this phase of the therapy, begins to take shape. A potential first draft could be formulated as follows, based on the information gathered so far:

The patient is a woman in her thirties who describes thoughts and fantasies about suicide, which arose after experiencing rejection from a man she thought was the prince of her dreams. When she experiences negative feelings, especially related to rejection by men, she tends to become self-destructive and suicidal rather than addressing her challenges and practicing self-care. This occurred recently, and it occurred when she was fourteen years old. Similarly, she experiences the same pattern when she perceives her friends possessing something she does not have, which arouses negative feelings. She attributes this pattern to a dysfunctional and loveless relationship with her mother, and she acknowledges that she has been hoping that a partner would serve as a remedy for the deficiencies in this relationship.

The other goal of this initial face was to reach an agreement on the nature of the problem. This has been achieved: The problem the patient wants help with is that she experiences suicidal thoughts in response to feeling rejected by men. Her goal is to address her challenges and practice self-care instead of becoming suicidal and self-destructive.

Note

1 This is what is called *associative networks* in cognitive theory of memory (Collins & Loftus, 1975).

Chapter 10

Agreement on the Therapeutic Task

Once the therapist and the patient have established the goal of the therapy, the next step is to reach an agreement on the specific therapeutic tasks required for the patient to successfully achieve their goal. This represents the second point in Bordin's (1979) definition of the working alliance (Chapter 8). In Intensive Short-Term Dynamic Psychotherapy (ISTDP), this agreement is closely related to the psychodynamic case formulation, which is based on Malan's (1979) two triangles. Complicated feelings in a given situation cause anxiety. To prevent experiences of these anxiety-inducing feelings, the patient turns to unconscious defense mechanisms that unfortunately create the very symptoms the patient is struggling with. When both the therapist and the patient have seen and understood this, it is relatively easy to understand that the task at hand is to become famil-iarized with the feelings, in order to alleviate the anxiety they may cause. When anxiety is reduced, there will no longer be any need for the defense mechanisms. If the case formulation is correct, the patient's symptoms should then disappear.

Malan's triangles describe processes that are more or less unconscious. When a patient seeks therapy, they are often not consciously aware of the mechanisms that cause their symptoms, nor the conflicts and driving forces lying underneath. In ISTDP specifically, and in psychodynamic therapy in general, one strives to modify these underlying unconscious driving forces that give rise to symptoms (Coughlin Della Selva, 2004). In order to establish an effective working alliance on which therapeutic tasks to carry out, it is crucial that the patient has a conscious hypothesis of the underlying driving forces that create their problems. Only when this point is reached can the patient provide informed consent to undergo the thera-peutic tasks, and the therapist can be certain that the patient is engaging in therapy out of their free will (Frederickson, 2013).

Once the nature of the symptoms and problems has been thoroughly inquired into (Please refer to chapter 9 and Table 9.1) and a goal has been agreed upon, the next step is to assist the patient in understanding the mechanisms that cause the pain. Agreeing on the therapeutic tasks is directly connected to agreeing on the mechanisms causing the difficulties. It is crucial for both the therapist and the patient to have a clear un-derstanding of the three corners of the triangle of conflict and how they relate to the patient's complaints. This mutual understanding can be challenging for a new ISTDP

DOI: 10.4324/9781003516217-13

therapist to achieve. As a therapist, you must skillfully be able to discern between the different corners of the triangle of conflict, and to be able to distinguish *the situation* from the basic, primary *feelings*. You need to be able to distinguish the *basic feelings* from the *anxiety* they evoke, and you must understand what a *defense mechanism* is. Finally, you need to understand how defense mechanisms and anxiety are related to the *symptoms and problems* the patient is grappling with.

There are several ways to acquire this skill. If you have read and understood the first part of this book, especially Chapter 4, you may have grasped the fundamentals. Chapters 12–15 of this book delve deeper into defense mechanisms, anxiety, and feelings, respectively. Books discussing feelings specifically, for example, that by Tone Normann-Eide (2020),[1] may also be helpful. Reading the books written by ISTDP therapists Patricia Coughlin Della Selva (2004) and Jon Frederickson (2013) will not only deepen your understanding of Malan's triangles but also provide valuable insight into ISTDP. Supervision of your own therapies by someone knowledgeable in ISTDP is incredibly valuable. If you are still struggling after all of this, you may need to see your own ISTDP therapist. At times, therapists may face challenges in distinguishing the corners of the triangle due to their own unresolved unconscious conflicts. These conflicts can be resolved if therapists themselves seek out therapy.

Why is it so important that the patient can see and separate the three corners of the triangle of conflict, including their relationship to the presenting symptoms and the triggering situations? This is because this understanding is closely associated with various symptoms, including depression and psychosomatic complaints (Davanloo, 1990; Fosha, 1988), as well as anxiety and difficulties with impulsivity (Coughlin Della Selva, 2004). If you struggle to distinguish the empowering and motivational aspects of anger from the tendency to weep, it may seem futile to let yourself experience anger: "Why should I be angry? I will start to weep, and when I do, no one will take me seriously!" In this case, the patient is unable to distinguish between *experiencing* the feeling of anger and *defending* against it by weeping. The adaptive function of anger is to ensure that we protect ourselves in situations where our integrity is challenged. If you let tears wash away the adaptive angry energy, self-protection becomes difficult, and it becomes challenging to establish healthy boundaries and assert oneself. A person who struggles with differentiating between grief and self-criticism will also face difficulties: "Why should I mourn and cry? It's weak, and I feel foolish!" This person struggles with differentiating between experiencing grief (emotional pain, lump in the stomach and throat, the urge to cry) and defending against this experience (telling oneself that it is weak and foolish to cry). If this is your perspective on mourning, and you have experienced a loss and are grieving, you will quickly end up depressed.

How to Distinguish the Corners of the Triangle of Conflict

Feelings

How can one learn to discern the corners of the triangle of conflict? First and foremost, it is crucial to understand which feelings are primary and adaptive, as these are the ones that patients need help in experiencing. There are different theories about which feelings are to be considered as primary.[2] Even within the ISTDP literature there is some disagreement about which feelings are fundamental (Abbass, 2015; Coughlin Della Selva, 2004; Frederickson, 2013; Kuhn, 2014). All of the above agree that anger, grief and guilt are important feelings. Of the remaining feelings, I have selected love, sexual feelings, joy and fear as those that you need to understand as therapist. These seven feelings are located at the bottom of the triangle of conflict (I/F), all of them serving important, adaptive functions for human beings.

By *adaptive functions*, I mean that these feelings provide us with fundamental information about our needs, as well as energy for self-care. However, this does not imply that every time these feelings are aroused in us, they always serve a direct adaptive function. You can, from time to time, experience anger, guilt, and sadness without them necessarily leading directly to anything constructive. However, if you have a conflicted relationship with these feelings and consistently suppress them, you will inevitably encounter difficulties. This is because, in many situations, they provide essential information and energy to help make healthy, self-caring choices.

Table 10.1 provides a comprehensive overview of the experiences associated with these feelings, what the related impulse is (what experiencing the feeling motivates you to do), and what the adaptive function of the feeling is. If you

Table 10.1 Overview of feelings, associated somatic components and impulses, and their adaptive functions

Feeling	Somatic component	Impulse	Adaptive function
Anger	Energy rising through the body from the stomach reaching the hands, increased pulse, physiological power, heat.	An urge to lash out, potentially violently, manifesting as a desire to strike, kick, bite, etc.	Self-care and self-protection, physically and psychologically.
Grief	Physiological pain, lump in the stomach and throat, pressure behind the eyes, production of tears, increased production of saliva and mucus.	An impulse to cry and sob, to seek solace, and a longing for comfort and support.	Reorganization: Acceptance of loss; to be able to reconnect with others.
Guilt	Pain and pressure in the chest and neck. Pain in the stomach. Can be very painful and cause difficulty in speaking.	Crying and sobbing. An impulse to apologize and repair the relationship with whom you have wronged.	Maintain community and connection with important others.

(Continued)

Table 10.1 (Continued)

Feeling	Somatic component	Impulse	Adaptive function
Joy	Warmth and lightness. Energy, vitality and spontaneity.	Impulse to smile and laugh, and a desire to create more joy. Motivation to facilitate positive experiences in the future.	Appropriate adaptation to the environment, motivation for self-sustaining behaviors.
Love	Experience of calmness, well-being, and often warmth and relaxation (typical for caring relationships). Warmth, excitement, energy and vitality (typical of romantic relationships—see also sexual feelings).	Impulses to do good for those you love. Desire for closeness and intimacy.	Ensure belonging to the community through the formation of strong emotional bonds.
Sexual feelings	Warmth, tingling and pleasure in the genitals and erogenous zones. Erect penis or moist vagina. Increased heart rate, heavier breathing and increased blood pressure.	Desire for sexual stimulation and satisfaction.	Quality of life. Pleasure alone and with others. Attachment to partner and reproduction of the species.
Fear	Tense muscles, increased blood pressure, increased heart rate, nausea, dizziness.	Fight, flight, freeze: Readiness for combat, the impulse to flee from danger, or to freeze and go blank in the face of unavoidable danger.	Ensure survival.

Sources: Normann-Eide (2020), Abbass (2015), McCullough Vaillant (1997), and Grünfeld and Almås (2021).

understand this table and can recognize these feelings in yourself and others, you have mastered an important skill as an ISTDP therapist.

All these basic feelings share a common feature: they motivate us to do something good for ourselves. These feelings inherently prompt us to act in ways that are directed outward, *toward the world*, and they motivate us to take care of ourselves.

Clinically, it also makes sense to include *pain* (Davanloo, 1990) and *pleasant feelings* (McCullough Vaillant, 1997). While these may not be considered primary feelings, it is often meaningful for the patient to address them. Patients go to great lengths to avoid pain and painful feelings. Frequently, patients find it easier to consciously acknowledge the presence of pain in general, as opposed to specific painful feelings like guilt and grief. Using the word "pain" thus provides a starting point for exploring these feelings. Being able to experience pleasant states like joy, enthusiasm, curiosity, calmness, and pleasure is an important outcome of therapy (McCullough Vaillant, 1997). Actually, reducing all these states down to the basic feeling of joy (Table 10.1) may seem oversimplified.

Anxiety

In addition to the seven emotions mentioned above, anxiety plays a particularly important role in ISTDP. I strive to make an effort to differentiate between anxiety and the feeling of fear. Fear is the feeling we feel when confronted with something genuinely dangerous, prompting us to flee and seek safety in order to survive. In ISTDP, anxiety is defined as the fear of internal states, such as feelings, which by themselves are not inherently dangerous. This understanding of anxiety can be traced back to Freud's (1936) second theory of anxiety. According to this theory, anxiety serves as a *signal* that our internal psychological equilibrium is under threat. In ISTDP, it is customary to discuss three *channels of anxiety*, which represent the primary ways in which anxiety manifests in the body. This categorization was developed by Habib Davanloo, based on his clinical observations. It aligns well with how the somatic, and the autonomic nervous systems (composed of the sympathetic and parasympathetic nervous systems), anatomically manifest fear (Frederickson, 2013). This tripartite channeling is described like this:

1 anxiety channeled into striated muscles (voluntary muscles, such as in arms and legs)
2 anxiety channeled into smooth muscles (muscles that operates automatically, such as the muscles of the digestive system and muscles surrounding blood vessels)
3 anxiety that manifests itself as cognitive and perceptual disturbances (resulting from hormonal imbalances and fluctuations in cerebral blood flow)

Table 10.2 provides an overview of typical physical symptoms associated with the different channels of anxiety, as well as their impact on learning and the potential benefits of therapy.

In ISTDP, the three channels of anxiety are commonly used to form hypotheses about the patient's anxiety level. The channels of anxiety provide information about whether the patient is operating within their window of tolerance (Nordanger & Braarud, 2014) and within *the proximal zone of development* (Vygotsky, 1978). If the patient squirms in the chair, sighs heavily, and clenches their hands

Table 10.2 Overview of anxiety channels, associated somatic components and symptoms, and implications for therapy

Channel of anxiety	Somatic component	Associated complaints	Implications for therapy
Striated muscles	Sighing—due to tightening of the intercostal muscles between the ribs. Hand clenching. Tension in large muscle groups such as shoulders, neck, and chest. Tension in the lips, jaw, and scalp. Bodily restlessness.	Pain and discomfort caused by tension in all kinds of voluntary muscles, such as in e.g., shoulders, neck, jaw, abdomen, pelvis (e.g., vaginismus) and scalp.	Regulated by the somatic nervous system which does not affect brain function, cognition, and learning.
Smooth muscles	Nausea. Sickness to the stomach. Dry mouth. Migraine (due to dilation of blood vessels in the brain).	Abdominal pain, nausea, diarrhea—often referred to as irritable bowel syndrome. Migraines. Fatigue, exhaustion. Somatic complaints without a physiological explanation, such as numbness, seizures, etc.	Regulated by the autonomic nervous system and may affect cognition, optimal brain functioning, and learning.
Cognitive and perceptual disturbances	Tunnel vision. Blurred vision. Dizziness. Difficulties concentrating. Confusion. Ringing in the ears.	Difficulties with perception and concentration. General and potentially extensive cognitive, relational and work/study-related challenges.	Regulated by the autonomic nervous system. Anxiety at this level affects cognition, optimal brain function and learning.

tightly, these cues are clear indications that the patient is experiencing activation, and suggest that they are somehow facing an underlying conflict (Freud, 1936). Since somatic symptoms in the striated muscles are regulated by the somatic nervous system, which cannot directly impact cognition, this observation reinforces the hypothesis that the patient is currently operating within their window of tolerance.

Consequently, learning can occur, allowing the therapist and the patient to proceed confidently with their therapeutic exploration. However, if the patient experiences symptoms of anxiety in smooth muscle (see Table 10.2) or displays signs of cognitive and perceptual disturbances, it indicates that the patient may be outside their window of tolerance. The therapist must therefore slow down the exploration or assist the patient in regulating their anxiety. These kinds of symptoms are caused by the autonomic nervous system (Frederickson, 2013), which *may* affect learning and cognition. For therapy to be effective, the patient needs to be cognitively functional and not excessively anxious to the point of impacting their ability to learn. If anxiety manifests in the striated muscles, it is reasonable to assume that these conditions have been met. However, if symptoms of anxiety are observed in smooth muscles, or if cognitive and perceptual disturbances are evident, the therapist should exercise heightened vigilance. In such cases, the patient's anxiety may be so severe that they cannot fully benefit from therapy unless the anxiety is effectively managed.

Sometimes it can be challenging to determine whether the feeling the patient is experiencing is a primary and adaptive emotion or if it is anxiety. In particular, differentiating between anger and anxiety can be challenging for both the patient and the therapist as they both involve tension in large muscle groups. A general rule is that primary feelings are designed to prompt action. This is a fundamental trait of adaptive emotions, like anger, which are experienced as *outward-directed*. In contrast, anxiety aims to restrain you, to halt your actions and withdraw. Anxiety is experienced as *inward-directed*, contrasting with the outward direction of anger (McCullough Vaillant, 1997).

Defense Mechanisms

Noticing the defense mechanisms used by a patient can sometimes pose a challenge. Some new therapists, therefore, choose to read up on the various specific defense mechanisms in order to prepare for this task.[3] As a new ISTDP therapist, my focus would not be on differentiating defense mechanisms or learning specific techniques to address each of them. The most vital aspect, as I see it, is to understand the *phenomenon* of defense mechanisms. If it is indeed true that "there are as many ways to defend as there are snowflakes or fingerprints" (McCullough et al., 2003, p. 86), then devising a strategy for each unique mechanism would present a significant and formidable task. Instead, if you have grasped the essence of the phenomenon, you will be adequately prepared. Defense mechanisms are the mechanisms that help us feel a little less anxious when facing the feelings associated with our inner conflicts. Simultaneously, they hinder our ability to truly access our thoughts, intentions, and feelings concerning a variety of matters, including important ones. One simple example is when we choose to overlook an irritating situation. It may provide temporary relief and help us avoid the discomfort of a potential conflict. However, in doing so, we fail to gather the necessary energy and motivation to resolve the issue and prevent its recurrence. Defense mechanisms serve as temporary solutions that only serve to delay the problem, offering short-term satisfaction but leading to long-term complications. It is crucial that your patients comprehend this concept.

What Is What?

It is important to note that our everyday language often fails to distinguish between the corners of Malan's triangles. This can be confusing at times, both for therapists and for patients. In everyday speech we use "I feel" to express a wide range of emotions, experiences, and opinions. In ISTDP, the use of "I feel" is specifically reserved for the seven primary feelings that have been discussed, which include anger, sadness, guilt, love, joy, sexual feelings, and fear. It is common to hear people say, "I feel criticized" or "I feel let down and rejected." Since criticized, failed, and rejected are not considered to be of the seven primary feelings, the expressions must represent something else. We say that we "feel" criticized, failed, and rejected when someone criticizes, fails, and rejects us. Hence, it is not a feeling—it is a depiction of the *situation* that elicits feelings: someone criticizes, disappoints, or rejects us. The typical feelings stirred up within us when we are criticized, let down, or rejected are anger and grief.

An example of this can be found in the therapy session with the Girl Who Wasn't a Princess. She recounts being mistreated by the man she was in love with, and I can sense an emotional reaction from her when talking about this. I wonder out loud if I perceive her correctly, and what kind of feelings are coming up.

T: Are there some feelings coming up again? I noticed that you start laughing when you talk about these things that sounds really painful.
P: I, yeah ....
T: What feelings are coming up right now as you remember this?
P: Um ... I guess kind of ... the absurdity of it ... Like, it was so bad! *LAUGHS*
T: Yeah, but that's not, that's not a feeling, that's the reality, isn't it? It was really bad.
P: Yeah.
T: It was absurd, so how .... When you remember this absurd reality ... how does that make you feel right now?
P: Um ... Well, it ... it hurts to remember it.
T: Of course, it does!
P: Yeah, and it's ... I mean ....
T: It's painful, isn't it?
P: Yeah, it is. *TEARS UP*

I ask about her feelings, and she answers "bad" and "absurd." Bad and absurd are not feelings; they describe the reality of the situation and how she was treated. When I show her this, she becomes more in touch with the painful feelings associated with being treated this way.

It is also common to say, "I feel like a foolish idiot," "I feel dumb," or "I feel it is hopeless." When looking at the list of feelings (Table 10.1), none of these statements are descriptive of the basic feelings. Rather, these are descriptions of what a person may *think* about themselves in a situation where they are criticized, let down, or rejected. You *think* that you were rejected because you are foolish, dumb, and an idiot, and you *think* that things are hopeless. Typically, adaptive feelings in such a situation are anger and sadness. These negative and self-critical thoughts act as defense mechanisms, preventing the experience of these complex yet adaptive emotions. The problem with these thoughts is that they often lead to symptoms, most commonly depressive symptoms.

An example of this is taken from the first session with the Girl Who Wasn't a Princess as well. She mentioned feeling angry toward the man who mistreated her. Considering that this situation triggered her symptoms, I'm curious to know how she has been dealing with her anger.

T: How did you deal with the FEELINGS? This anger?
P: I thought there was something wrong with me, I guess. Or that I hadn't been good enough.

Confronted with the adaptive feeling of anger, which is meant to provide her with the strength to protect herself and possibly escape, she thinks that there is something wrong with her. This misconception is an important factor contributing to the Girl Who Wasn't a Princess's problems. Thinking that something is wrong with her serves as a defense mechanism against feeling anger toward the man. By convincing herself that there is something wrong with her, she no longer has a reason to react with anger toward others. This strategy is highly effective in disarming any self-serving reactions: I should not react; there is something wrong with me; the other person is right.

The Girl Who Wasn't a Princess

In order for the Girl Who Wasn't a Princess and I to reach an agreement on the therapeutic tasks, it is crucial that we develop a solid hypothesis regarding the underlying mechanisms of her challenges. Only by doing so can we reach a consensus on the pertinent and necessary therapeutic measures. Understanding the root causes of her challenges provides the foundation for finding effective solutions. Hence, we must continue working on the psychodynamic case formulation.

The process of reaching an agreement on the goal and establishing a shared understanding of the problem is conducted simultaneously. The topics are divided into two chapters to make the teaching process clearer, but they are not separate therapeutic projects. In practice, these two therapeutic tasks complement each other and shed light on one another.

The following excerpt is from two minutes into the first session. The Girl Who Wasn't a Princess has just revealed that she reached out for therapy because she felt

"very suicidal" and self-destructive. These symptoms emerged early in the cohabitation, and she speaks of receiving criticism and being confused by mixed signals
from him. Nevertheless, they continue to be part of the same academic group and
maintain regular social interactions.

T: *SPEAKS SOFTLY*[4] Well, that sounds really complicated! There has to be a
lot of mixed feelings about this.

P: Yeah, there's a lot of mixed feelings about it... *LOOKS AWAY AND SIGHS*

P: *LOOKS SAD AND LOOKS AT ME AGAIN*

T: Ah.... Okay.... Is it ... can you experience some of them right now?

P: Um... *SIGHS AND LOOKS AWAY*

T: *SPEAKS GENTLY* Are there feelings coming up right now as you start talking about it?

P: Well ... yeah ... I think so, I think it's something where ... um ... *BECOMES
SILENT AND HOLDS HER BREATH*

T: What kind of feelings are you experiencing, right now, as you talk about this?

P: I guess ... *HESITATES AND LOOKS AWAY* Regret that I got into it in the
first place ... um ....

T: Mm.

P: Because now it's like I wish I could move on from it! And I find it really, really
hard to move on from um ....

T: Mm.

P: Because it was just ... it was an incredibly ... personal ... *SIGHS* When
things got bad between us, there were a lot of very personal judgments
from him coming toward me and ... um ,.. he sort of ....

T: Like, he evaluated or judged you ....

P: Yeah, yeah ... *SIGHS*

T: You must have some reactions to that?

P: Well, I just took everything he said as the truth and I think that was the thing
... um ....

T: Mm. That was a part of the problem?

P: Yeah, well I really liked this person and I think, um, when you sort of idealize
someone ... then they say something about you and you just accept it. And the
things he said about me and then continues to say about me ... um ... when
we talk with each other are just .... They're not ... accurate?! To myself?!
LAUGHS

T: Mm, mm?

P: Um .... But I still ... I take it seriously, and always take it really personally and
so it's just ....

T: *SPEAKING SOFTLY* Mm, can I ask you why? You say that he has these
personal judgments, you idealize and take it as the truth even though you say
that it's not accurate.

P: Um ... *SIGHS*

T: That's sort of like ... uh ... what's the word ... contradictory....

P: Yeah. **NODS, SMILES AND LOOKS AT ME**
T: It's conflicting ....
P: Yeah.
T: "It's not accurate but I take it as a truth."
P: Well, I guess ... with him ... I don't really know how things could have gotten so bad ....

Beginning the therapy, my initial goal was to swiftly formulate hypotheses about the root causes of her suicidal inclinations. Additionally, I sought to ascertain if this patient could derive benefits from short-term dynamic therapy. The applicability of this therapeutic approach to her case hinges on the ability to interpret her struggles through a psychodynamic case formulation. If we consider Malan's triangles as a true representation of her situation, she is undergoing emotional responses triggered by the man's personal judgments. These reactions are distressing (A) for her, prompting her to put up defenses (D). As per the theory, it is these defenses that give rise to the symptoms.

Distinguishing the Corners of the Triangle of Conflict

I start by mentally adding the relevant content to the corners of the triangles. This involves seeking her reactions (i.e., feelings) to her circumstances. Her lack of specific answers at this stage is not unexpected. As per psychodynamic theory, she is grappling with an *unconscious conflict* that poses challenges. It is natural that she has not got conscious answers to all my queries at the onset of therapy. However, she does share her *thoughts* on the man's statements, agreeing with him. This agreement, rather than a reflection of her feelings toward his judgments, serves to suppress her reactive feelings toward his negative behavior. This approach provides a temporary solution: by concurring with him, she sidesteps a potentially difficult and confrontational discussion, and avoids dealing with complex emotions.

Yet, agreeing with personal judgments, which she internally disagrees with, is self-destructive. As you might recall from earlier sections, resorting to mechanisms that offer short-term solutions but create long-term problems is indicative of a *defense mechanism* (D). Thus, her uncritical acceptance of his assertions becomes a defense against experiencing reactive feelings.

The Girl Who Wasn't a Princess reveals that she *likes him very much*, indicating positive feelings (love). The complexity of enduring harsh treatment from a loved one stems from the necessity to reconcile two opposing feelings toward the same individual. Her dialogue during our conversation suggests that she finds this reconciliation challenging and discomforting. As she discusses this emotional dilemma, her sighs and visible stress become apparent. Within the framework of ISTDP, such sighs and restlessness are interpreted as physical manifestations of anxiety, with the anxiety being directed into striated muscles (refer to Table 10.2). This is visually represented in Figure 10.1. Drawing from the data gathered during the session, I am beginning to form a psychodynamic case formulation, based on Malan's triangles.

Symptoms
Self-destructive and "very suicidal"

Thinking: Agree with the
judgments, even if they are   *Defense* ←—————————— *Anxiety*   *SIGHS*
not right   D   A   *RESTLESSNESS*

Situation: —————————————→   I/F
                                 Impulse/Feeling
Personal judgments   —————→   *UNKNOWN FEELING*
She likes him very much ——————→   Love

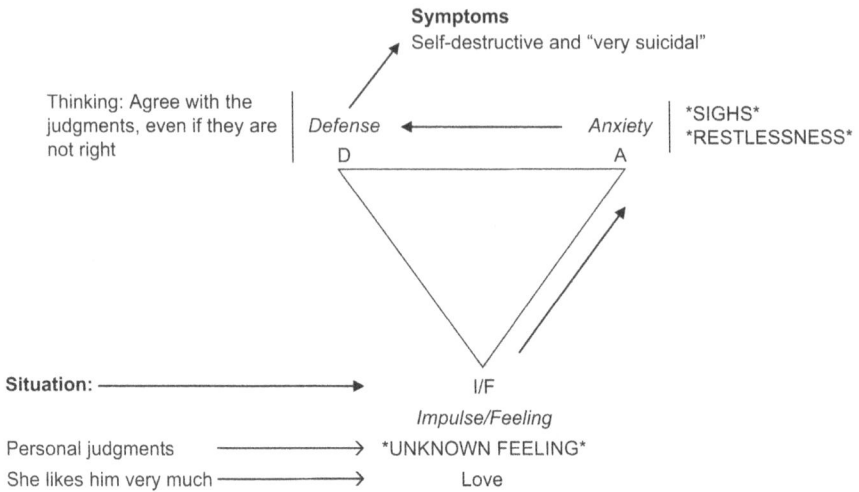

Figure 10.1 The Triangle of Conflict applied to the case of The Girl Who Wasn't a Princess

By visualizing the triangle depicted in Figure 10.1, I have initiated the process of fostering a mutual comprehension of her challenges. I am transparent about my thoughts and seek her agreement to ensure we share the same perspective. This mutual understanding will serve as a framework that guides our joint exploration of her difficulties. I strive to clarify *the situation* when I mention that "he evaluated you, judged you" and "he has these personal judgments." I repeatedly inquire about her feelings and responses to these events. In my queries, I distinctly separate the event from her reaction. This distinction aims to help her differentiate between the *situation* and the *feeling/impulse* that arises as a result of the situation. I am already assisting her in recognizing her conflict: she is accepting as truth something she believes to be incorrect. I am attempting to pique her curiosity about why she is doing this. From the beginning, my goal is not only to gain a comprehensive understanding of her problem (refer to Chapter 9) but also to foster an understanding of the mechanisms that contribute to the problem.

The subsequent passage from the therapy is derived from the twelfth to thirteenth minute of the initial session (portions from these initial minutes are also reiterated in Chapter 9):

T: So, what happened here, if we try to sum up …. On, like, a little bit of a higher level …. He sends out mixed signals. He flirts with you, and at the same time, talks about this other girl.

P: Yeah.

T: And obviously you have some reactions to that. And it confuses you. And somehow, again, the solution becomes suicide. Is that correct?

P: Yeah.

T: That your way of avoiding these mixed feelings that … these feelings … that his mixed signals are triggering in you … is going to thoughts about suicide? Is that a way to see it?

P: I think it was that it was always there in my house. So, I was being assessed in this romantic way. And it was confusing. And I didn't know what was going on. And there was no escape from it. And nobody else saw it happening, that was the other thing!

I strive to assist her by elucidating the causal chain of events as I comprehend them (refer to Figure 10.2). He emits mixed signals (*the situation*), to which she responds (*impulse/feeling*). However, instead of acknowledging these reactions, she finds herself contemplating suicide (*the outcome of self-destructive defenses like turning angry impulses inward*). I inquire, "Is this a way to see it?" Her response suggests that we *do not* have a mutual understanding of the situation. Her attention is diverted elsewhere. She narrates the details of the house, that she was assessed, that she could not escape, and the fact that no one else witnessed the incidents. All these elements describe *the situation*: She informs me about her location (the house), the actions of the other person (assessed her), that she could not escape (she had no alternative accommodation), and her solitude (no one else saw it happening).

Internal Focus

Psychotherapy cannot alter the situations that trigger her problems. The sole aspect I can assist the Girl Who Wasn't a Princess with is her emotional response to situations, ensuring she does not resort to suicidal or self-destructive tendencies when her feelings surface. This will equip her to better handle any future instances of mistreatment. In the preceding paragraph, her focus is on external factors: events that occurred in her life. The only sphere where we can effect change is her internal world, which is how she *processes* the external. As long as she remains fixated on past events and the actions of others, we will not be able to aid her in resolving her inner psychological challenges.

In the following section, I persist in aiding her in structuring her difficulties. Utilizing Malan's triangles as a foundation, I construct a psychodynamic case formulation. My aim is also to guide her focus toward what I can actually assist her with—that is, her *internal* experiences. Without a mutual comprehension that this is our primary concern, we lack the groundwork for therapy. Achieving this shared understanding can be swift or gradual; both scenarios are perfectly acceptable. The crucial aspect is to reach an agreement on the therapeutic goals and tasks, and a psychodynamic case formulation that hypothesizes the interrelation between them.

P: Because … it did get progressively worse. After he …. I confronted him about that, and he said that he *did* want to date me. And then … later on that he didn't, and then still wanted to be friends. And so … I was trying really hard to be friends with him, but I didn't really know how …. And it obviously wasn't working and he obviously didn't like me … anymore… *INCREASINGLY MAKING MORE GESTURES*. Even in a friendly way. And then that was the thing where I did … I got progressively angry, because I was so frustrated that he was saying he wanted to be friends and then obviously avoiding me or obviously like … looking at me, angry, and I hadn't seen him smile in months. And it was in my house and he wasn't like …. It was obvious, looking back. *SIGHS*

T: So obviously a whole lot of feelings here.

P: A lot of feelings! *LAUGHS*

She starts to recognize that his actions evoke feelings within her. She recalls experiencing anger and frustration as a result of his behavior. The ability to articulate this feeling, a natural and healthy response to such treatment, is a positive step. Her speech becomes more assertive, and her gestures increasingly animated. She appears to become progressively angry during our session when discussing this matter. However, the key question arises: Does she permit herself to experience anger and harness the energy from this feeling to establish healthy, self-protective boundaries? Or does she resist this feeling, and if so, what could be the potential outcome of such a defense?

T: And how did you deal with them? Of course there was a lot of feelings, but how did you deal with them?

P: I talked to the roommates about it … because I had some excellent, really, really supportive roommates. And I talked to some of my friends about it, but HE … wouldn't … like, he didn't talk to anybody!

T: But … but, how did YOU deal with them?

P: I tried to get help. And I tried to ask other people, like, how do I get this person …. Like, how can we be friends? You know, I'm trying!

I inquire about her approach to managing her feelings, specifically how she internally copes with her anger toward him. Her response revolves around her practical actions. The fact that she confides in friends is a positive indication, demonstrating her effective relational strategies.[5] However, her discussions with them primarily concern how she can get this individual to be her friend. She seeks guidance on altering HIM, not on managing her own feelings or determining what would be beneficial for her. Once again, her attention is externally directed, focusing more on the events that transpired. She does not concentrate on herself, her own feelings, or how she can utilize the signals and energy from these feelings for self-care.

Turning Anger Toward Oneself

T: How did you deal with the FEELINGS? This anger?

P: I thought there was something wrong with me, I guess. Or that I hadn't been good enough.

T: Uh huh. So, facing this anger, you thought that there was something wrong with you?

P: Yeah.

T: You're angry at him. And then you start thinking that there's something wrong with you. Is that correct?

P: Yeah.

T: Right. And also ... you're angry at HIM, then you start thinking about killing YOURSELF.

P: Yeah.

In this part, she begins to focus on herself, which I see as a positive progression. However, a familiar pattern resurfaces: He mistreats her, and she feels anger toward him. So far, so good. But her approach to managing anger is to think that the problem lies within HER, thereby avoiding the experience of the feeling. What is initially a feeling directed at him is internally transformed into self-criticism. This method of avoiding anger, by directing it toward oneself, often results in depressive symptoms (Town et al., 2022). She employs a defense mechanism that involves accepting responsibility for issues that are not her fault (refer to Figure 10.2). Consequently, her interpretation of the poor treatment she receives is that there is something wrong with her, and that she isn't good

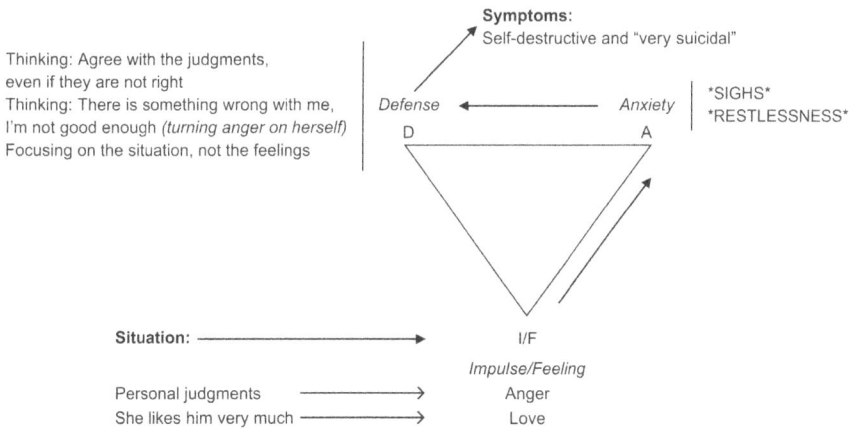

Figure 10.2 The Triangle of Conflict applied to the case of The Girl Who Wasn't a Princess

enough. This way, she does not need to feel anger toward others for their actions; she blames herself.

Figure 10.2 encapsulates the therapeutic process to this point. She employs a variety of defense mechanisms, all of which prevent her from actively and healthily addressing her feeling of anger toward this man she is fond of, yet who mistreats her. The result of this is a self-destructive and suicidal tendency.

Agreement on the Consequence of Defense Mechanisms

At this phase of therapy I have formed a distinct hypothesis linking her struggles, which brought her to therapy, to how she treats herself and how she avoids her feelings. However, it is not sufficient for me alone to hold this hypothesis. It is crucial for her to also embrace it. Our goal is to reach mutual agreement on the therapeutic tasks. To accomplish this, we need to agree on the underlying mechanisms causing her difficulties.

Does SHE comprehend the impact of avoiding her feelings in such a manner? If she does, could this understanding motivate her to make a change?

T: How does that work out for you?
P: Well, if somebody says they want to be friends with you and ... you ... continue under that assumption. And then they continue not to like you.
T: Can I ask you something?
P: Yeah.
T: How does it work for you? When you're angry at someone who's treating you in this way that you obviously don't like?
P: I don't think I realized how angry I was until after it was over.
T: How does it work for you, to like, when you're angry at him, you start thinking that there's something wrong with you. And when you were angry at him, you start thinking about committing suicide. How does that strategy of avoiding anger work out for you? How is that? What's the result of going that way?
P: I don't know.
T: Does it work out?
P: I don't know how that happens.

The Girl Who Wasn't a Princess does not provide a clear answer about the effectiveness or outcome of her avoidance. However, she still offers valuable insights. She is unable to comprehend the mechanism at play, and she does not understand how it happens. Before we delve into understanding her actions, it is crucial that we share a common hypothesis about the problematic mechanism at play, and its consequences. If she is satisfied with believing that something is wrong with her, and she considers her strategy effective, then I have no right to argue with her. She has the freedom to self-criticize. And why should we investigate the origin of a mechanism if she does not perceive it as problematic or undesirable?

I strongly believe that she does not actually think her current approach is working out well for her, but she lacks a conscious realization of how she is treating herself. The defense mechanism, which involves accepting blame for others' mistreatment of her, has remained unconscious until now. As I discussed in Chapter 4, defense mechanisms have often been adaptive at certain stages in life, helping to manage challenging feelings. Therefore, my aim is to assist her in recognizing these mechanisms and understanding their impact on her present life.

T: What happens inside of you when you start thinking that there is something wrong with you? That it's your fault?
P: I guess ... it was also that it was ... just ... this denial of my feelings and what I was going through.
T: Mm-hmm!

Once more, the Girl Who Wasn't a Princess avoids the question. Despite my repeated inquiries about the internal impact of thinking that something is wrong with her, she remains silent on this issue. However, the information she does share is valuable. I attentively listen to her, all the while noting that she does not fully grasp the link between her defense mechanism and her symptoms (Figure 10.2). It is crucial for her to understand this connection if she is to eventually find the motivation to cease her self-critical thinking. Simultaneously, she acknowledges that she has denied her feelings and what she has gone through. And isn't this the core of the matter? She has been mistreated and has refused to acknowledge this fact. In fact, she has done the exact opposite: She has turned a blind eye to the poor treatment she received and internalized his justification that it was her fault.

Trusting Oneself

The Girl Who Wasn't a Princess recounts how the man would dismiss her as dramatic every time she tried to discuss issues in their relationship. He even conveyed this perception to their mutual friends. At first, she agreed with his viewpoint, but looking back, she realizes that her reactions were not dramatic at all. Now, a few months later, and in the therapeutic environment without his influence, she still struggles to assert that his accusations were unjust and that she was in the right. Despite numerous opportunities, she consistently resists affirming that her conduct in the situation was entirely appropriate.

T: And how do you deal with that? When he says you're causing drama and you say that it's wrong, you don't agree. You're not causing drama. You're not making drama.
P: Yeah.
T: How do you deal with that? He says that, and you don't agree. Like internally, like emotionally, how do you deal with that?
P: Internally, emotionally, at the time with him ....

T: Right now.
P: Huh? Right now?
T: Right now.
P: *LAUGHS*
T: How do you deal with that? When you're sitting here, right now?
P: I think it's dumb. I think it's … it's ….
T: What is dumb or who is dumb?
P: *ANSWERS QUICKLY* He's dumb.
T: He's dumb.
P: *HESITATES* It's dumb of me to get this upset about it.

She realizes that she is being held responsible for actions she did not commit. This realization forms the crux of her predicament. By accepting criticism without question, she has overlooked and doubted her own feelings. In our therapy session, I challenge her to pay attention to her feelings and how she manages them in the present moment. Her initial response is *IT* is dumb, and then *HE* is dumb. However, she soon reconsiders and decides that it is dumb of *HER* to get this upset. Instead of recognizing and accepting her feelings and responses, she finds fault with them, thinking it is dumb of her to become so upset.

A Shared Understanding

I recapitulate our conversation, aiming to confirm whether we agree that her coping strategies are causing her difficulties. In the upcoming excerpt, I have detailed her body language to illustrate how her interest and seriousness progressively intensify throughout the passage. Even though I pose my question multiple times, it is always done in a composed manner and with a soft tone.

T: But does it upset you?
P: Yeah, it does because….
T: Okay, so that's reality. It does upset you.
P: *LAUGHS EXASPERATEDLY AND NODS* Yeah, it does.
T: Yeah. Yeah, so it's a bit interesting here. Let's just stop a little bit for a while. Because you say that you're angry at him.
P: *LOOKS AWAY* *MOVES RESTLESSLY*
T: But you think that it's your fault. You say that you're angry at him, but it's you who's going to die.
P: *LOOKS AWAY*
T: You say that you're upset about it, but it's dumb, even though you *are*. So do you see that when we're talking about these negative reactions toward him, you're angry at him, but somehow, it's back onto you.
P: *NODS SLOWLY*
T: And this is what you do, isn't it? When you sit here talking about this, and right now it's dumb, and all the way here, he does things that you don't like.

He accuses you of things, he keeps you at a distance, he sends you mixed signals, and obviously you have a lot of feelings toward him for doing that. But somehow, it's about you. It goes back onto you. Do you see what I mean?

P: *LOOKS SERIOUSLY AT ME* Yeah.

T: How does that strategy work out for you? When you're angry at him, you take it back onto you. How does that work out for you?

P: *SIGHS*

T: Does that help you?

P: *SHAKES HER HEAD AND LOOKS SERIOUS* No.

T: How does it make you feel? You're angry at him, and then you take it back on yourself.

P: *SIGHS*

T: How does that work out for you?

P: *SIGHS* I mean, it doesn't work out. It's not a good strategy.

The Girl Who Wasn't a Princess finally recognizes these mechanisms. She expresses her understanding verbally and also demonstrates it through her body language, indicating that she takes it seriously. She maintains eye contact, speaks earnestly, and her laughter has ceased. She admits, "I mean, it doesn't work out. It's not a good strategy." She acknowledges the repercussions of her self-treatment and realizes its imprudence. This is a crucial initial step toward agreeing on goals and tasks. If she wants to avoid becoming depressed and self-destructive, she must stop avoiding her feelings.

Figure 10.3 encapsulates the insights we have gathered and agreed upon thus far. The diagram illustrates the conflict she encountered with the man she lived with (represented by the C-corner of the triangle of person), and the conflict that surfaced during our session (denoted by the T-corner of the triangle of person).

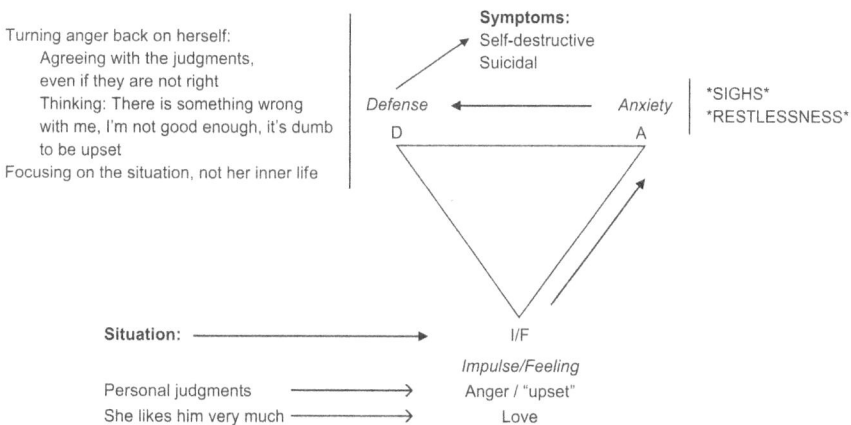

```
                                        Symptoms:
Turning anger back on herself:          Self-destructive
    Agreeing with the judgments,        Suicidal
    even if they are not right
    Thinking: There is something wrong  Defense ←———————— Anxiety    *SIGHS*
    with me, I'm not good enough, it's dumb    D                A     *RESTLESSNESS*
    to be upset
Focusing on the situation, not her inner life


    Situation:  ————————————————→    I/F
                                      Impulse/Feeling
    Personal judgments    ————————→   Anger / "upset"
    She likes him very much ————————→ Love
```

Figure 10.3 The Triangle of Conflict applied to the case of The Girl Who Wasn't a Princess

I am providing a summary for the Girl Who Wasn't a Princess, and I am curious if we have reached an agreement regarding our joint course of action.

T: And obviously he was sending all these mixed signals. And it had really affected you, it triggered a lot of emotions. And you tried to figure it out. But instead of trusting yourself and leaving him right there, you started doubting yourself ... like, attacking yourself .... Getting into this self-destructive pattern .... Like, even the most self-destructive, committing suicide .... Even though you didn't do it.

P: Yeah.

T: Is this something that we should take a closer look at? This way that you avoid your negative feelings? That you don't .... You start to, like, not trust yourself .... Getting into this negative self-destructive mode? Instead of facing your feelings and trying to figure it out and trust yourself? Is that something that we should have a look at right now?

P: I think so. Yeah.

T: Right.

P: Yeah.

T: Please tell me if there's something in that .... If it's not precise enough. That's how it seems to me. That there is something .... That there's something about the way you treat your feelings ....

P: Yeah.

T: When you get angry ... and it gets back ... back onto you. And it's been that on quite a few occasions, also with this guy when you were 13–14. Even sometimes with your friends as well.

P: Yeah.

We have successfully completed the initial stage of alliance building. We agree on the nature of her symptoms, specifically suicidal and self-destructive thoughts. The alternative to these thoughts is self-trust and making choices that promote self-care when faced with complex feelings. This is the goal she aspires to achieve. Our joint effort will involve a detailed examination of how she processes negative feelings and discovers new coping strategies. As therapy progresses, and we address situations triggering her symptoms, it will be understandable for the Girl Who Wasn't a Princess when I inquire about her feelings. If it becomes challenging to explore these feelings and new defenses emerge, we have our groundwork established. I often remind my patients: "Our purpose here is to understand how you manage your feelings, right? We observed in our first session how you avoided your feelings with these self-destructive thoughts, and it seems to be happening again. Are we still on the same page?" This mutual comprehension serves as a crucial safeguard against potential alliance disruptions and misunderstandings in future therapy sessions.

Psychodynamic Case Formulation

While we were working on shared understanding of goals and of therapeutic tasks, we developed a psychodynamic case formulation, drawing from Malan's two triangles. This formulation is not something I jot down and share; it is a product of our collaborative effort. For a therapist's learning process, it might be beneficial to put such case formulations into writing. A written case formulation for the Girl Who Wasn't a Princess might appear as follows:

The Girl Who Wasn't a Princess is a woman in her thirties who turned to therapy due to suicidal thoughts. These thoughts surfaced when living with a roommate she initially adored, believing him to be the prince of her dreams. In the early stages of their relationship, he was very caring. They even shared the experience of having been seriously ill. However, he eventually started treating her poorly and became judging toward her. His behavior made her angry, but amid these mixed feelings toward him, she doubted her own perception of reality and accepted his criticism instead. She sought validation from others rather than trusting herself, often thinking something was wrong with her. Her self-destructive thoughts included contemplating suicide with a knife. She experienced similar, albeit less intense, symptoms when interacting with friends who possessed things she lacked. The first time she experienced suicidal symptoms was when she was thirteen to fourteen years old after a boy rejected her. She harbors long-standing thoughts that a relationship with a man should remedy a difficult life, as portrayed in princess stories. She has hoped that a man's love will make up for the love she lacked from her mother, with whom she has a strained relationship. We have agreed to work on how she manages her feelings, so she does not have to resort to self-destructive defense mechanisms, and to understand why she treats herself this way.

One Last Comment

The therapy examples I have discussed are not meant to serve as a *step-by-step guide* for developing a dynamic case formulation or establishing agreement on goals and tasks. Rather, they illustrate certain *principles* rooted in psychodynamic theory that the therapist should apply adaptively during this stage of therapy. The exact path you take to reach your destination is not as crucial as actually getting there. Moreover, the journey you undertake should also foster a strong therapeutic bond, a topic we will delve into in the following chapter.

Notes

1 Unfortunately, as of July 2024, this book is still only available in Norwegian.
2 If you understand a Scandinavian language, I highly recommend Tone Normann-Eide's overview of different theorists' perspectives on primary feelings (Normann-Eide, 2020, pp. 30–31). Obviously, there are different perspectives on this topic.

3 Both Blackman (2004) and Frederickson (2013) have extensively explored the topic of defense mechanisms.

4 I have included additional descriptions to illustrate the body language and tone of voice in this excerpt. These additions aim to emphasize that the dialogue exudes a serene, tender, and courteous tone. It may seem confrontational when you read that I ask the same question multiple times, and in a way it is. It is therefore vital to ask in a manner that conveys respect and empathy toward the patient, which is something I consistently strive for in this excerpt.

5 In Chapter 6, we delved into research illustrating the connection between possessing social networks and maintaining sound mental health. The Girl Who Wasn't a Princess not only has friends but also actively engages with them.

Chapter 11

Therapeutic Bond and Trust

The task of defining a solid therapeutic bond is by no means a straightforward one, and outlining how it can be established is equally challenging. Bordin refrains from providing a precise definition of a therapeutic bond. Instead, he describes it using expressions like "the human relationship between therapist and patient," "liking or disliking each other," "trust," and "attachment" (Bordin, 1979, p. 254). Therefore, a therapeutic bond can be understood as a significant relationship between individuals, characterized by trust and positive feelings. Bruce Wampold (2017) posits that an effective therapy's foundation is an initial therapeutic bond comprising three elements: trust, understanding, and expertise. Consequently, Bordin and Wampold employ somewhat similar terms when discussing the therapeutic bond.

Jan Smedslund, a Norwegian psychologist and professor emeritus at the University of Oslo, is recognized for his development of the *Psycho-Logic*. This approach presents what he terms commonsense psychology, which is "the psychology we all know tacitly and use in everyday life. This psychology is embedded in ordinary language and is acquired by everyone in the process of becoming socialized into a culture" (Smedslund, 1988, p. VII). Using *Psycho-Logic*, Smedslund (1997) defined several key psychological terms, including the concept of *trust*. I assert that the definitions and portrayals of the therapeutic bond provided by both Bordin and Wampold are entirely encapsulated within Smedslund's examination of the concept of trust. Therefore, if we follow Smedslund's line of thought, the therapeutic bond fundamentally boils down to a matter of *trust*.[1] Rognes (2002), based on Smedslund's Psycho-Logical analysis, outlines five conditions that are both *necessary* and *sufficient* for a patient to trust the therapist. These five conditions are:

1 The patient believes that the therapist *cares* for the patient.
2 The patient believes that the therapist *understands* the patient.
3 The patient believes that the therapist has *own-control*.
4 The patient believes that the therapist has *self-control*.
5 The patient believes that the therapist has the relevant *know-how*, knowledge or expertise to help.

DOI: 10.4324/9781003516217-14

Smedslund's concepts of *care* and *understanding* encompass the significance of positive feelings and genuine human connections, as emphasized by Bordin. Wampold underscores the significance of expertise and understanding along with trust. Smedslund's analysis suggests that these elements are integral to the concept of trust, rather than being distinct entities. Hence, I propose that if a therapist cultivates trust by meeting Smedslund's five conditions, it is reasonable to believe that a strong therapeutic bond has been established.

Certain terms, like the distinction between *own-control* and *self-control*, require more detailed explanations to be fully understood. Smedslund (1997) conducted an analysis rooted in the inherent Psycho-Logic of these terms, and I will proceed to clarify these terms based on his analysis. However, what is even more crucial is understanding what you, as a therapist, can do to help the patient gain a sense of trust, thereby fostering a strong therapeutic bond. In this endeavor, the Girl Who Wasn't a Princess will once again prove to be a valuable resource.

Care

Rognes (2002), drawing on Smedslund (1997), defines *care* as when the therapist wants the patient to feel good in the long term and guided by the therapist's best judgment. This necessitates the therapist keeping track of how the patient is doing, offering help when the patient is in pain, and experiencing satisfaction or dissatisfaction in response to the patient feeling good or bad, respectively. The opposite of caring is indifference and hostility, which are both detrimental and incompatible with trust.

Thus, care extends beyond mere warmth, empathy, and compassion. It involves a clear communication from the therapist that they desire the best for the patient, and their dissatisfaction when this is not achieved. This approach deviates from the psychoanalytic principles of abstinence (Killingmo, 1997) and neutrality (Gullestad & Killingmo, 2019), which primarily encourage non-judgmental reflection over a definitive therapeutic stance. Smedslund's definition of care aligns with the therapeutic stance of Habib Davanloo (1990), the founder of Intensive Short-Term Dynamic Psychotherapy (ISTDP). Davanloo advocates for the ISTDP therapist to adopt a clear and explicit position on what is healthy and what is not, and to convey this to the patient. The ISTDP therapist, driven by the best interests of the patient, expresses discontent when these are not met, without any attempt to conceal this sentiment.

The Girl Who Wasn't a Princess

What does this look like in a practical context? In the therapy segments detailed in Chapters 9 and 10, I point out several instances where the Girl Who Wasn't a Princess engages in self-destructive behavior. This stems from my commitment to the patient's well-being and my discontent when this is not achieved.

From my perspective, making the patient aware of their destructive behaviors and ensuring they fully comprehend them is an act of care: it is only when the patient recognizes these harmful behaviors that they can begin to address them. This approach is evident in multiple parts of my dialogue with the Girl Who Wasn't a Princess.

The Girl Who Wasn't a Princess found herself under criticism from her romantic interest, who accused her of being dramatic. Aware of her tendency to accept criticism without scrutiny, I encouraged her to actively consider the validity of these accusations. I am not indifferent to her tendency to unquestioningly accept his assertions, even when they contradict her own beliefs.

T: Did you do that? Did you cause drama?
P: I didn't try to! *LAUGHS*
T: Did you?
P: I didn't try to!
T: Did you cause drama?
P: Yeah, no, I didn't try to. I mean, I think there's sort of the inherent drama of, like, roommates liking each other. That's always going to go poorly. And then we were locked down, sort of, together .... But I was in so much pain and it was just at the very end, to be told, like ... I've hated this and you've been mean to me, and you're causing drama.
T: Did you cause drama?
P: No! *GESTICULATES EMPHATICALLY AND LEANS BACK*
T: No, you didn't! So he was accusing you of something that you didn't do.
P: *LAUGHS* Yeah. And this still happens .... Apparently, so .... *LAUGHS*

Assisting the patient in actively opposing destructive mechanisms also demonstrates care. In the following section, which was also discussed in the preceding chapter, I encourage her to actively consider the implications of her self-treatment. When she responds vaguely, I do not relent, but gently and compassionately challenge her vagueness.

T: Yeah. Yeah, so it's a bit interesting here. Let's just stop a little bit for a while. Because you say that you're angry at him.
P: *LOOKS AWAY* *MOVES RESTLESSLY*
T: But you think that it's your fault. You say that you're angry at him, but it's you who's going to die.
P: *LOOKS AWAY*
T: You say that you're upset about it, but it's dumb, even though you *are*. So do you see that when we're talking about these negative reactions toward him, you're angry at him, but somehow, it's back onto you.
P: *NODS SLOWLY*
T: And this is what you do, isn't it? When you sit here talking about this, and right now it's dumb, and all the way here, he does things that you don't like.

He accuses you of things, he keeps you at a distance, he sends you mixed signals, and obviously you have a lot of feelings toward him for doing that. But somehow, it's about you. It goes back onto you. Do you see what I mean?

P: *LOOKS SERIOUSLY AT ME* Yeah.

T: How does that strategy work out for you? When you're angry at him, you take it back onto you. How does that work out for you?

P: *SIGHS*

T: Does that help you?

P: *SHAKES HER HEAD AND LOOKS SERIOUS* No.

T: How does it make you feel? You're angry at him, and then you take it back on yourself.

P: *SIGHS*

T: How does that work out for you?

P: *SIGHS* I mean, it doesn't work out. It's not a good strategy.

A fundamental tenet in ISTDP is the therapist's active opposition to the patient's destructive tendencies while accentuating the positive. This principle aligns with Smedslund's (1997) definition of care and is a crucial element in establishing a strong therapeutic relationship.

Understanding

Rognes (2002), drawing on Smedslund (1997), defines *understanding* as a consensus on what is equivalent with, what follows from, what contradicts, and what bears no relevance to the patient's statements. The perception of being understood by the therapist is crucial for establishing trust and a strong therapeutic bond. Without this, the therapist's interventions may seem arbitrary and disconnected from the patient's therapeutic goals.

In ISTDP, shared understanding is utterly essential and foundational, as I have demonstrated repeatedly in Chapters 9 and 10. The focus of these chapters is fostering a mutual comprehension of the goal, the mechanisms that generate the problems, and the necessary steps for resolution. A key technique involves consistently reflecting back to the patient your understanding, while simultaneously inviting corrective feedback. In ISTDP, this technique is known as *recapitulation* (Abbass, 2015).

The Girl Who Wasn't a Princess

In Chapters 9 and 10, I presented numerous instances of *recapitulations*, a few of which I will revisit here. The shared characteristic of these examples is that I encapsulate my comprehension of her narrative and verify if our understanding aligns.

Example 1:

T: So, what happened here, if we try to sum up .... On, like, a little bit of a higher level .... He sends out mixed signals. He flirts with you, and at the same time, talks about this other girl.

P: Yeah.

T: And obviously you have some reactions to that. And it confuses you. And somehow, again, the solution becomes suicide. Is that correct?

P: Yeah.

T: That your way of avoiding these mixed feelings that ... these feelings ... that his mixed signals are triggering in you ... is going to thoughts about suicide? Is that a way to see it?

Example 2:

T: How did you deal with the FEELINGS? This anger?

P: I thought there was something wrong with me, I guess. Or that I hadn't been good enough.

T: Uh huh. So, facing this anger, you thought that there was something wrong with you?

P: Yeah.

T: You're angry at him. And then you start thinking that there's something wrong with you. Is that correct?

P: Yeah.

T: Right. And also ... you're angry at HIM, then you start thinking about killing YOURSELF.

P: Yeah.

Time and again, as also demonstrated in the *care* example, I make clear that I have understood her reason for seeking therapy—a struggle with self-destructiveness. I consistently convey that I have heard her and have understood the link between her challenges and the defense mechanisms she employs. I share my insights in a manner that allows her to either refute or refine them. This mutual understanding is vital for her to trust me and for us to establish a strong therapeutic bond.

Own-Control

Rognes (2002), drawing on Smedslund (1997), defines *own-control* as the therapist's capacity to act or abstain from acting according to their own will, irrespective of others' desires. In the absence of own-control, those who lack understanding or care for the patient can control the therapist's actions, which is incompatible with trust.

Own-control plays a crucial role in fostering trust for a multitude of reasons. A significant factor is that numerous therapists—at least in the authors' native country, Norway—operate within a public healthcare system that is under immense strain, with resources that do not match the demands of the tasks at hand. It is reported by many therapists that therapeutic decisions are often dictated not by their professional evaluations but rather by resource availability (Nordland et al., 2022). For patients to trust their therapists, they must perceive that the therapists are not controlled by resource limitations and can make independent decisions rooted in their care and understanding.

It is equally crucial that the patient perceives the therapist as not being controlled by the patient's desires. This might seem odd at first, particularly in a healthcare system, like that of Norway, where user involvement is key. However, in most instances the patient is unaware of the mechanisms causing their issues. Chapters 1 and 2 addressed the fact that unconscious mechanisms often underpin the patient's problems. Chapter 4 highlighted how the patient frequently attempts to evade what is painful, and Chapter 3 outlined how all of this will also manifest in the therapist-patient relationship. If the patient senses that the therapist is unable to make autonomous decisions and allows themselves to be directed by the patient, the patient will not trust that the therapist can manage transference phenomena helpfully. Consequently, the therapist will be controlled by *both* the self-destructive and healthy wishes of the patient.

Consider a situation where a therapist, to evade a difficult conversation, chooses not to confront the patient about their excessive use of sedative medication. The therapist makes this choice, even though they are aware that it could lead to less effective therapy outcomes. In essence, the therapist allows the patient's wishes to control their actions, even though it is fundamentally detrimental to the patient's well-being.

In the session with the Girl Who Wasn't a Princess, there are numerous instances where I did not sanction her unconscious efforts to obscure matters and thereby evade crucial, health-enhancing experiences. In the *care* segment, the example shows that I maintained attention on her detrimental mechanisms, even though she sidestepped the subject by not responding to my inquiries, and clearly found it distressing.

Example 1:

T: Did you do that? Did you cause drama?
P: I didn't try to! *LAUGHS*
T: Did you?
P: I didn't try to!
T: Did you cause drama?

Example 2:

T: Yeah. Yeah, so it's a bit interesting here. Let's just stop a little bit for a while. Because you say that you're angry at him.
P: *LOOKS AWAY* *MOVES RESTLESSLY*
T: But you think that it's your fault. You say that you're angry at him, but it's you who's going to die.
P: *LOOKS AWAY*

My priority was not to be controlled by her diversions and unease; instead, I maintained my attention on what I deemed significant. This is a demonstration of *own-control*, which is crucial for building trust and a strong therapeutic bond. Displaying own-control can sometimes seem confrontational to the patient. Hence, it is vital that the actions involving own-control are not stand-alone but are embedded within a framework of understanding and care, with shared goals and a shared understanding of therapeutic tasks.

Self-Control

Rognes (2002), drawing on Smedslund (1997), defines *self-control* as the therapist's ability to act or abstain from acting in line with their reflective and normative wants and beliefs rather than their personal and unreflective ones. This implies that the therapist possesses the self-control to do what is right, acting intentionally rather than impulsively. A therapist who acts impulsively and irresponsibly is necessarily detrimental to the patient.

This holds significance on multiple levels. A therapist who, amid their own doubts about the therapy's progression, impulsively and without reflection alters their therapeutic stance without the patient's comprehension and agreement, will seem to lack self-control. This could manifest as the therapist switching the therapy model and implementing techniques from cognitive behavioral therapy unplanned. Alternatively, the therapist might start discussing their own challenges in an effort to build rapport through self-disclosure.

Consider another scenario where an ambitious therapist becomes frustrated with the patient for sidestepping a crucial topic in therapy. If the therapist *impulsively* voices this frustration instead of collaboratively investigating with the patient the reasons for their avoidance, it exemplifies a lack of *self-control* and can lead to trust issues.

A clear instance of deficient self-control causing direct harm to the patient is when a therapist enters into a romantic or sexual relationship with their patient. The therapist, in this case, acts impulsively on their personal, unreflective wants: sexual feelings. Regrettably, such behavior is alarmingly prevalent. Research indicates that between 4% and 10% of all healthcare professionals have engaged in sexual interactions with current or former patients. While these figures are not exclusive to psychotherapists, they nonetheless highlight the magnitude of the issue (Health Professions Regulatory Advisory Council, 2011).

Know-How

Rognes (2002), drawing on Smedslund (1997), defines *know-how* as the pertinent knowledge and expertise concerning the problem, coupled with the capacity to address challenges that surface in connection with the problem. The therapist needs to instill belief in their ability to assist the patient with the problem they bring to therapy. Absent this belief, the patient's trust in the therapist will be lacking.

How does a therapist demonstrate their expertise, and how can it be ensured that the patient perceives the therapist as having relevant know-how? In their analysis of *facilitative interpersonal skills* in therapists, Anderson et al. (2009) underscored aspects such as verbal fluency, the ability to manage their own feelings, communication skills, the ability to forge alliances, and a clear focus on the problem, as elements linked to improved therapy outcomes. This suggests that concentrating on establishing shared goals and agreement on tasks (Bordin, 1979) aids in building a strong therapeutic bond. The capacity to articulate and present matters verbally also appears to be crucial. Wampold (2017) notes that a common trait of effective therapists is their skill in convincingly explaining the origin of the problem, and how this is directly tied to the solution of the problem.

In Chapters 9 and 10, I have elucidated the process of fostering mutual understanding by concentrating on the problem at hand, and that of illustrating the link between the mechanisms causing the problems and their respective solutions. Generating a common understanding of the problem, fostering a psychodynamic case formulation that illustrates the problem's mechanisms, and—based on this—developing a shared understanding of the therapeutic tasks at hand, demonstrates relevant know-how. If all of this is effectively communicated, the path to demonstrating relevant knowledge and expertise becomes straightforward. This is vital for building trust and a robust therapeutic bond.

Therapeutic Bond and Trust

I propose that the third element of Bordin's definition of a therapeutic alliance, the therapeutic bond, aligns with Smedslund's (1997) concept of trust. This alignment provides a clear depiction of the actions therapists need to undertake in order to cultivate trust and thereby establish a robust therapeutic bond. This surpasses the simple display of warmth, empathy, and the nurturing of positive feelings: it encompasses therapeutic actions that instill in patients the feeling of having discovered a place where they can obtain help from a therapist who possesses the requisite knowledge and appropriate qualities.

In Part II, I have illustrated the formation of a therapeutic working alliance, drawing on Bordin's (1979) definition. I have also demonstrated the creation of a psychodynamic case formulation, grounded in Malan's (1979) triangles. This forms the cornerstone of all short-term dynamic therapies. A strong alliance and a shared[2] case formulation chart the path for the therapeutic journey. When challenges surface along the way, the course remains steadfast, enabling both parties to recall their destination and the initial plan on how to reach it. This shared understanding lays a solid foundation for the journey to proceed as seamlessly as possible. Despite its vital importance, a solid alliance is merely the initial phase of the process. The next part of the book delves into *how* to accomplish the patient's goals.

Notes

1 I owe my understanding of this connection to Waldemar Rognes (2002), former associate professor at the Norwegian University of Science and Technology (NTNU). His insightful series of lectures on the therapeutic relationship, delivered as part of the master's program in clinical psychology at NTNU in Trondheim, Norway, enlightened us on this subject.
2 When I use the word *shared*, I am speaking of a mutual understanding that has been collaboratively developed to comprehend the patient's challenges. It is not about the therapist crafting a theory to eventually present to the patient as a final verdict.

Part III

Alliance-Guided Short-Term Dynamic Cooperation

T: Is this something that we should take a closer look at? This way that you treat your negative feelings? That you don't … You start to, like, not trust yourself … Getting into this negative self-destructive mode? Instead of facing your feelings and trying to figure it out and trust yourself? Is that something that we should have a look at right now?

P: I think so. Yeah.

We have reached agreement on goals, outlined the therapeutic tasks, and fostered a relationship rooted in trust. Now we're prepared to delve into the work. The forthcoming chapters explore how to navigate defense mechanisms, anxiety, and feelings, all crucial to helping the patient achieve their therapy goals. While each of these three therapeutic elements has its own dedicated chapter, they are not isolated phenomena. They are intertwined, as illustrated by Malan's triangle of conflict. It's meaningless to consider defense mechanisms without the presence of anxiety and feelings. These three elements are manifestations of an underlying, unconscious conflict that complicates lives and generates symptoms. Even when the attention is on one corner of the triangle, you're concurrently working with the other two, given their inseparable connection. This understanding underscores the complexity and interconnectedness of the therapeutic process.

DOI: 10.4324/9781003516217-15

Chapter 12

How to Do Defense Work

Getting Acquainted with Your Defense

Defense mechanisms primarily function as automatic, unconscious reactions, serving as the patient's immediate response to situations that stir up anxiety-provoking feelings. The use of these mechanisms isn't a deliberate choice, but rather instantaneous reactions that have been ingrained over time. There is, however, a silver lining: If the patient gains awareness of these mechanisms and recognizes that there are alternative responses that lead to less suffering, it becomes possible to reduce the automaticity of these reactions and chart a new path. The unconscious can be brought into consciousness, allowing for a departure from old strategies that once dominated their life.

For an individual to successfully set aside ingrained and unconscious defense mechanisms, assistance is needed. The process of altering these defense mechanisms is pursued through three specific objectives (Coughlin Della Selva, 2004):

1 *Identification* of the defense
2 Clarification of the *function* of defense
3 Examination of *the consequence* of defense

First, the patient must first identify their defenses. This means they need to *consciously* recognize their use of a specific defense mechanism. Indeed, altering something you're not aware of is a formidable task! They also require guidance to comprehend why they resort to these defense mechanisms, which is essentially to avoid feelings that provoke anxiety. Then the patient needs assistance to understand that these defense mechanisms have negative consequences. If the defense doesn't result in any problems, there's no motivation to cease its use. It's only when the patient becomes aware of these three facets of their defense that they can make an informed choice about whether they wish to continue using it.

Once the patient becomes acquainted with their defense mechanism, it becomes evident that the defense is an active effort made by the patient. It's not merely a spontaneous occurrence, but an action taken by the patient to avoid confronting something challenging. Naturally, it is crucial to acknowledge that discarding old

DOI: 10.4324/9781003516217-16

coping strategies can be a difficult and often painful process. However, it is only when you realize that you have a choice that you also gain the possibility to opt for a new approach. The ultimate aim of defense work is for the patient to realize that they can take control and alter how they manage their feelings.

These are the three sub-goals of defense work. While the sections are numbered in a sequence that is commonly followed, it's not a *requirement* to proceed in this order. The psychodynamic dialogue is flexible, with the *objective* being to achieve a comprehensive understanding of the three aspects of the defense work. This understanding can be attained in various ways and doesn't necessitate a step-by-step procedure.

1. Identification of Defense

The patient requires assistance to recognize their use of defense mechanisms. After all, altering a mechanism that one is unaware of is impossible. The therapist might pose a question like, "Do you notice that you laugh when discussing this tragic loss?" when the patient laughs while sharing a painful experience. The therapist could also ask, "Do you notice that you call yourself stupid when you recount his poor treatment of you?" This helps the patient understand that they tend to criticize themselves in situations where others have behaved poorly. By asking, "Do you notice that you view everything as hopeless when you talk about your boss's criticism?" the therapist assists the patient in recognizing their inclination to give up rather than confront difficult feelings in a challenging situation. Before the therapist can aid the patient in letting go of harmful defense mechanisms, both need to clearly recognize their presence.

2. Clarification of the Function of Defense

Once the patient *recognizes* the use of a defense mechanism, the subsequent step is to comprehend the *reason* behind its use—that is, its *function*. The defense mechanism represents merely one corner of Malan's triangle of conflict. The patient resorts to defense because they encounter feelings that induce anxiety, and the role of the defense mechanism is to keep these feelings at bay. It is crucial for the patient to acknowledge this, not only to understand themselves and their problem-causing mechanisms, but also to grasp the alternative to employing this defense. Given that the defense mechanism suppresses feelings, the alternative is *not* to suppress them, but rather to experience them.

The patient has recognized their tendency to use laughter as a defense mechanism when discussing sad topics. A typical follow-up from the therapist then might be: "What happens to the sad feeling when you laugh at it?" The goal of the therapist is to guide the patient toward understanding that using laughter in response to sadness is a way to suppress and distance themselves from their feelings. For a patient who realizes that they resort to self-criticism when mistreated, a possible follow-up question could be: "What happens to your anger toward the person who mistreated you when you label yourself as stupid?" The therapist seeks to help the patient understand that self-criticism and self-blame are strategies to avoid experiencing feelings of anger. This understanding is crucial because feelings of anger are a natural and healthy response to being mistreated.[1]

3. The Consequence of the Defense

Once a patient becomes aware of their defense and understands its function, it's important for them to also see the negative consequences of this defense. If there are no negative outcomes from the defense, there's no reason to stop using it.[2] Defense mechanisms have been a long-standing method for the patient to reduce anxiety. The alternative to using these mechanisms is to face difficult, anxiety-provoking feelings, which requires a compelling reason. One such reason could be the patient's realization that the defense mechanism is causing problems, preventing them from reaching the life or therapy goals they aspire to.

Therefore, the therapist aims to explore the consequences of the patient's defense. For a patient who tends to laugh off their sadness, a pertinent question might be: "How does this affect you? And how will your therapy progress if you continue to laugh away your feelings?" For a patient who self-criticizes when treated poorly, it would be appropriate to ask: "How does this affect you? What are the consequences of criticizing and blaming yourself for being mistreated?" In order to foster a willingness to let their defense mechanisms go, the patient needs to understand that they lead to negative outcomes. They must realize that laughing things off hinders their process of grieving and moving on in life. If they laugh at their feelings in therapy, they won't receive the help they are seeking. They need to understand that if they blame themselves for things beyond their control, they risk becoming depressed and stuck in challenging situations.

Becoming Acquainted with Defense Mechanisms

Patients need to realize that they are employing defense mechanisms, understand that these mechanisms serve the function of dampening feelings causing anxiety, and recognize the negative consequences of these mechanisms. These three sub-goals contribute to *acquainting the patient* with their defense mechanisms (Coughlin Della Selva, 2004). Only when this comprehension is established can the patient provide informed consent to cease using their defense mechanisms. If a therapist challenges a patient to stop using their defenses before achieving all three sub-goals, it could jeopardize the working alliance. It is unreasonable to expect someone to abandon a significant behavior without clearly understanding what they've been doing, recognizing its detrimental effects, and identifying a suitable alternative.

The Man Who Worried About His Heart

The Man Who Worried About His Heart was a young man who sought therapy due to health anxiety. He began experiencing chest pains around the time the COVID-19 pandemic hit Norway, sparking fears of a potential heart problem. In the ensuing nine months leading up to his therapy, he underwent a series of medical examinations, both urgent and scheduled. He reported feelings of tightness in his chest, breathing difficulties, and occasional discomfort and pain in his hand. No physical issues were found during the medical examinations. Upon starting therapy, he had a degree of awareness that his chest tension was rooted in psychological factors. Yet, the possibility of a severe physical condition remained a concern, causing him to worry significantly about potential heart defects.

In the treatment of the Man Who Worried About His Heart, it was promptly agreed that his primary issue was health anxiety. Even though he acknowledged that his chest tightness was a symptom of anxiety provoked by psychological factors (refer to Table 10.2 for an overview of physical symptoms of anxiety), he remained profoundly worried about its physical causes. My hypothesis suggested that his focus on physical explanations prevented him from understanding the psychological root cause of his problems. His preoccupation with physical illness thus served as a defense mechanism, keeping anxiety-inducing feelings unconscious. Each time he experienced tightness of the chest, he was gripped by the fear of a serious illness. This fear effectively diverted his attention from the psychological aspects causing his tension. Since he didn't orient his focus toward the psyche, the feelings that arose stayed beyond his conscious perception. This encapsulates the concept of unconscious feelings.

When the COVID-19 pandemic began, something sparked a dormant conflict within him, kindling feelings tied to this conflict. These feelings caused anxiety. Instead of trusting the doctors who assured him of his physical health, he believed there was an issue with his heart. His pursuit of physical explanations kept his feelings unconscious and obstructed his understanding of the *actual* situation. This defense mechanism resulted in him experiencing health anxiety and repeatedly undergoing medical examinations. This hypothesis is illustrated using Malan's triangle of conflict in Figure 12.1.

The Three Sub-Goals of Defense Work

To reach a consensus on our therapeutic tasks (refer to Chapter 10), we need to grasp the mechanisms causing the issues. When the Man Who Worried About His Heart observes that his symptoms manifest during the session, it provides an opportunity to examine these mechanisms in real time. Events that transpire in other aspects of life also occur in conjunction with the therapist in *the transference* (refer to Chapter 3). This presents a unique opportunity to become acquainted with and understand his symptoms and mechanisms.

P: It's a bit tighter in the chest *right now* *LAUGHS*!

T: It's getting a bit tighter right now! Great that you notice it! So let's have a look at it, then!

P: Yes.

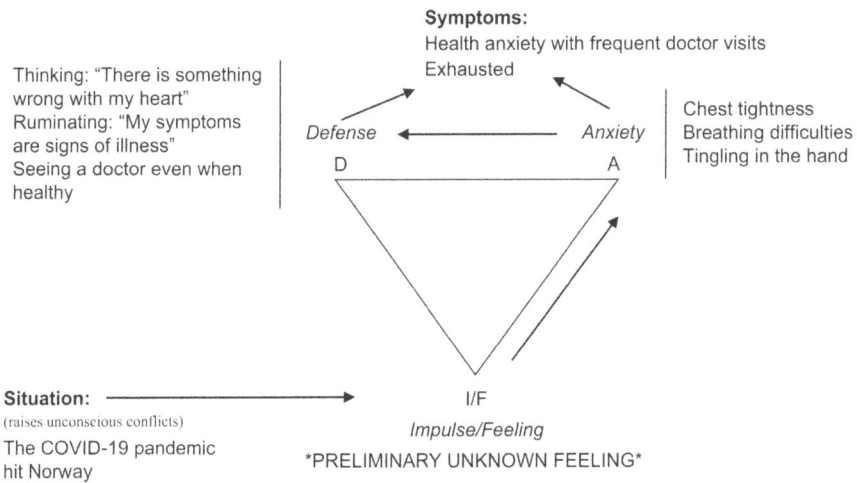

Symptoms:
Health anxiety with frequent doctor visits
Exhausted

Thinking: "There is something wrong with my heart"
Ruminating: "My symptoms are signs of illness"
Seeing a doctor even when healthy

Defense ⟵ Anxiety
D   A

Chest tightness
Breathing difficulties
Tingling in the hand

Situation: ⟶ I/F
(raises unconscious conflicts)
The COVID-19 pandemic hit Norway

Impulse/Feeling
PRELIMINARY UNKNOWN FEELING

Figure 12.1 The Triangle of Conflict applied to the case of the Man Who Worried About His Heart

T: Because it's interesting—here we are, wondering whether it's psychological. And as we talk about it, the symptom gets worse.

P: Yes.

T: So I wonder what is being triggered inside of you right now … that makes you anxious, and that tightens your chest? What is it about sitting here, talking to me about this right now…

This passage is from the initial therapy session, immediately after he recognized becoming anxious while discussing his challenges. He observes that the symptoms he experiences during the session mirror those he encounters when he suspects heart issues. This prompts him to reflect on his approach to managing mental health concerns:

P: I haven't really considered it at all, psychological issues and such. It's not something that happens to me, sort of.

T: Mmm.

P: So, I'm not familiar with it, that that's kind of the, yeah … the code …. To look into that, sort of.

T: So, you're saying that you have little experience thinking about yourself in psychological terms.

P: Yes. Or I've been thinking very coldly about myself, in a way …. Things have gone so well for me that such things shouldn't actually bother me.

The Man Who Worried About His Heart realizes that he hasn't engaged in psychological thinking. He has not directed his attention toward feelings, thereby evading a psychological perspective. This is the function of defense mechanisms: they divert attention from what is distressing and anxiety-inducing. He also harbors a belief that he should not be psychologically distressed, given his achievements in life. This belief further helps to shift the focus away from his internal world, serving as another defense mechanism.

Given that he can discuss this, he reveals that he can notice his defenses. This is a positive development: He can identify the defense (the first sub-goal of the defense work) when he realizes that he is seeking physical explanations instead of psychological ones. The function of the defense (the second sub-goal of the defense work) is to keep complex feelings at bay as they trigger anxiety. He recognizes this as well. But does he understand the consequences of this (the third sub-goal)? Does he realize that this manner of thinking and focusing leads to his difficulties? He conveys that he recognizes his tendency to set high standards for himself, that he grapples with finding answers, and that he is short of understanding.

T: So, how is it to not understand?
P: Well, then you have no answers.
T: No, you don't.
P: So, I notice ... when I'm about to sleep. That's when it's the worst. It becomes a bit difficult to fall asleep. When I think about .... Well, putting the spotlight on the body and, sort of .... When focusing on it, it becomes impossible not thinking about breathing. It becomes ... breath manually ... It gets so ... uncomfortable. Then there's ... a bit of despair that I don't get a definitive answer.

He starts to recognize the consequences of his defenses: His search for physical reasons behind his symptoms, trying to control his breathing, and ruminating that he shouldn't struggle mentally, all compound his challenges. He is left feeling lost, unable to make sense of the situation, which again leads to fear and symptoms of depression, as well as sleep becoming elusive. His defense mechanisms are indeed causing him problems.

When the therapist and patient collaboratively identify the defense, grasp its function, and discern the consequences of its application, the patient generally begins to harbor a distaste for his defense: They discern that the use of the defense mechanism culminates in unfavorable results. What was previously an unconscious defense and an automatic process has now transitioned into the sphere of consciousness. The patient *has become acquainted* with their defense mechanism, and their drive to abstain from employing it escalates. But what unfolds when the patient now strives to curb the (previously) automatic defense mechanisms? According to psychodynamic theory, individuals utilize defense mechanisms to suppress complex feelings and the anxiety these provoke, as depicted in Malan's triangle of conflict. If this theory holds true, the Man Who Worried About His Heart should either connect with his feelings or experience heightened anxiety. In this instance, it's the latter that occurs:

The Anxiety Increases When He Doesn't Use Defense

T: How is this for you? If we look at your hands now, what is happening in them?
P: They are tight! *LAUGHS*
T: Hmm. Your knuckles are turning white. You're squeezing pretty hard, aren't you?
P: Yes.
T: So, your hands are a bit tense?
P: Yes.
T: Your chest is tense as well, isn't it?
P: Yes, a bit.
T: Are there other places where you feel tense? Like your neck or shoulders?
P: *LAUGHS* Yes.
T: Are you more tense now than when you arrived?
P: Yes, absolutely.
T: So, we've talked about what's going on: your difficulties and problems, and how you understand them. We see that it is causing tension. Somehow, we're managing to … make you more tense by talking together. By talking to a psychologist …
P: Yes.
T: … inquiring into whether this is psychological, and we see that you get symptoms.
P: Yes.
T: Somehow, we are onto something here, don't you agree?
P: Mm.

So far, Malan's (1979) theory has proven accurate. When he ceases to employ the defense mechanisms mentioned and instead starts to explore the psychological realm, he experiences an increase in anxiety: He feels tension in his chest, neck, and shoulders, and his hands become clenched. Even though this is uncomfortable for him, it is a positive sign for therapy. The anxiety serves as a signal (Freud, 1936) that he is nearing the complex underlying feelings that are important to address in psychodynamic therapy. The symptoms of anxiety he describes are also indicative of anxiety being directed into striated muscles (Figure 10.2). This form of anxiety activation does not interfere with cognition and learning, allowing us to proceed safely with the therapeutic process (Frederickson, 2013). All signs point to him being within his window of tolerance (Nordanger & Braarud, 2014).

While we understand that anxiety serves as a signal, and even when all signs suggest that the patient's level of anxiety is manageable, it's often challenging for us, as therapists, to take actions that heighten our patients' anxiety. Our instinct is to alleviate their pain, not amplify it! At this juncture, it's crucial to remember that change, by nature, is uncomfortable. Our role as therapists is to accompany our patients through this discomfort, facilitating healing on the other side. This means we must accept that our patients may experience increased anxiety during the process. For the Man Who Worried About His Heart, it's vital that he experiences anxiety during the session, enabling him to comprehend the root of his issues. The fact that his symptoms can be triggered through conversation provides compelling evidence that the tensions he experiences are not of physiological origin.

Feelings and Defenses

My supposition is that anxiety-inducing feelings have been stirred up as we've discussed his issues while simultaneously aiding him in identifying his defenses. I'm curious if this holds true and whether he can observe and acknowledge this process. A common observation in ISTDP is that the patient's anxiety will diminish when they permit themselves to experience their feelings (Abbass, 2015). Consequently, I inquire about his feelings:

T: What feelings arise as we talk about these difficulties that have plagued you for almost a year?
P: It's strange. It's a bit like … I can't see a solution to it.
T: But these are thoughts, right?
P: Yes.
T: "I can't see a solution to my problems."
P: *LAUGHS* Yes.
T: Right. It seems like, this is a tendency of yours:
P: Yes ….
T: Rather than paying attention to your feelings, you lean toward your thoughts: "I can't see a solution."
P: Yes.

When I inquire about his feelings, he responds with his thoughts. Concentrating on thoughts rather than paying attention to one's feelings serves as a defense mechanism. This type of defense might be somewhat challenging to comprehend. Indeed, his statements are accurate: he doesn't instantly see a solution to his problem! However, *thinking* that he can't see a solution, without making an active effort to seek a solution or to comprehend his feelings, results in him not making an attempt to recognize his feelings. Consequently, a new defense emerges that he needs to be acquainted with. This is a predictable occurrence. Very few patients rely solely on one single defense mechanism to cope with their feelings. When they let go of one defense, another typically surfaces that requires attention.

Hence, we are embarking on another cycle with the three stages in addressing the newly surfaced defense. I have clarified to him that he resorts to his thoughts (sub-goal 1: identification) rather than his feelings (sub-goal 2: function). I am curious if he recognizes the consequences of this defense:

T: Mm. And how does it affect you, when you start thinking: "I can't see a solution"?

P: It's hopelessness, in a way. It becomes a bit like ... I feel tired, kind of ... That it's kind of not ...

T: Mm. Right.

He can discern that the statement "I can't see a solution" is a thought (sub-goal 1). He also understands that this thought results in a sense of hopelessness and feeling tired (sub-goal 3). Recently, he concurred that thinking like this was a method to evade the underlying feelings (sub-goal 2). He's beginning to get acquainted with this thought defense, and I'm curious if he's prepared to let it go. Consequently, I encourage him not to succumb to hopelessness, and I observe attentively to see if he manages to do so:

T: So, what feelings are underneath, if we don't succumb to hopelessness? If we shouldn't give up already. We've only been trying for a little while.

P: Yes. Well, it's ....

T: What feelings are coming up right now? What are you feeling inside of you—right now?

P: Right now, I feel sad. *LAUGHS*

T: Mm.

The Man Who Worried About His Heart effectively combats hopelessness and dispels the thoughts that hinder his feelings. Upon doing so, he becomes aware of his sadness. However, a defense mechanism used previously in the session re-emerges—he laughs. This laughter serves as a defense mechanism, cushioning the intensity of the sadness he feels. Now, it's crucial to acquaint him to this defense mechanism as well. This is achieved by once again concentrating on the three sub-goals of defense work: assisting him in identifying it, comprehending its function, and acknowledging the adverse consequences of its use.

T: Do you notice yourself laughing?

P: *NODS*

He can identify his defense (sub-goal 1).

T: You mention that you're sad, yet you laugh. Do you have any thoughts on why you do that? Can you comprehend why you laugh when you've just stated that you're sad?

P: I'm not really sure.

T: Does your sadness increase or decrease when you laugh?

P: I reckon it decreases a bit.

T: That's what I was thinking too. So, in some way, is this a method for you to alleviate your sadness?

P: *NODS*

He also grasps the function of the defense mechanism (sub-goal 2), which serves to ease his feelings of sadness. It's unclear if he's aware of the consequences of this defense (sub-goal 3), and it would have been appropriate to inquire about this at this juncture. However, for some reason, I refrained. Instead, I opted to provide a summary and share *my* perception of the consequence—that is, it diverts us from identifying the source of his challenges. Therapy is typically most effective when the therapist assists patients in uncovering insights on their own, rather than pre-scribing them. Yet, in this instance, I find myself somewhat impatient and eager to impart my understanding:

T: What do you believe happens to your feelings when I inquire about them, and you respond with thoughts of hopelessness? How does that affect you? What do you think you are doing to your emotional accessibility when you start thinking as I ask about your feelings?

P: I suppose I distance myself from them.

T: That's what I thought as well. Is that a habit of yours? Is this the coldness you mentioned earlier; that you distance yourself from your feelings?

P: Yes, actually.

T: Mm. Could you consider participating in an experiment where you don't distance yourself from your feelings? For us to understand the psychological aspects of what's making you anxious, right now? Because, as long as you keep distancing yourself from your feelings and who you are, it becomes somewhat challenging to figure out? Would you agree?

P: Yes.

T: Mm. So if you don't laugh this off. If you don't distance yourself from it…

P: Yes.

T: What do you feel then?

P: Well, I don't know. I just became incredibly stiff! *LOOKS UNCOMFORTABLE*

Once more, it's evident that as he becomes acquainted with his defense, by recognizing the defense, understanding its function, and acknowledging its consequences, his anxiety escalates, manifesting as him becoming incredibly stiff (anxiety in striated muscles; refer to Table 10.2). If the psychodynamic hypothesis holds true, this is because he approaches his challenging feelings more closely when he refrains from thinking hopeless thoughts or laughing at his feelings.

The Result of Effective Defense Work

To assist him in acknowledging his feelings and comprehending what provokes his anxiety, I once again inquire about his feelings. The fear of the unknown is a common human trait. Hence, it's crucial for him to grasp what's happening within him; that it is his own feelings that are causing him fear.

T: What kind of feelings did you notice in that moment just before it hit you? What did experience as your body stiffened?
P: Well, I don't know. I can't seem to pinpoint it.
T: No? Mm. Is it difficult to comprehend?
P: Yes, I lack the words to describe it somewhat.
T: Did you notice any physiological sensations? Behind your eyes or elsewhere in your body… Your throat?
P: I did get a lump in my throat.
T: You got a lump in your throat. I see.
P: And I recognized it from… a symptom when I… Yes, from a prior instance, sort of.

The Man Who Worried About His Heart tears up, gets a lump in his throat, and his voice carries a tone of tension.

T: Are you noticing a tightening sensation in your throat, right now?
P: Yes.
T: What is the sensation in your throat? Behind your eyes?
P: It feels like … all the way up here …. It's as if …. Yes, I can …. Yes …. Yes, yes. *LAUGHS*
T: Mm. Okay.
P: *LOOKS SURPRISED*

He pauses, realizing that he is *laughing*. Our defense work is starting to show results, and he's becoming *acquainted with his defenses*. In the past, he would instinctively and unknowingly laugh off his feelings, but now he's aware of this laughter and makes an effort to suppress it. He's now in a position to consciously decide whether he wants to continue dismissing his feelings with laughter. This is the ultimate goal when working with defense mechanisms. The task is to assist patients in understanding their defenses, enabling them to make an informed decision about whether to continue using them.

T: Did you notice what just happened?
P: Yes, I did!
T: What just happened? By the way, it's great that you noticed that!
P: Yes! Well, I smiled and …. Yes.
T: What do you observe when you smile?

P: It kind of relieves me. It sort of takes … Yes …. It alleviates …

T: Yes. And then you said "take"… Can you complete the sentence you started there?

P: It takes the load off …. It doesn't become so … serious anymore, in a way. And that's … not right. Mm.

T: Okay, so you're not here to laugh it off and not take it seriously?

P: No, I'm not.

The Man Who Worried About His Heart has become well acquainted with his defense mechanism, and he is committed to taking his emotions and therapy seriously. He recognizes that laughter serves as a defense (sub-goal 1), understands that laughter lightens the experience of sadness (sub-goal 2), and realizes that the consequence of this is a lack of seriousness toward his feelings (sub-goal 3). It appears that we have successfully achieved the objective of our defense work.

Invitation, Encouragement, and Challenge

Once the patient gains a clear understanding of their defense mechanisms, including their function and consequences, it opens up a new chapter in therapy. The therapist can start to *invite, encourage* and *challenge* the patient to let go of their defenses and instead, embrace the alternative: experiencing their feelings. A strong alliance is established, characterized by a mutual agreement on the therapy's goal, the approach to achieve it, and a solid bond. Such an alliance allows the therapist to challenge the patient to address their defense mechanisms without causing any confusion or misalliances. The mutual understanding is robust, enabling the patient to comprehend why the therapist is challenging them. However, transitioning to this phase prematurely, a common mistake when the therapist is overly enthusiastic, can lead to misunderstandings and potential alliance disruptions.

Davanloo (1990) referred to the techniques in this phase as exerting *pressure* toward experiencing feelings and *challenge* to abandon the defense. However, I find it more fitting to describe it as an *invitation* and *encouragement* to experience feelings. The term *pressure* might imply that the therapist is pushing the patient into something, possibly against their will. My actual intention is to invite and challenge the patient to follow through on what they have expressed a desire to do. Concurrently, as I invite the patient to experience feelings, I challenge them to let go of the defenses they have acknowledged they no longer wish to employ.

Invitation to Feel Feelings

The Man Who Worried About His Heart went to visit his grandmother during a particularly rough period. He had hoped that a change of surroundings would help him escape the discomfort he was experiencing. Contrarily, he found himself shedding tears in her presence. As he recounts this episode, his eyes fill with tears and his voice carries a strain. I make an effort to encourage him to embrace the feelings that are visibly surfacing. My voice is gentle as I strive to connect with his sadness. The essence of my message, which is challenging and encouraging, needs to be delivered within a context that is empathetic, warm, and understanding.

T: *SPEAKING IN A GENTLE VOICE* It appears there's a new wave of it right now.
P: Yes, mm.
T: Now, you have an opportunity to take it seriously, allow it to pass through, and not hold it back.
P: Yes.
T: It seems incredibly exhausting to constrict your throat like this.
P: Yes! *LAUGHS*
P: *CATCHES HIMSELF LAUGHING*
P: It's astonishing! It happens automatically!

Our work on his defense has been fruitful. He has come to understand that laughter is not a productive way to handle feelings, and he is making a conscious effort to stop this mechanism from functioning automatically and outside his awareness. Consequently, I *invite* him to explore an alternative to defense, which is to *experience* his feelings. I facilitate this by directly encouraging him to allow his feelings to surface, through communicating in a gentle and empathetic manner, and by clarifying the difference between the act of defending and the experience of feeling.

T: *GENTLE VOICE* A lot of feelings have been surfacing here. Yet again, you're holding back, distancing yourself from them, and trying to simplify things.
P: Yes.
T: But then, it's the same thing that's coming up, as it was with your grandmother.
P: Yes. Yes.
T: So, the question is, are you going to allow yourself to feel this? It's been exhausting!
P: Yes, it's been exhausting *SIGHS*
T: It seems like it's just below the surface. The question is, should you hold it back once more?
P: Ugh...
T: Are you going to distance yourself from it, or are we going to take an honest look at it together ... if we're going to ... let it out, sort of, get rid of it. You and I. Together! So you don't have to bear it all alone!
P: *SIGHS* Yes ... That's true. *SIGHS* Yes ....

Challenge to Set Defenses Aside

We have arrived at a juncture where, despite his awareness of his defense mechanisms, he continues to employ them. Merely *inviting* feelings falls short, hence I *encourage* him to set his defenses aside. I *challenge* him to refrain from using these mechanisms that we've acknowledged as harmful to him. It is of utmost importance that you don't pose such a challenge without prior thorough defense work, ensuring the patient is well acquainted with their defenses.

T: So, if you don't go to your thoughts.
P: Yes.
T: Don't laugh it off—just take an honest look at who you are underneath. Who are you, really, deep down?
P: Mmm. Yes ....
T: Because it is happening right now .... These phenomena, right now, with pain and tension...
P: Mmm.
T: ... in your throat, in your chest. I guess you notice it in that muscle across here, as well. Has it become even more tense?
P: Yes, all of it. Now I'm starting to get this ... numbness in my hand and I sometimes experience that in the evening.

Strange sensations in his hand were among the symptoms he was afraid of, leading him to seek therapy. He had assumed it was an indication of heart disease. Now, it emerges during our session as we focus on experiencing feelings. Its occurrence during the session allows me to clarify that this is a byproduct of anxiety and psychological defenses, not a symptom of heart issues. And once again, it becomes evident that he requires additional rounds of defense work before he can fully let it go:

T: And somehow, we have managed to give you heart problems just by talking for half an hour.
P: Yes. *SMILES*
T: Right. So how do you interpret this numbness right now? What do you think caused the numbness? Is it the heart? Is there something wrong with your heart?
P: No.
T: How certain are you that there is nothing wrong with your heart, right now?
P: I should be 100 percent sure, but I'm not.
T: So logically, you are 100 percent sure, but if you were to be completely honest, then?
P: Yes, no, then I'm still a bit ... It just doesn't feel right, somehow! *VOICE CRACKS* *TEARS COMING*
T: Okay! *SPEAKING WITH A GENTLE VOICE* So here's an opportunity to just let it out. If you're not going to keep this inside any longer .... Here comes a wave .... There are lots of tears that want to come out ....
P: Oh .... *SOBBING*

Over a period of roughly thirty minutes, I assisted the Man Who Worried About His Heart in identifying his defenses, comprehending their function in repressing his feelings, and recognizing their contribution to his symptoms as he persistently pondered over physical causes for what were in reality anxiety symptoms. Once this was understood, I repeatedly *invited* him to experience his feelings and *challenged* him to relinquish the defense mechanisms he had now become acquainted with. Following a brief detour to thoughts of an actual heart condition, which he no longer believes in, the tears flow: The Man Who Worried About His Heart sobs in waves for several minutes. We have achieved the intended result when doing defense work: the patient identifies them, decides to let them go, and instead gives themselves permission to feel their feelings.

Significant Occurrences Unfold When Feelings Are Felt

I remain silent, only providing comforting sounds as he cries. As the wave of grief recedes, I voice my curiosity about his anxiety. The theory posits that when you permit yourself to experience your feelings without restraint, it should lead to a sense of relief. It's vital for the therapeutic alliance that he acknowledges this link. If feeling feelings leads to lessened anxiety, it's essential for him to comprehend this connection clearly.

T: How is your chest feeling right now?
P: It's a little better, actually. It's a bit strange.
T: And how is your hand?
P: My hand is still a bit stiff.
T: So, your chest feels a bit better, but your hand is still a bit stiff.
P: Yes. It has loosened up a bit.
T: It has loosened up?
P: Yes, it has.
T: Right. How do you interpret that? That it loosened up when you let all of this out?
P: Well, it's like the faucet is shut, sort of. The pressure increases.
T: And when you turn the faucet off, it tightens all around. The pressure increases.
P: Yes.
T: Mmm.
P: It's so strange .... Because ... I've thought about it before ....
T: Yes, I suppose you have.
P: Like, resisting feelings and such, as a general problem.
T: Mmm.
P: That I'm a bit ... cautious and ... I ruminate over everything before I do it. Like ....
T: Mmm.
P: Yes .... But I somehow didn't think that it ... could go so wrong, somehow.

As he opens the faucet, the tension in his chest subsides. He becomes aware that he has frequently suppressed his feelings, a fact he has acknowledged before. This strategy has proved beneficial for a significant duration, but why has it turned problematic recently? It is clear that he has protected himself from the painful feelings of grief, but what has provoked these feelings in him in the first place? I remember him stating at the onset of the session that everything started when COVID-19 reached Norway, which leads me to inquire further:

T: It seems that something happened when the coronavirus pandemic hit, which caused it to stop functioning.

P: Yes .... I had .... I'm not certain of its relevance ....

T: Well, I'd suggest we trust your associations.

One of Davanloo's (1990) significant clinical findings was that the insights patients share immediately after openly expressing their feelings are particularly vital in illuminating their challenges. As the feeling is experienced, defenses have receded, granting the patient greater access to previously unconscious content. I bear this in mind when I invite him to voice whatever is present in his mind.

The Man Who Worried About His Heart conveys that his social circle is rather restricted, with he and his friends primarily keeping to their own company. He also describes himself as not being particularly inclined toward social activities. At the same time, he has felt the lack of a wider network but hasn't discovered the right opportunity to broaden it. He goes on to mention that he met someone through his work, and after a series of text messages, she suggested they go to a seminar together.

P: And then, sort of ... it was sort of a big moment ... Because, sort of .... Yes!

T: So, she asked if you wanted to accompany her to the seminar?

P: To the seminar, yes, and it was like ....

T: Like a date?

P: Uh .... Like .... She wanted me to be there. And it was, sort of, really nice.

T: Yes, of course it was!

P: Because until then, we had been, sort of... It seemed like we both wanted to be friends, at least. And that was sort of nice, but we were both very shy, and sort of .... But it was, sort of, the first time she wanted me to be around, and it was very nice.

T: Of course it was. It must have felt great!

P: It did! And just like that—and then: Covid. It was then. It was actually right then! I don't know, it didn't affect me that much immediately... But I've kind of thought about it since. That somehow... Covid has put everything on hold... And somehow...

T: So you met a girl who you connected with... You describe yourself as not very social, or an introverted guy ... who had mostly stuck with the people you knew from before. And then you get a really good connection with a girl who is a bit like you. That must have given you quite a bit of hope and expectations...

P: Yes, it kind of seemed like it was... Now it's happening!

T: What was happening?

P: That somehow… A social life, in a way, which is beyond…
T: Have you missed that? Did you miss that?
P: Yes!

This was what had happened when the COVID-19 pandemic struck Norway: For the first time, the Man Who Worried About His Heart had met a girl who was somewhat similar to him, and they were planning to meet. This was an exciting prospect, not only for the potential of gaining a girlfriend but also for the opportunity to broaden his social network. However, just before their first meeting outside of work, Norway went into lockdown due to the pandemic, and the seminar they were due to attend was canceled. They no longer saw each other at work, and both were too timid to advance the relationship. For a young, introverted man, this was a significant loss that inevitably led to grief. As we would later discover, he had spent his entire life concealing his true feelings and trying to lift the spirits of those around him. Therefore, he kept his feelings to himself. But the loss of potential love, along with all the other social losses brought about by the pandemic, meant that this strategy was no longer effective. The pressure mounted when he turned the faucet off. The grief persisted, and instead of grieving, he became anxious about the feeling. Instead of recognizing symptoms like breathing difficulties, chest tightness, and hand tingling as anxiety, he interpreted them as signs of a heart problem. This was an effective distraction from the actual feelings, but it had a downside: He ended up worrying and obsessing over physical problems, leading to what could be termed health anxiety (refer to Figure 12.1). Once the Man Who Worried About His Heart became acquainted with his defenses via *the three sub-goals of defense work*, I could safely invite him to experience his feelings and challenge him to abandon the defenses he now recognized as harmful.

Although this chapter has primarily centered on dealing with defense, it is evident that we also had to address both his anxiety and his feelings. Naturally, this is the case, as defense mechanisms are a result of feelings that provoke anxiety. These phenomena cannot be handled separately. The therapist must dynamically engage with all three corners of Malan's triangle of conflict to help the patient free themselves from the strategies that are creating problems.

Notes

1 Here, it's crucial to differentiate between *feelings* of anger and angry *behavior (aggression)*. Feeling angry is an internal, physiological reaction that provides us with the energy needed for self-care. On the other hand, aggressive behavior refers to *actions* that are mostly inappropriate, both for the individual exhibiting aggression and for their surroundings.

2 Certain defense mechanisms do not lead to issues and are thus not a focal point in therapy. The therapist's interest lies in the defense mechanisms that either generate or sustain the symptoms that prompted the patient to seek help.

Chapter 13

Restructuring Defenses

For most patients, the process of relinquishing deep-seated defense mechanisms is not as immediate as it was for the Sweet Child and the Man Who Worried About His Heart. The underlying conflicts and the feelings they evoke are typically so distressing, anxiety-inducing, and complex that they continue to be avoided, even when there's a conscious desire not to do so. When patients find themselves in circumstances that stir up these latent internal conflicts, they instinctively fall back on their customary defense mechanisms. These mechanisms, due to their familiarity and sense of security, seem like the appropriate response when anxiety levels escalate. Within the framework of psychodynamic theory, this phenomenon is referred to as the defense mechanisms being *ego-syntonic* (Coughlin Della Selva, 2004), implying that these mechanisms are perceived as important, appropriate, and an aspect of one's identity.[1]

Many patients have long depended on their defense mechanisms, and it requires more than mere *intellectual understanding* to set them aside. In practical terms, this implies that the therapist will repeatedly observe the patient grappling with the symptoms that brought them to therapy. Although it can be distressing to witness the patient experiencing symptoms, it also presents a chance to address their challenges. Every time a symptom surfaces, it offers an opportunity to comprehend what sparks the difficulties, to explore the corners of the triangle of conflict, and to assist the patient in discovering alternatives to their well-known defense mechanisms.

In Intensive Short-Term Dynamic Psychotherapy (ISTDP), this process is known as *restructuring* or *restructuring of regressive defenses*,[2,3] and it involves repeated exploration of situations that trigger symptoms while acquainting the patient with the corners of Malan's triangles (Davanloo, 1990). This technique is crucial for patients with depressive symptoms, psychosomatic symptoms like pain, irritable bowel, and migraines, or those who react impulsively to their feelings (Coughlin Della Selva, 2004). The patient needs to clearly and distinctly comprehend the differences between the corners of the triangle of conflict. Without this understanding, mechanisms that generate symptoms are activated automatically and unbeknown to the patient. If the therapist *invites* feelings and systematically *challenges* defenses before this understanding is established, it can lead to an increase in symptoms.

DOI: 10.4324/9781003516217-17

In this case, the therapist has not assisted the patient in altering the symptom-generating mechanisms, turning the therapy into a symptom-inducing situation, much like other life situations. During the learning process of ISTDP, it is beneficial to devote ample time to this phase and opt for the restructuring technique more frequently rather than too infrequently. Effective restructuring also aids in establishing a clear and shared understanding of the patient's complaints, leading to a robust psychodynamic case formulation.

Grasping the specific phenomena that can be placed on each corner of the triangle of conflict, and how the corners interact and potentially lead to symptoms, is an essential aspect of what is known as possessing a robust *ego-adaptive capacity* (Ten Have-de Labije & Neborsky, 2012), or more simply put, high *capacity* (Kuhn, 2014). This concept also encompasses that the patient recognizes that past experiences with significant individuals influence the present, as demonstrated by the *triangle of person*, and that they manage feelings, anxiety, and defense in a healthy manner.

The Girl Who Wasn't a Princess sought therapy due to her intense suicidal thoughts. She attributed these thoughts to winter and to a man with whom she shared a flat, fearing the return of these thoughts in the upcoming winter. She perceived her symptomatic improvement over the months leading up to therapy as a result of the arrival of summer and distancing herself from the man. However, she had limited insight into the fact that the man and the winter were merely *triggering situations*, not the actual *cause* of her suicidal thoughts. The root cause of her suicidal thoughts was of course psychological, as she evaded the anxiety-inducing feelings triggered by the situation. She did this by employing defense mechanisms that involved directing anger and aggressive impulses toward herself through self-criticism and contemplating suicide. As long as she holds the belief that the man himself is the cause of her suicidal thoughts, her natural response will be to avoid the man and places they commonly frequent. This becomes complex when they both study the same subject and are part of a small social group. Given her initial understanding, she is faced with the choice of either avoiding significant places in her life, or experiencing suicidal thoughts. An alternative for her, which she is beginning to understand (see Part II), is to constructively deal with the feelings that arise when she encounters him.

Struggling to distinguish the corners of Malan's (1979) triangle of conflict, in terms of both cognitive comprehension and practical implementation, is at the heart of numerous psychological issues. I will provide some examples to illustrate how this may manifest.

Mixing the Corners of the Triangles

Example 1:

A man seeks therapy, burdened by depression and pain, coupled with numerous extended periods of sick leave. He shares that his workplace is rife with conflict, which negatively affects him. His energy drains and he experiences pain in his shoulders and back when he is at work, leading to his frequent sick leaves. His condition improves when he is not at work, and he expresses a wish for disability benefits. The patient believes that his pain and fatigue are *directly* caused by his work environment, and thus, he should steer clear of it.

Workplace conflicts stir up complex feelings within him, as he finds himself feeling angry when individuals he appreciates contribute to a negative environment. His upbringing in a home filled with conflict and aggressive behavior has led him to associate anger with anxiety and discomfort. Unconsciously, he equates *feeling* angry with *acting* aggressively, which complicates and intensifies his anxiety when he experiences angry impulses. This anxiety results in tension and pain in his striated muscles, particularly in his shoulders and back (refer to Chapters 10 and 14 for more on anxiety). The pain is draining, and he expends considerable energy ruminating over potential workplace scenarios. He frequently contemplates his negative role in the conflicts, which further contributes to his exhaustion and insecurity. The patient attributes his exhaustion to his job. However, the true sources of his tiredness are his constant anxiety, physical pain, worries, and negative self-perception. His job merely serves as the triggering *situation* for these feelings. Refer to Figure 13.1 for further details.

As long as he views his job as the single cause of his problems, a therapist won't be able to assist him. The scope of a therapist's assistance is confined to managing psychological issues. In this particular case, it involves handling feelings tied to

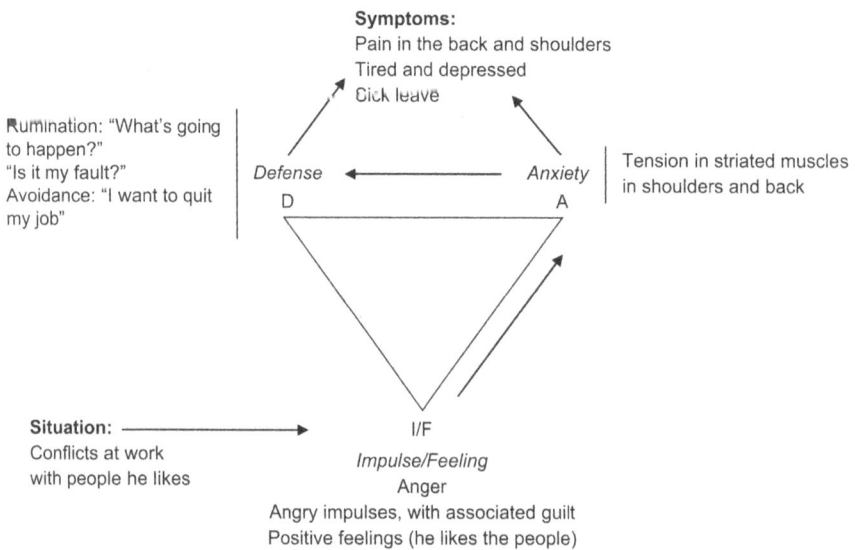

Figure 13.1 The Triangle of Conflict Applied to a Patient Experiencing Work-Related conflicts

work conflicts without becoming overwhelmingly anxious or avoiding the situations that trigger these feelings. It is essential for him to acknowledge this in order to give informed consent for therapy and to develop new psychological skills for effectively dealing with work conflicts.

Example 2:

A woman seeks therapy, feeling depressed following the birth of her first child. Her general practitioner has diagnosed her condition as perinatal depression. She expresses thoughts of regret about becoming a mother and admits to not having affection for her child. She has experienced weight loss, has feelings of restlessness and stress, and has difficulties with sleep and maintaining basic hygiene. She believes that there is an inherent flaw within her, leading her to conclude that she should not have become a mother.

The arrival of her child has stirred a multitude of feelings within her that she finds challenging to manage. The child keeps her awake during the night, and she spends most of her waking hours nursing. Her body has undergone changes, her hormones have heightened her sensitivity, and her life has been completely transformed. She had envisioned herself being filled with joy and an overwhelming sense of maternal love when the child was born. Contrarily, the child triggers feelings of anger and aggressive impulses in her, which subsequently provoke a sense of guilt ("One shouldn't wish to get rid of one's child!"). She grieves over the changes to her body and the loss of her previous freedom. All these experiences are intensified due to sleep deprivation and hormonal fluctuations.

Coming to terms with these negative feelings is particularly challenging for her, given that her own mother didn't seem overly enthusiastic about motherhood. Throughout her life, she has attempted to bring joy to her mother by suppressing her own needs and rather focusing on the needs of others. This approach has served her well thus far, as those around her have valued her attentiveness and her knack for making them feel good. However, this strategy is proving ineffective now when she urgently needs to prioritize her own needs. She must embrace the assistance offered to her and actively seek support, such as asking her husband to care for the child at night or requesting her mother to babysit, enabling her to socialize with friends or take a shower. This contradicts her life's narrative so far, where she has prided herself on her self-sufficiency.

All of this unfolds within this woman, yet she remains unaware of it on a conscious level. Instead, she harbors the belief that there is an inherent flaw within her. She needs help to understand that having children has stirred up intense mixed feelings, and that it is possible to experience these feelings without being overwhelmed by them. If she can acknowledge this internal occurrence, she will no longer believe that she is flawed or that she mirrors her mother. This is illustrated in Figure 13.2.

What she perceives as an unavoidable link between motherhood and depression is actually about how she manages the feelings that come with being a mother.

Symptoms:
Depression
Weight loss, lack of
sleep, poor hygiene

Thinking "There is something wrong
with me"
Ignoring basic needs
(food, sleep, and hygiene)
Avoids asking for assistance so she can
attend to basic need
Trying to handle motherhood without help

Defense ←——————— *Anxiety*
D   A

Anxiety in smooth muscle,
manifesting as nausea,
lethargy, palpitations, etc.

Situation: ————————→
Becoming mother of a child, which keeps
her awake at night and requires a lot of
attention. Her body and her life
has changed significantly.

I/F
Impulse/Feeling
Anger (toward the child)
Guilt over the anger
Grief
Love (toward the child)

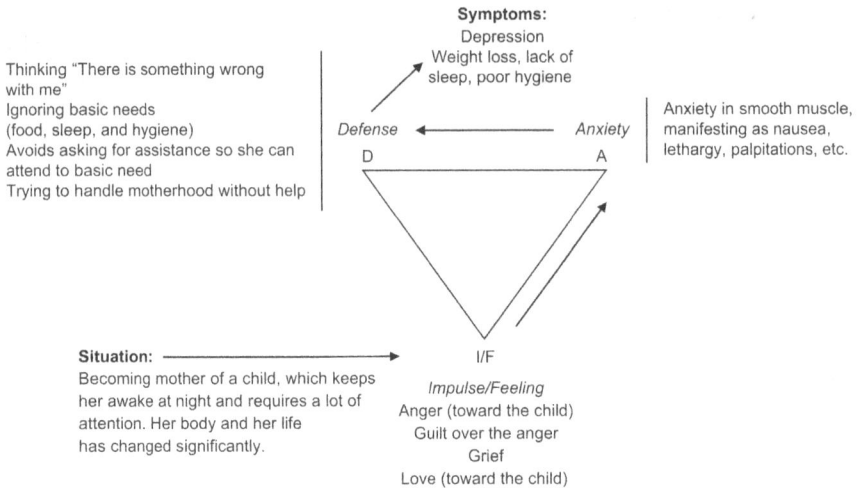

Figure 13.2 The Triangle of Conflict Applied to a Patient with Perinatal Depression

The task in psychotherapy is to aid her in discerning this difference, and then helping her navigate these feelings. This doesn't negate the potential benefits of other strategies, such as medication, advice from a proficient health nurse, or a supportive social network. However, these interventions fall outside the purview of psychotherapy.

How to Restructure

In the initial phases of therapy, the therapist endeavors to comprehend the mechanisms contributing to the patient's challenges, as detailed in Chapter 10. This exploration will clarify if the patient is confusing the corners of the triangle of conflict. This confusion is particularly prevalent among patients with psychosomatic issues (as in example 1), depressive disorders (as in example 2), and impulsivity problems, such as the Girl Who Wasn't a Princess. Their difficulties are directly tied to the blending of situations, symptoms, and the three corners of the triangle of conflict. The primary focus of the therapy's initial phase is to assist the patient in distinguishing these elements. Consequently, the patient's comprehension of the origins and reasons for their problems needs to be *restructured*.

The Goal of Restructuring

The goal of restructuring, as outlined by Coughlin Della Selva (2004), can be broken down into three sub-goals. The *first* sub-goal involves making the patient aware of the defense mechanisms that give rise to their symptoms, a concept previously discussed in Chapter 12. However, when patients possess egosyntonic defense mechanisms, which they perceive as integral to their personality and identity, they require help through *restructuring*. In such cases, the therapist minimizes the use of the technique of *challenge* (refer to Chapter 12) to deter the patient from relying on harmful defenses. Instead, the therapist aims to foster a gradual process where the patient *progressively places less trust in their defenses*, marking the *second* restructuring sub-goal. The *third* and final sub-goal of restructuring is to help the patient feel less anxious about the underlying feelings. The issue of separating the corners, which forms the crux of the patient's suffering, is often deeply ingrained and closely tied to the patient's identity. This lack of distinction contributes to the patient's anxiety.

The Steps of Restructuring

Restructuring is a process that unfolds gradually and repetitively, guiding the patient step by step toward achieving these three sub-goals. The time frame for this achievement varies among patients; for some, it may be a swift process, while for others, it may necessitate numerous sessions. The process involves systematically, one symptom-generating episode after another, clarifying the corners of the triangle of conflict (1), gradually exposing the patient to the underlying feelings and impulses (2), and subsequently summarizing the insights gained from this process (3) (Coughlin Della Selva, 2004). Please refer to Table 13.1.

1. Clarifying the Corners of the Triangle of Conflict

The restructuring process begins by identifying specific instances in which the patient's issues have become apparent. These instances should be so explicit that it becomes evident who was involved, what transpired, and the time and place of the occurrence. The episode's description should be detailed enough for you, as a therapist, to create a vivid mental image of the event, akin to reading a captivating book by a renowned author. Often, patients find this level of detail challenging. The act of being specific stirs up the feelings linked to the situation, and these are the very feelings that the patient tends to resist. However, the more lucid the example, the higher the likelihood of the patient deriving benefit from the restructuring

Table 13.1 Restructuring

Restructuring
1 Clarifying the corners of the triangle of conflict
2 Gradual exposure to the underlying feelings
3 Summarizing the process

process. Therefore, it is crucial that the patient is assisted in clarifying the situation's details.

Once you have a specific and well-defined example, you start guiding the patient to recognize how the different corners of the triangle of conflict come into play. Which elements of the patient's experience are feelings? Which experiences manifest as anxiety symptoms? Which actions of the patient serve as defense mechanisms? How do all these elements connect to the patient's initial complaints? The therapist attentively listens to ensure the patient comprehends this and provides empathetic and instructive clarification when the different corners become entangled.

2. Gradual Exposure to Feelings and Impulses

As the patient gains a deeper understanding of the components of the triangle of conflict and begins to see the mechanisms that underlie their symptoms, the therapist seizes the opportunity to acquaint the patient with the activated feelings. With each specific example, the therapist's objective is to progressively enable the patient to experience a slightly greater portion of the somatic component of the feeling and to help them to connect with the associated impulse (refer to Table 10.1). This systematic and gradual exposure will eventually empower the patient to fully tolerate their feelings and impulses. This process demands perseverance and patience from the therapist. It is tempting to hasten the restructuring and intensify the exposure in an attempt to help the patient as swiftly as possible. However, for a patient who struggles to differentiate between the corners of the triangle of conflict, this haste can lead to an increase in symptoms. It is futile to build a house without first laying a solid foundation, as it will inevitably collapse sooner or later. Effective restructuring lays a strong foundation upon which to construct the therapy.

3. Summarizing the Process

Throughout the restructuring process, the therapist periodically pauses to recapitulate the progress made. The objective is to assist the patient in cognitively *understanding* the ongoing events while concurrently *experiencing* their feelings. Once the patient has succeeded in feeling a certain feeling, the therapist aids them in comprehending their experience. This parallel process of experience and insight is vital for accomplishing the restructuring goals. The process resembles a spiral where cognitive clarification is followed by gradual exposure to experience, and then a summary to intellectually integrate the experience. Subsequently, preparation begins for a new spiral, involving either the same episode or a different one. The therapist and patient navigate through numerous episodes, drawn from both current situations (C) and interactions with the therapist (T). It is vital for the patient to identify the repetition of the same phenomena across different situations.

Navigating through this process may not always be as straightforward as it appears. As a therapist, there are a few considerations to bear in mind: If you find yourself at a standstill during the exploration of an episode, it's often beneficial to request another example, ideally from a different corner of the triangle of person. If discussing the challenges that surfaced during the therapy session becomes too demanding, you can shift the exploration to an incident from the patient's daily life, or the other way around. During a phase of restructuring, it is generally advisable to steer clear of episodes from the past (P). This is because the feelings tied to significant individuals from the patient's early life, such as parents and siblings, are typically more intense and complex, thereby inducing more anxiety. These scenarios can be deferred until the patient has distinguished the corners of the conflict triangle and understood the mechanisms that contribute to their presenting problems.

The Girl Who Wasn't a Princess

The Girl Who Wasn't a Princess, introduced in Part II, encountered difficulties in distinguishing the corners of the triangle of conflict. Despite numerous attempts to clarify the links between her defense mechanisms and symptoms, she continually returned to her initial belief that something was inherently wrong with her. Furthermore, the Girl Who Wasn't a Princess was grappling with issues that were both of a depressive and impulsive nature. According to Davanloo (1990), these characteristics indicate the need for restructuring. The following example illustrates the process of restructuring. It begins with repeated clarifications of the elements of the triangle of conflict (refer to point 1, Table 13.1), followed by a gradual exposure to feelings (refer to point 2, Table 13.1), and concludes with a summary of the process (refer to point 3, Table 13.1).

Clarifying the Difference Between Situation and Feeling

The Girl Who Wasn't a Princess shared several episodes where she tried to initiate a dialogue with Sean, the man she shared a flat with. Her intention was to understand the essence of their relationship and to confirm if they were truly in a romantic relationship. Sean, however, did not provide her with any definitive answers, and it was apparent that the situation was not entirely as she had envisioned. This was challenging for her, particularly because she had initially held high hopes for their relationship, partly due to their similar life experiences. She recounts numerous occasions when she strived to decipher his intentions and gain clarity. As she narrates these incidents, tears fill her eyes and she appears truly sad.

T: Can I ask you something? How does that make you feel right now? It seemed like there was a wave of emotions coming up right now. Is that correct?
P: *LOOKS THOUGHTFUL* Yeah.
T: What are you experiencing right now? What are you feeling right now?

P: I feel like … I did my best.
T: Yeah, you did that. That's what you *did*.

    The Girl Who Wasn't a Princess looks sad as she recounts her numerous attempts to repair her relationship with Sean. Earlier in our session, we had decided to focus on her feelings (as discussed in Chapter 10), leading me to inquire about how she feels. However, instead of expressing what she *feels*, she describes what she *did*, specifically that she *did her best*. This is *the situation* that triggers her feelings: the understanding that despite her utmost effort, Sean did not respond in kind, which brings her sadness. I acknowledge this by clarifying, "Yes, you did that. That's what you *did*." After underlining this point, I once again inquire into feelings. This is the process of restructuring; it starts with clarification (point 1, Table 13.1) and then moves on to gradual exposure to feelings (point 2, Table 13.1).

Exposure to Feeling and Clarification of Defenses

T: But what do you feel about that? When you sit here with me and you realize you tried … You tried to do your best…
P: Just sad. *LOOKING SAD*
T: You're sad, right?
P: Yeah. *NOT LOOKING SAD ANYMORE*

    The Girl Who Wasn't a Princess states that she is sad, and for a fleeting moment, her demeanor reflects this feeling. For a brief moment, she is exposed to her feeling of sadness. We are in the early stages of the restructuring process, and I understand that it will take time for her to fully experience her genuine feelings. So far, I am content with the progress. She has grasped the clarification between situation and feeling, and acknowledges her sadness. During this phase of restructuring, I choose not to persistently challenge her to let go of her defenses, as I did with the Man Who Worried About His Heart in Chapter 12. Instead, I accompany her through her narrative, illuminating the corners of the triangle as they appear to me (step 1), and attempt to gradually expose her to her feelings (step 2).

Clarifying the Difference Between Anxiety and Anger

The Girl Who Wasn't a Princess continues to elaborate on her relationship with Sean:

P: I tried to make it better and *it's* still bad. *MAKES GESTURES* Like I, I still have a bad relationship with this person, and I tried! And he didn't try at all. And he doesn't think he did anything wrong at all! *SPEAKS MORE STRONGLY*
T: How does that make you feel? Toward him?
P: Angry. *SIGHS* *LAUGHS*

The Girl Who Wasn't a Princess states that she's angry. She is cognitively aware of the feeling she is experiencing, and identifying the feeling is an important objective to reach (refer to Chapter 15). Another key aim is for the patient to be capable of somatically experiencing the feeling, which is why the patient is gradually exposed to the feeling during restructuring. Feelings are physiological experiences, not merely cognitive processes (refer to Table 10.1). Allowing oneself to feel anger physically provides the strength and energy that The Girl Who Wasn't a Princess truly requires to look after herself. She comprehends that she is angry, and thereby clarifies the feeling corner of the triangle of conflict independently. The subsequent step for her is to be gradually exposed to the physiological activation that the anger induces (refer to Table 13.1):

T: How do you experience that anger right now? How do you experience this anger toward Sean right now? Because … he didn't try. You tried!

P: I'm ….

T: How do you experience it, physically in your body? This anger toward Sean.

P: Here. In my chest.

T: What do you notice there?

P: Um, in my chest …. Here, on my sternum.

T: How does it …. How does your chest feel?

P: Tight.

T: Tight. Tight, like in a strong way or like in an anxious way?

P: In an anxious way.

I aim to expose her to the experience of her anger, physically within her body. The Girl Who Wasn't a Princess senses tightness in her chest, and a tight feeling of strength and power in the chest is a common sensation when one is angry (refer to Table 10.1). However, it is not strength that she is experiencing at this moment. She observes that her chest feels tight, but in an *anxious way*. She conflates the somatic experiences of anger and anxiety, which results in her confusing the I/F corner and the A corner of the triangle of conflict. As long as she equates the uncomfortable feeling of anxiety with anger, it is understandable that she shies away from her anger. Consequently, I shift from exposure and clarify what I have observed:

T: So when you …. When I ask you about how you experience this anger toward Sean, you get anxious.

P: *NODS* Yeah.

T: So there's something about this anger that makes you anxious.

P: Yeah.

I clarify (step 1) that she is feeling anxious about her anger, aiding her in distinguishing between feelings (I/F) and anxiety (A). She now recognizes, at least temporarily, that she is experiencing *both* anger and anxiety.

Further Clarification of Defenses

The process of restructuring unfolds in a spiral manner, involving numerous repetitions. The clarification of one phenomenon invariably leads to the need for clarification of another.

The Girl Who Wasn't a Princess continues to share her thoughts about the potential reactions of others if she permits herself to feel her anger. Despite the fact that it is only me and her in the therapy room, and our conversation is centered solely on her *feelings* rather than her *actions*, she starts to think that others won't validate her anger. This thought leads her to distance herself from her feelings, serving as a defense mechanism characterized by negative thinking and focusing externally when faced with feelings. I proceed to clarify this (step 1).

P: That … I'm alone in being angry. And that I don't have anyone who really understands my level of being angry about it. And then, I'm still so upset about it.

T: Yeah. And then, and then you said, "No one would understand. If I tell people they won't believe me."

P: Yeah.

T: Right now … Right now, these are thoughts. And what are, what are the meta … uh, message from these thoughts?

P: Um…

T: "No one can understand. If I tell them they won't believe me." These are thoughts, these are your thoughts about yourself. You put … other people in there, but these are thoughts.

P: Yeah.

The Girl Who Wasn't a Princess has *thoughts* about others' potential lack of understanding. As we engage in restructuring, with the goal of clarifying the different corners of the triangle of conflict, I elucidate that these are negative thoughts she harbors that belittle her feelings. Consequently, this serves as a defense against feelings.

T: And what is the meta-message of these thoughts? Can you hear that?

P: My feelings about it aren't valid.

T: Right. You can't trust yourself.

P: *SPEAKING CLEARLY* Yeah!

T: Don't trust your feelings. Other people … "I need external validation."

P: Yeah!

T: "I can't trust myself." See what I mean?

P: Yeah.

The Girl Who Wasn't a Princess acknowledges that she is *thinking* that her feelings lack validity. To enhance the clarity of this understanding, I am providing a

Thinking: "No one will really
understand"
"No one will believe me"   *Defense* ◄─────────── *Anxiety*   *SIGHS*
My feelings are not valid   D   A   Tightness in her chest
I need external validation   (Anxiety in striated muscles)

Situation: ───────────────►   I/F
Sean didn't try to sort   *Impulse/Feeling*
things out   Anger

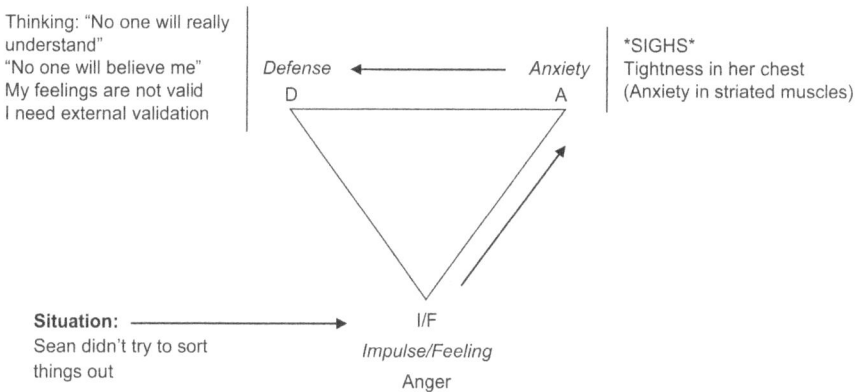

Figure 13.3 The Triangle of Conflict Applied to The Girl Who Wasn't a Princess

summary of her statements. She lacks trust in herself and her *inner* experiences, relying on others for *external* validation (refer to Figure 13.3).

First Grief, Then a Wish for External Validation

The Girl Who Wasn't a Princess comes to realize that she is devaluing her feelings. If she truly embraces this realization and acknowledges the significant difficulties this devaluation has brought upon her, it will be a painful truth to face. As my goal is to expose her to her feelings (step 2), I proceed to ask:

T: So, how does it feel? To see that?
P: *TEARS UP, LOOKING SAD**
T: Right now? What feelings are coming up right now?

For a fleeting moment, she experiences a feeling of sadness, a consequence of recognizing her long-standing pain and lack of self-trust. This experience is a healthy sign, indicating the emergence of self-care. It also grants her a brief exposure to the feeling of sadness. In ISTDP, experiencing sadness upon realizing that a defense has been harmful is regarded as an indicator that you're on the right path. However, at this stage, this feeling is allowed to remain for just a few seconds before new thoughts emerge:

P: I'm upset that I'm still so bothered by this.
T: Is it okay to be bothered about it, or is that a self-critical thought?
P: I think it's okay to be bothered by it, but it's just that it's been so long now that
       … it's harder and harder to reach out to other people about it, because now the
       message I get from others is that you just need to get over it. Because it's not
       going to get better.

T: How do you find that?
P: I hate it. I hate it.
T: Oh, of course you do.
P: Because I don't think it's easy to get over.
T: Right. So if we face reality, you *are* bothered.
P: Yeah.

Previously in the session, we addressed her tendency to devalue her feelings. Once more, she is questioning her feelings—specifically, if it's acceptable to still *be bothered* and harbor feelings related to an event from a while ago. Concurrently, the thought that she relies on the approval of others resurfaces.

T: Are you going to let yourself be bothered? Is it okay to still be bothered?
P: Is it? *LOOKS SAD*
T: Now you're asking for an external validation.

Instead of relying on her own judgment, she turns to *me* for reassurance. I clarify that she is seeking validation from me, not from within herself. We have just discussed her tendency to seek validation from others, and she gets the point: She claps her hands and affirms that it's okay to still be bothered by it.

Clarification of Defenses

T: So then the next question is, are you going to allow yourself to … feel what you feel, be who you are, being bothered with the things that you are bothered with? Let's look at how you deal with it. But first of all, is it okay for you? Are you allowed to have your reactions the way your reactions *LAUGHS* react?
P: Yes. It's okay.
T: It's okay.
P: Yeah.
T: Are you sure?
P: Well, no … I'm …. Because not everybody gets this obsessed about things! Or at least that's the way that I've been made to feel by … the other people involved, or my friends who ….
T: Right.
P: Sean definitely doesn't feel like it's okay that we're still bothered, that I'm still bothered!

Again, her thoughts gravitate toward how others perceive her, overshadowing her own perspectives. It is crucial for her to recognize this pattern. During her relationship with Sean, she didn't give due importance to her feelings, leading to major problems as she remained in a harmful relationship.

T: Do you notice what you're doing right now?
P: Talking about how other people feel about my feelings.
T: Right.
T: How does that work for you? When you're having these mixed feelings ....
P: *NODS THOUGHTFULLY*
T: You're having feelings that are painful and you don't quite understand .... And you start thinking about what other people think about it. How does that work for you?
P: *SHAKES HEAD* Yeah, that's not helpful. *LOOKS SERIOUS*

I assist her in realizing that, instead of acknowledging her true feelings, she is repeatedly focusing on the perceptions of others. She does not trust her own evaluation of the situation, but seeks confirmation from the other person. Sean didn't provide this, and it is unlikely he will in the future. This mechanism leaves her extremely susceptible to those who mistreat her.

Summarizing the Process

We have arrived at a crucial juncture in the restructuring process, where she recognizes that her existing strategy is unproductive. After repeated clarifications of her quest for external validation, she now understands the harm in this approach. Clarification (step 1) and gradual exposure to feelings (step 2) have led to new insights. To reinforce these insights, I choose to provide a summary of our current understanding.

T: So let's just look at what we saw here ... because you were talking about you being angry at Sean.
P: Yeah.
T: First of all, you got sad because you said, "I tried. I tried to figure it out. I offered to leave. I tried to have us talk about it." And then you said, "I'm angry because he didn't. He didn't try."
P: Yeah.
T: And then you get anxious, and then you started thinking about all these ... these external things. Doubting your own feelings, saying that it's not okay to feel what you feel. Other people say this and that ....
P: Yeah.
T: So first there was anger. Then there was anxiety. And then there were all these avoidance strategies, like, distancing you from the internal dilemma.
P: Yeah. *NODS*
T: Making it an external dilemma.
P: Yeah.

Ruminating external factors
Doubting feelings
Thinking: It's not okay to
feel what I feel
Thinking: Others will not
validate my feelings
Turn the internal dilemma
into an external

Defense ←————————— Anxiety
D   A

Sighs
Tightness in the chest
(Anxiety in striated muscles)

Situation: ————————————→   I/F
"I did the best I could"   Impulse/Feeling
Sean didn't try to mend the
relationship   Grief

Angry

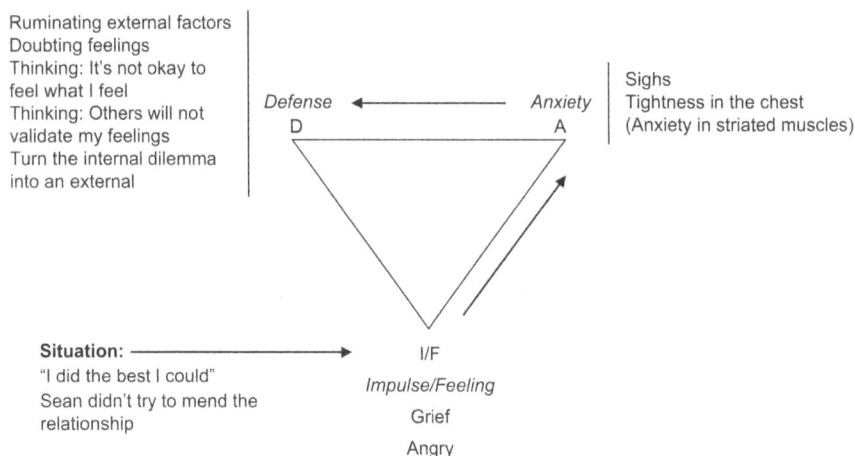

Figure 13.4 The Triangle of Conflict Applied to The Girl Who Wasn't a Princess

In this section, I articulate what is encapsulated in Figure 13.4. I visualize the triangle of conflict and strive to explain its content in simple, everyday language. Such a summary serves as a form of closure for a cycle of restructuring.

A New Cycle of Restructuring

A sign of progress in the restructuring process is when patients start to gain fresh insights and a deeper understanding of their problems. Even though my summary in the preceding paragraph provided a form of closure to the restructuring process, there are still numerous cycles to complete before we cross the finish line. The Girl Who Wasn't a Princess has realized that she is attempting to address her *internal* emotional conflicts by transforming them into something *external*. This newfound understanding leads her to spontaneously comprehend more about her own tendencies toward suicidality:

P: And I think that is … part of why I wanted to kill myself, also, is to do it in front of other people.

T: Right.

P: Be like, I …. This was so bad. Here! Now you can see!

T: Right. Like, rather than keeping it like an internal emotional battle inside of you. How to deal with this painful thing ….

P: Yeah. And to sort of prove, I mean …. When I wanted to kill myself, it was always in a way where … um … he would find out about it fairly quickly after. Yeah. If not to be the one to find the body.

T: And how would he feel then? When he found your body?

P: Oh, God, I don't even know. I guess, ideally, he would feel bad or guilty, but like, I didn't …. *SIGHS*

T: So somehow this fantasy was about making him feel bad or guilty, right?

P: No, I think the fantasy was about making him feel my emotions and the depth of them. Because it was so … so invalidating. And to be told all the time ….

T: You wanted him to feel the way you did.

P: I wanted him to feel how intensely bad he made me feel.

Clarifying the Difference Between Impulse and Defense

"An eye for an eye, a tooth for a tooth." This principle often applies to retaliatory anger. Your wish is for the person who has caused your anger to feel the same feelings that you have experienced. When she becomes angry with Sean, she notices the impulse to inflict pain on him. However, her fantasies of retaliation also involve self-harm, and it is crucial that she grasps this. She wants him to experience the pain he has caused her. But instead of validating this impulse and fully allowing herself this human *desire* for revenge, she fantasizes about self-sacrifice in the same act. As she indulges in a revenge fantasy, she simultaneously defends herself against it by redirecting the anger toward herself. I attempt to clarify this for her (step 1, Table 13.1):

T: So obviously there are some feelings toward him. Wanting him to feel bad, right? When you're angry at him?

P: Yeah.

T: But somehow, rather than truly feeling these impulses of wanting to make him feel bad … to feel the way you felt … you, like, have to sacrifice yourself at the same time, at least in fantasy.

Gradual Exposure to Anger

Experiencing feelings of anger toward Sean, without simultaneously directing them at herself, is challenging for her. She requires a step-by-step encounter with her feelings, allowing her to bear them. This *gradual exposure* takes place within the context of a specific example of a particular symptom-inducing event. For the example to be deemed specific, it needs to be detailed within the setting of a certain time and place, as will be demonstrated in the following paragraph:

P: Because he … told me he liked me and then within a couple of days, I broke up with the person I was dating. And then the night after we broke up, Sean and I watched a movie and … it was in my room. And the first time he kissed me, he also tried to have sex with me …. And it was very fast. And … it was very …. I didn't …. It was going very fast. And at one point he said that he couldn't start dating me then, because it was too soon after he'd broken up with his last girlfriend. And so he wanted me to wait ten days until February started, because then it would have been a full month since he broke up with his ex. And then that would have been sort of a respectful period ... for him from his point of view. And I said, okay. That's cool. We won't do anything for ten days. But can I .... Can we still, like, can I still kiss you? And then I said that I wouldn't have sex with him. I told him to stop trying to take my clothes off, please.

T: Okay. So he was having this, what's the English word, celibacy? He was not going to date someone for ten days, but still he tried to have sex with you?

P: Yes. Yeah.

T: Well, how do you feel toward him for that? For doing that?

P: I feel very used about that. I felt very, like, he tried me out.

T: But that's not your feeling. That's what he did.

The terms "used" and "he tried me out" are not descriptors of feelings (refer to Table 10.1). However, they provide a lucid depiction of his actions; that he was using her and trying her out. I clarify this to her, and she realizes that these very actions are the source of her anger. She promptly connects with her anger, which is one of the key objectives of restructuring.

P: No. No, no, no. He treated me like, he treated me like ... *SPEAKING AGI-TATEDLY* I wasn't somebody he would have to continue seeing. And he continues to treat me like someone I'm not, someone, like not someone he has to continue seeing. *MAKING GESTURES* And that's the thing that really pisses me off about it, is because ... it's a classmate! Like, we have to continue seeing each other!

The Girl Who Wasn't a Princess speaks faster, more energetically, and her hands move in expressive gestures. Anger is an activating feeling, causing energy to flow through the body and into the hands. It appears that this is her current experience, so I inquire if she can direct her attention to this sensation. Can she permit herself to both feel and observe this energy? If so, it will provide a valuable exposure to the physical experience of the feeling.

T: And how do you experience that you're pissed off, right now? How do you experience ....

P: Because I ....

T: How do you experience it physically in your body? Not because, but how do you experience it?

P: Well, I feel, I feel .... *MAKING HAND GESTURES*

T: What do you notice in your hands right now? What is it? What are your hands doing right now?

P: This! *LAUGHS* *GESTURES ANIMATEDLY*

T: Uh huh. How do you feel? What do you notice in them?

P: Tense. It's like I feel the need to move.

Her energy is palpable, her hands are animatedly engaged, and she acknowledges their energizing tension. Every indication suggests that she connects to her anger, allowing herself to be exposed to the experience of this feeling.

Exposure to Angry Impulses

Each feeling, including anger, carries behavioral impulses (as seen in Table 10.1). For healthy anger management, it is necessary to withstand this activation at the *impulse level*, feeling *the urge* to react toward the individual one is angry at. These *impulses of anger* are a natural and harmless internal event that can be observed, experienced, and talked about.

Chapter 15 introduces a commonly used ISTDP technique, referred to as *portrayal* of feelings (Kuhn, 2014). This technique is designed to assist patients in fully experiencing feelings and impulses, including those of anger. However, it is premature to apply this technique to the Girl Who Wasn't a Princess. Our current focus is on restructuring her defenses to prevent an automatic reaction of self-attack when she encounters feelings of anger. If I encourage her to portray these feelings too soon, it could escalate the self-attack.

At the same time, it is crucial for the Girl Who Wasn't a Princess to understand that the impulses in themselves are not dangerous. When faced with the *impulse* to make Sean experience the same pain that as she has felt, she turns this impulse inward, imagining her own death. Yet, she voices fantasies of slapping him, shouting at him, and scaring him, thereby showing her anger. It's vital for her to learn to distinguish between her impulses directed toward him and the self-destructive mechanisms directed at herself. However, talking about these fantasies is difficult for her, because when she does, she pictures him in her mind, revealing her anger to him:

P: He looks scared.
T: Uh huh. How does that make you feel?
P: Satisfied.
T: Mm, so what happens then?
P: *SIGHS* Um ....
T: You've cornered him. You scared him.
P: Well, if it happens .... I guess this is the point where it's almost impossible for me to consider this in the absence of other people. Because I know that this would be an unacceptable thing to do in real life.

Summarizing the Process

She has permitted herself to experience her anger to a certain extent, along with the impulses that come with it. We have achieved one of the restructuring goals, namely, exposure to feelings. However, we are not entirely done. She once again becomes anxious about her feelings (evident from her deep sigh), and withdraws. She resorts to a defense mechanism that we have observed before, where she desires validation from others to acknowledge her own feelings. I conclude that this is as far as we can come in this cycle, and that it's time to recap our progress. This allows her to integrate her experience of anger and impulses with cognitive comprehension, a desirable outcome in the restructuring phase (step 3, Table 13.1).

T: Yeah. But right now this, this is the way you treat your anger, right?

P: Yeah.

T: Instead of experiencing your full ... the full amount of anger, you start to doubt yourself. You say, I can't feel what I feel. It's not acceptable to feel this.

P: Mm. Yeah.

T: The question is .... Because we've seen this happen before. When you get angry, you stop believing in yourself, stop trusting yourself.

P: Yeah.

T: And instead of validating yourself internally, you turn to external validation, right?

P: Oh. Yeah.

T: And right now you have these impulses that you would never act on in real life, right?

P: Yeah.

T: So these are your feelings, and there are impulses. And at this point right now, when you were telling me about, like, "I'm cornering you" ....

P: Yeah.

T: "I'm making you scared and I feel satisfied."

P: Yeah.

T: You said, "I have to stop here and get external validation."

P: Yeah. *APPEARS SERIOUS*

The Girl Who Wasn't a Princess not only confirms but also expresses through her body language that she understands. Yet, she is faced with a predicament, a predicament that is common to many. She fails to grasp that feelings can simply be experienced, without any need for intervention. She doesn't understand that Sean's unchanging nature will continually stir up feelings within her, and the decision she faces is whether to permit herself to experience these feelings.

P: *SIGHS* But it's kind of hard to, um .... 'Cause I don't get anything out of feeling these feelings at this point. Because it's not going to get fixed, just knowing the person.

T: So then the question is: Do you feel it? You said you're not going to get anything out of it, but the question is: Is there this rage toward him? Is there this really strong anger toward him or not?

P: Yes.

T: How does it work for you when you avoid your anger with self-criticism, saying that you can't trust yourself ...? Going for external validation instead of accepting yourself just as you are?

P: Mmm.

T: How does that work out for you? You said that it's not, you're not going to get anything out of feeling it, but let's face it, you *are* feeling it!

P: *NODS*

T: And how has it been to … deal with the feelings the way you've been doing?

P: *SIGHS HEAVILY* It hasn't let me move on from this. I'm stuck in it.

To progress beyond an emotionally challenging situation, you must permit yourself to experience the feelings you genuinely have. The Girl Who Wasn't a Princess is currently acknowledging this reality. Her use of these defense mechanisms, which she has now become acquainted with, has hindered her from moving on. She is stuck in it.

In the restructuring phase, when working with patients like the Girl Who Wasn't a Princess, patience is a virtue for a therapist. The understanding and clarity that exist at a certain point may gradually diminish. The goal is to incrementally enhance the understanding and capability to manage feelings differently. One clarifies, exposes feelings, and summarizes repeatedly. It's akin to ascending a spiral staircase. The journey doesn't proceed directly upward, and such a trajectory shouldn't be anticipated. You have to go through round after round, and with each cycle, the capacity and comprehension of the process gradually increase.

How Did the Girl Who Wasn't a Princess Progress?

The therapeutic process for the Girl Who Wasn't a Princess extended slightly beyond twenty sessions. As we journeyed through the therapy, the complexities of her distinct situation with Sean became increasingly clear. Both had endured the hardship of a life-threatening illness, making their fall-out particularly challenging for her. Another layer of complexity was unveiled when she shared her mother's struggles with her maternal role. From a young age, the Girl Who Wasn't a Princess was told by her mother that she was manipulative and caused her pain. Children, when told they are in the wrong, naturally attempt to rectify their actions. The Girl Who Wasn't a Princess was no exception. She took her mother's criticism to heart, believing there was something inherently wrong with her. This experience was reflected in her relationship with Sean. The strategy she adopted as a child to maintain her bond with her mother, which involved agreeing with her and striving to change, proved to be harmful in her adult life. This strategy, once a survival mechanism, now became a source of harm.

Over the course of therapy, she gradually came to terms with the complex feelings she harbored toward Sean, toward their mutual friends, toward her mother, and toward me. Instead of resorting to self-destructive behavior, she gradually learned to experience these feelings. We followed the same therapeutic approach outlined in this chapter, using a range of specific examples to help her distinguish between the corners of the triangle of conflict, gradually exposing her to her feelings and subsequently reflecting on our therapeutic progress. This process proved beneficial for her. By the end of therapy, she had experienced the longest period in her life without suicidal contemplations. The goal we set at the beginning of therapy was achieved. How does she understand this outcome?

P: Well, I think … um … kind of recognizing that the people who have been some of the most harmful have also been people dealing with issues that would make them harmful to maybe anybody. It's not me specifically.

T: It's not about you.

P: It's not about me.

T: Who is it about?

P: It's my mom and all of her stuff and Sean who has harassed people in the past, and we know this.

T: And he has his issues.

P: He has …. All of them, yes …. Any.

T: So it's them, not you.

P: Yeah.

In the beginning of our first session, we discussed a significant mechanism where she would assume responsibility for situations that weren't caused by her. This pattern has now been altered. She is now able to attribute the blame appropriately to those who are truly responsible. Importantly, she does not vilify these individuals. Instead, she comprehends in a nuanced manner that their actions stem from their own personal issues.

P: And then also just to …. I guess, catching myself when I start thinking … what do other people think of me, obsessively.

Once more, she mentions a mechanism that we pinpointed and addressed in our initial session: her inclination to ruminate over the opinions of others. She has started to become aware when she engages in this behavior, and then deliberately stops herself.

T: What is it that you and I have done that has helped you?

P: For me, I think … um … being comfortable with being angry at people has really helped. To say, like, that this thing that this person has done … has made me mad. And I don't feel bad for being mad about it. It is …. Whatever it was, was bad.

T: Mm.

P: So …. That actually …. That's the thing that I think about a lot now after I leave is … like … when stuff upsets me, to actually be upset about it.

T: Because what was your …. What was your way of dealing with it, rather than being mad at people?

P: To assume that they were right for doing whatever they've done. And that I deserved whatever it was.

T: Yeah, because that's back to the first thing again. Deserving, that it's your fault. Like, you were deserving these bad things.

P: Right.

T: And if you don't deserve it, then obviously you're angry!

P: I haven't really *done* anything because of being angry. I haven't gotten into arguments or things like that. But I think not …. It's that idea of feeling bad for feeling a bad emotion. I don't do that anymore.

The Girl Who Wasn't a Princess has undeniably made remarkable progress, and the fruits of our joint endeavors are evident. She now possesses a new, experiential understanding of how to handle herself, others, and her feelings. This understanding is cognitive as well, allowing her to remember these insights when faced with new challenges in the future. She has successfully met the restructuring goals outlined at the start of the chapter. She has gained insight into her mechanisms, relies far less on defense mechanisms, and no longer feels anxiety about her feelings. Consequently, her symptoms have also vanished.

Notes

1 In the previous chapter, we observed the Man Who Worried About His Heart making a deliberate effort to curb his laughter in response to feelings. His defensive use of laughter was ego-dystonic, contrasting with ego-syntonic, implying that the defense mechanism was perceived as foreign and erroneous.

2 Regression and regressive defense are traditional psychodynamic concepts that are not within the scope of this book to explain in detail. Regressive defenses encompass depressive and somatizing defenses, as well as defenses that involve impulsive acting-out (Frederickson, 2013). Davanloo (1990) devised the restructuring technique specifically for managing these types of defenses.

3 Diana Fosha (1988) and Patricia Coughlin Della Selva (2004) have also provided insightful perspectives on restructuring, making their works valuable in comprehending this technique.

Chapter 14

How to Do Anxiety Work

Anxiety Is a Signal

While fear is a feeling that arises when we encounter genuine danger in the *external* world, anxiety is a feeling that surfaces when we confront what frightens us *within* ourselves (Frederickson, 2013). Thus, experiencing anxiety serves as a signal (Freud, 1936) that we are nearing internal psychological conflicts that are distressing.

Just as a metal detector begins to beep when nearing a hidden metal object underground, with the beeping intensifying as one draws closer, anxiety similarly signals when you are approaching what is complex within you, with the signal strengthening the closer you come. The aim of psychodynamic therapy is to identify, unearth, and process inner, unconscious conflicts, making the signal of anxiety crucial. Anxiety points the way toward what is significant, complex, and painful. This is demonstrated by Malan's 1979 triangle of conflict, which also forms the basis for understanding symptoms in ISTDP (refer to Chapter 5): due to unresolved, unconscious internal conflicts, feelings evoked by specific situations will lead to anxiety. This anxiety can lead to the symptoms that bring the patient to therapy, such as stomach issues and physical pain. The patient's defense mechanisms, employed to lessen their anxiety, can also result in symptoms. By exploring the nature of the patient's anxiety, its triggers, and how it is managed, a significant part of the task of developing a case formulation is accomplished.

When a patient feels anxious during a therapy session, it is therefore a positive sign. It indicates that they are discussing something complex and challenging, which is crucial for resolving internal conflicts. A patient who is calm isn't confronting the painful issues that brought them to therapy in the first place. This can be a tough truth for many therapists, both new and seasoned, to accept. They hope to create positive experiences for the patient, and it is obviously uncomfortable for the patient when they inquire into painful and difficult matters. The question then arises: Should the conversation continue to focus on this distressing topic that the patient is also trying to evade?

Indeed, this question can be answered affirmatively, but it comes with certain conditions. The first condition is the necessity of a mutual agreement that the set

DOI: 10.4324/9781003516217-18

goal can be reached by addressing these distressing and anxiety-provoking topics. Hence, it is necessary for a working alliance (see Part 2) to have been formed. Without this shared understanding, it would not make sense for the patient to face challenging issues. The second condition is that the patient's anxiety must be at a level they can handle. If the patient is overwhelmed by anxiety, little change will occur. Against expectations, if a change does take place, the anxiety would likely feel so intolerable that the patient might drop out of therapy.

The research summarized by Ecker and colleagues (2013) indicates that enduring change happens only when the patient is emotionally mobilized. If the patient undergoes corrective experiences while their inner conflicts are triggered, a process Ecker refers to as *reconsolidation*, takes place. This implies an *actual change* in the feelings tied to a specific memory, suggesting that the patient does more than just learn *how to cope* with their challenges. Therefore, for the patient to realize substantial transformation through therapy, they must engage with what is painful and complex, and, in this state, encounter a new and corrective experience.

This chapter explores how to discern when a patient is experiencing an optimal level of anxiety for facilitating change, how to foster such a level of anxiety, and how the therapist can intervene when the patient's anxiety escalates beyond a manageable limit.

The Zone of Proximal Development

In ISTDP, the therapist consistently aims to engage with the patient at their highest level of functioning, and to fully utilize the patient's resources (Coughlin Della Selva, 2004). By doing so, the intensity of the therapy increases, leading to a reduction in the duration of the therapy course. Consequently, this also lessens the period of the patient's suffering.

Lev Vygotsky (1978) studied children's learning. He claimed that a clear distinction exists between what children are able to learn on their own and what they can learn when interacting with more capable others. For instance, a three-year-old can comfortably ride a tricycle on their own, but when the time comes to transition to a larger bicycle, they need a certain degree of challenge introduced by someone else. This challenge should be adapted to the child's capabilities, such as presenting a bicycle with training wheels, and must be executed appropriately by the individual who introduces the challenge. Vygotsky referred to this method of appropriately challenging as *scaffolding*. A competent helper constructs a scaffold around the individual who requires assistance, enabling them to develop securely.

Vygotsky referred to the space between what one can learn independently and what one can learn when suitably challenged by more skilled individuals as *the zone of proximal development*. This zone represents a person's *learning potential* at any given moment. The zone is dynamic and evolves with each new learning experience. To maximize learning, it is beneficial to be challenged at the outermost boundary of the zone of proximal development. Of course, the challenge must be realistic. A three-year-old would be at risk of serious injury if asked to ride an adult's racing bike. However, by pushing the boundaries of a person's learning potential, significant learning can take place. An ISTDP therapist aims to challenge the patient at the farthest edge of the development zone, while striving to be a proficient therapist who provides a robust *scaffold* for the patient.

In practical terms, this involves dedicating as much time as possible during a therapy session to addressing situations that generate symptoms. The aim is to work in a manner that prevents the patient from resorting to defense mechanisms that either produce symptoms or impede the therapeutic process. The collaboration should be marked by mutual understanding, a strong alliance, and an empathetic stance from the therapist. By doing so, the patient will end up experiencing complex feelings, leading inevitably to anxiety. This anxiety serves as a signal that you're on the right track. As demonstrated by Ecker et al. (2013), the most substantial change takes place when the patient is activated. Concurrently, the therapist seeks to ensure that the anxiety is manageable, not excessively elevated, and does not obstruct the therapy. If these conditions are met, the patient will operate at the outer edge of the *zone of proximal development*, maximizing the effectiveness of the therapy.

What Is Anxiety?

To help the patient work within the zone of proximal development, the therapist needs to discern when the anxiety is at an optimal level and when it surges excessively. To do this, the therapist needs a thorough understanding of the concept of anxiety as it is used in ISTDP.

In everyday life, we use the term *anxiety* in various ways. Anxiety can refer to a minor discomfort causing little disruption, similar to a teenager feeling "super anxious" about the task of cleaning the toilet. This discomfort, linked to a disliked chore, is referred to as anxiety. On the other hand, a person who has been on disability benefits for two decades and rarely leaves their home might also state that they are grappling with anxiety. We also use different forms of the term anxiety to describe *what* we fear, such as social phobia, fear of spiders, fear of heights, or fear of flying. Moreover, we use the term anxiety when we discuss *thoughts*, such as worrying by repetitively thinking about future events (Borkovec et al., 1983). We talk about anxiety *disorders* like generalized anxiety, panic disorder, and PTSD (WHO, 1992). In existential psychology (Yalom, 1980), existential anxiety is seen as the universal fear that everyone experiences when dealing with life's big questions, such as the meaning of life, the inevitability of death, and our psychological isolation from others. The term anxiety is thus used in a broad range of contexts and ways in daily life.

In contrast, ISTDP offers a distinct definition of anxiety: anxiety is the *physiological* activation that happens in the body when facing *internal* conflicts (Frederickson, 2013). This activation is regulated by the somatic and autonomic nervous systems, the same systems that alert us when we are facing an objectively dangerous situation, known as *fear*. This activation does not depend on conscious awareness and is a system that has been present in our evolution since ancient times (Kardong, 2012). When discussing anxiety in ISTDP, we do not refer to *triggers*, *thoughts*, or *behaviors* that occur at the *same time* as the anxiety.

Given that anxiety is defined as *physiological* reactions deeply rooted in our evolution, it follows that anxiety can be triggered without our conscious knowledge. Thus, anxiety is *unconscious*. We may not always recognize that a stomachache could be a result of anxiety. It requires us to focus our attention on the stomach and comprehend the underlying cause-and-effect relationship to acknowledge that this physical sensation is a sign of anxiety.

In this context, anxiety is defined in a way that allows us to operationalize it as a *signal*. This signal refers specifically to the physiological responses of anxiety that the patient experiences within their body. The therapist pays attention to the *observable* responses and shares these observations with the patient. Furthermore, the therapist encourages the patient to focus on the internal physiological responses of anxiety that are not visible to the therapist. This joint effort aids in making the initially unconscious and physical anxiety conscious. In collaboration, the therapist and patient construct a psychological anxiety detector. This detector signals when the patient is nearing the underlying conflict and indicates whether the level of anxiety is manageable.

In the realm of trauma theory, the process is referred to as determining the patient's window of tolerance (Ogden et al., 2006). The objective is to identify the patient's optimal level of activation, the state where they are most receptive to therapy. Anxiety can take two forms: one where the body enters a state of overactivation or *hyperarousal*, and another where the body goes into a shutdown mode, termed *hypoarousal*. The patient's window of tolerance is situated between these two states. This notion bears a close connection to the understanding of anxiety activation in ISTDP. Refer to Figure 14.1 for more details.

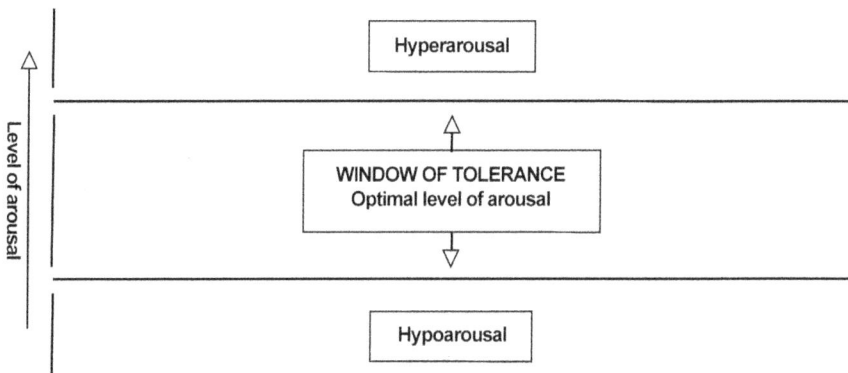

Figure 14.1 Window of Tolerance

Source: Adapted from Nordanger & Braarud (2014) and Ogden et al. (2006).

Channels of Anxiety

By carefully monitoring the patient's anxiety level, the therapist can recognize when the patient's anxiety exceeds their window of tolerance. Habib Davanloo identified three customary categories of anxiety (Frederickson, 2013). Referred to as anxiety channels in Davanloo's terminology, these categories have shown their worth in guiding therapeutic interventions. They provide rules of thumb to determine when the patient is in the zone of proximal development with a manageable level of anxiety, and when they are not. These rules of thumb, developed by Davanloo, are based on the close examination of therapy video recordings and clinical experience. Still, they correspond closely with the physical symptoms that the activation and deactivation of the autonomic nervous system generate (Frederickson, 2013).

The three channels of anxiety, introduced briefly in Chapter 10, were termed by Davanloo as anxiety in *striated muscles*, anxiety in *smooth muscles*, and anxiety manifesting as *cognitive and perceptual disruptions*. A summary of these is provided in Table 14.1, which is largely identical to the table presented in Chapter 10.

The Brain Exerciser

The Brain Exerciser, a forty-year-old physiotherapist, sought therapy due to his prolonged absence from work. He had encountered several instances of severe confusion while treating his patients, which eventually became so pervasive and distressing that it prevented him from performing his job. For many years, he had experienced sporadic mild confusion, which usually subsided when he engaged in brain exercises, such as mentally solving math puzzles. His symptoms severely worsened after a colleague disparagingly discussed a patient who chose to maintain contact with her father, despite being sexually abused by him. As a child, the Brain Exerciser was coerced into performing sexual acts on an older cousin named Gunnar. As an adult, Gunnar played a significant role in the family, complicating their relationship. The Brain Exerciser had kept the abuse a secret until he discovered that his younger brother had been subjected to the same abuse. In an effort to support his younger brother, he disclosed the abuse to his closest relatives.

From the outset of the initial session, it was evident that the patient's disorientation was triggered by recollections of the abuse he had endured, grappling with articulating his thoughts and frequently losing his train of thought. The therapeutic goal, mutually agreed upon by the patient and therapist, was to gradually face the memories of the abuse and the associated feelings, and to learn to manage these feelings without being overwhelmed by them. The anxiety experienced by the Brain Exerciser will serve as illustrations of how Davanloo's three anxiety channels unfold in the therapeutic setting.

Anxiety in Striated Muscles

One potential way anxiety can be channeled, according to Davanloo, is into the *striated muscles*. These muscles, also known as skeletal muscles, are under *conscious*

Table 14.1 Overview of anxiety channels, associated somatic components and complaints, related defense mechanisms, and implications for therapy

Channel of anxiety	Somatic component	Associated complaints	Implications for therapy	Typical defense mechanisms
Striated muscles	Sighing—due to tightening of the intercostal muscles between the ribs. Hand clenching. Tension in large muscle groups such as shoulders, neck, and chest. Tension in the lips, jaw, and scalp. Bodily restlessness.	Pain and discomfort caused by tension in all kinds of voluntary muscles, such as in e.g., shoulders, neck, jaw, abdomen, pelvis (e.g., vaginismus) and scalp.	Regulated by the somatic nervous system which does not affect brain function, cognition, and learning.	Isolation of affect: Defense mechanisms that hinge on efficient cognitive processing. These mechanisms are observable as relatively advanced thought processes, and can be modified or halted upon gaining awareness of them. For example: intellectualization, rationalization, trivialization, detachment, passivity, etc.
Smooth muscles	Nausea. Sickness to the stomach. Dry mouth. Migraine (due to dilation of blood vessels in the brain).	Abdominal pain, nausea, diarrhea—often referred to as irritable bowel syndrome. Migraines. Fatigue, exhaustion. Somatic complaints without a physiological explanation, such as numbness, seizures, etc.	Regulated by the autonomic nervous system and may affect cognition, optimal brain functioning, and learning.	Repression and somatization of psychological difficulties: these are typically less successful than isolation of affect in mitigating discomfort, and they usually result in more significant issues.

(Continued)

Table 14.1 (Continued)

Channel of anxiety	Somatic component	Associated complaints	Implications for therapy	Typical defense mechanisms
Cognitive and perceptual disturbances	Tunnel vision. Blurred vision. Dizziness. Difficulties concentrating. Confusion. Ringing in the ears.	Difficulties with perception and concentration. General and potentially extensive cognitive, relational and work-/study-related challenges.	Regulated by the autonomic nervous system. Anxiety at this level affects cognition, optimal brain function and learning.	Projection and Splitting: Defense mechanisms characterized by their primitive cognition and absence of subtlety. They influence the capacity of reality testing and can to a greater or lesser extent impact daily functioning.

control and are responsible for our skeletal movements. The term *striated* comes from their appearance when viewed under a microscope, where they show a striped or *striated* pattern. The *somatic nervous system* is responsible for controlling these muscles (Betts et al., 2022).

Davanloo noted that patients experiencing anxiety often display specific behaviors. They may fiddle with their thumbs and fingers, show restlessness in their arms, move uncomfortably in their seats, and feel tension in their chest, shoulders, neck, and even scalp. These behaviors are all controlled by voluntary muscles, muscles we can consciously control if we choose to. A prominent indicator of anxiety being channeled into striated muscles is when the patient sighs. This sighing occurs because the intercostal muscles (Betts et al., 2022), the muscles between the ribs, contract. To alleviate this constriction, we automatically and unconsciously take a deep breath and sigh. The activation of this anxiety channel can often be visually observed. Signs such as sighing, fiddling with the thumbs, and bodily restlessness suggest that anxiety is being channeled into the striated muscles.

Through extensive video analysis over the years, Davanloo found that patients who were activated in this manner were engaging in discussions about psychologically significant topics that also induced anxiety. These patients appeared to derive benefit from therapy. Davanloo concluded that as long as the patient exhibited symptoms of anxiety channeled into striated muscles, it was safe to delve deeper into the explored topics, and progress in therapy could be anticipated. In the realm of trauma theory, this would be interpreted as the patient being within the window of tolerance (Ogden et al., 2006). From Vygotsky's (1978) perspective, the patient is in the zone of proximal development. The activation of anxiety in striated muscles is a positive sign for the therapeutic process, providing a green light to continue focusing on the current topic.

Davanloo's understanding is grounded in clinical observations and *experiential* knowledge. However, his observations can also be explained from a neurological standpoint. As noted earlier, the somatic nervous system controls the striated muscles. This nervous system *exclusively* controls this muscle type and lacks mechanisms to impact cognitive or emotional processes. When a patient exhibits anxiety, manifested through the activation of voluntary muscles, there's no evidence of mechanisms at work that could influence cognition.

Patients who channel their anxiety into striated muscles often employ defense mechanisms rooted in sophisticated cognitive functions. They intellectualize, rationalize, distract, and trivialize to avoid facing uncomfortable feelings. These defense mechanisms are controlled by the cortex, specifically our brain's frontal lobe (Abbass, 2015). In psychodynamic therapy, the outcome of using such defenses is termed *isolation of affect* (Kuhn, 2014). This means that while feelings are available for conscious examination, defense mechanisms establish an "insulating gap" between the cognitive and somatic aspects of the feeling. As long as these defenses maintain this separation, the feelings remain cognitively *isolated* from the somatic experience of the feeling. When a therapist observes this type of defense mechanism, it signals that the patient's cognition is functioning effectively, and learning can take place.

The Brain Exerciser

The Brain Exerciser sought therapy as his confusion intensified, triggered by the similarities between the abuse he endured and that suffered by a patient at his workplace. This comparison stirred up difficult feelings and anxiety within him. At this juncture in the session, the discussion revolves around the distinction between experiencing abuse from a father versus a cousin. The patient maintains an upright posture in the chair, meets my gaze directly, and articulates his thoughts with clarity.

P: But the father is an adult, and ... and more of a carer than a cousin is. And Gunnar *[the cousin]* was much younger, you see?
T: How old was Gunnar?
P: He was 16, I think ... 15–16, and I was about 8–9 years old then. But when it happened to Hans *[the younger brother]*, he was an adult. Or a young adult. I guess he was ... 26, I think. So he was an adult then.
T: So, he groped Hans, your little brother, and he was 26 years old.
P: Yes...
T: He was 16 years old, a youth, and he made an 8–9-year-old boy perform sexual acts on him.
P: *SIGHS* Yes ... but....

At this point in our conversation, the Brain Exerciser's anxiety is channeled into his striated muscles. He sits up straight in his chair, expressing his thoughts with clarity, and *sighs* when I recap the actions of his cousin. Both his posture and sighs indicate the activation of his voluntarily controlled muscles. Moreover, he demonstrates clear thinking and *intellectualization:* By *reflecting and discussing* how the abuse he endured was less severe than that experienced by another, he distances himself from his own experiences. Consequently, he employs defense mechanisms that necessitate sound and relatively intricate cognition. These kinds of defense mechanisms correlate with anxiety channeled into striated muscles (refer to Table 14.1). There are no indications that his anxiety levels are excessively high or that his learning is adversely impacted at this juncture. We can confidently proceed with our agreed exploration of his negative experiences.

P: Yes, I completely agree with you. However, I still feel that it is more serious when the father is involved.
T: Yes, definitely. I agree.
P: Yeah. Okay....
T: It is perhaps a bigger betrayal.
P: Yes, I think so.
T: At the same time .... The woman with her father ... was a patient of yours, where you were in a professional role. Your cousin is your cousin! And the boy was you! The question here is actually about what is stirred up inside of you when you, somehow, face this trigger ....

P: *LOOKS AT ME* *FIDDLES WITH SOME PAPER*
T: ... the reminder of the complexity of having been a victim of abuse.

The Brain Exerciser meets my gaze, fiddling with his fingers. He is capable of clear thought and can engage in a discussion with me about the parallels and distinctions between the instances of abuse. He establishes a strong connection, and the voluntary controlled striated muscles allow his fingers to discharge his unease and anxiety. The signs suggest that his anxiety continues to be channeled into his striated muscles, providing me with a green light to delve deeper into our exploration.

P: It's really strange *SIGHS* ... because I also believe that we, as a family, should have talked about it.
T: Mm.
P: But we never did. I never did, directly. *LOOKS DOWN*.
T: No, you kept it within you.
P: I sort of talked about it, because I told ... *MAKES GESTURES*... first my uncle, and then he informed my parents.
T: Did that happen a long time after?
P: No, it was, like, the next day. He told my dad, and then we had a conversation...*ACTIVELY MOVES HANDS, FIDDLES, SPEAKS IN A STRONG AND CLEAR VOICE*
T: But this was when Hans was also abused [*several years later*]?
P: Yes, it was during that time. I hadn't told anyone before that.
T: So you've kept it to yourself for a long, long time ....
P: *TEARS UP* Yes, I've kept it to myself for a very long time. And I was really conflicted ... about what I should do ....

The Brain Exerciser is able to articulate the conflict between validating his own feelings and defending his cousin with clarity. He communicates in coherent sentences, shows no signs of confusion (which is the symptom he is seeking help for), and exhibits physical signs of anxiety such as sighing, moving, and fidgeting. His voice is clear and distinct, and his defense mechanisms involve *thinking* about what happened. All of these observations indicate that his *anxiety is being channeled into his striated muscles*. As long as the anxiety remains within this system, it is reasonable to anticipate that learning can occur. He is within his zone of proximal development and his window of tolerance as he discusses the pain of concealing the abuse.

Anxiety Channeled into Smooth Muscles

Davanloo's second channel of anxiety is the discharge of anxiety into smooth muscles. These are muscles that cannot be consciously controlled, and they work automatically. They are found in various parts of the body, such as the digestive system (including the bladder and intestines), the respiratory tract, the heart, the muscles surrounding blood vessels, the internal genital organs, and the eye. These muscles have the ability to cause their organs to either open or contract. As a result, they can create urges related to the bladder and bowels, regulate the blood supply received by different organs by affecting the blood vessels, and affect the experience of breathing by impacting the airways. These muscles are referred to as *smooth* due to the absence of stripes found on striated muscles, giving them a smooth appearance when viewed under a microscope. These muscles are controlled by the autonomic nervous system, which is responsible for controlling automatic and unconscious bodily processes (Betts et al., 2022).

The contraction or relaxation of smooth muscles can lead to a range of somatic sensations. For instance, activity in the smooth muscles of the guts can cause diarrhea or constipation, frequent urination, nausea, and acid reflux. Constriction or dilation of blood vessels can cause sensations like cold hands and feet or a flushed face or neck. Rapid expansion of blood vessels in the brain can trigger symptoms of a migraine. Given that the heart is a smooth muscle, changes in heart rate can be triggered through this channel of anxiety.

When anxiety is channeled into this system and remains at a high level for a long time, it can lead to significant physical health issues. The individual might suffer from gastrointestinal disturbances, including chronic diarrhea and irritable bowel syndrome. It can also trigger migraines. It is common for individuals to go through numerous physical examinations to account for these symptoms, often turning to psychotherapy as a final attempt to comprehend and address their health concerns.

Davanloo's (1990) studies on patients showing symptoms linked to smooth muscle activation revealed that their physical complaints could possibly worsen if the therapist failed to demonstrate specific care, such as being thorough during the restructuring process (see Chapter 13). Their potential to benefit from the therapy was entirely dependent on extensive restructuring.

Smooth muscles are controlled by the autonomic nervous system, including the sympathetic and parasympathetic systems (Betts et al., 2022). The primary function of these systems is to regulate the body's arousal levels. *Hyperarousal* occurs from to high arousal, while *hypoarousal* results from too low arousal, as detailed by Ogden et al. (2006). This nervous system *may* influence blood pressure and the blood flow to the brain, which can subsequently affect the functionality of the cortex. If symptoms of anxiety channeled into smooth muscle are observed, this could potentially indicate that cognitive processing, which is vital for successful psychotherapy, is impaired. Spotting this type of anxiety during therapy acts as a yellow traffic light. As a therapist, it is essential to remain vigilant, ensuring that the patient doesn't experience potentially severe physical symptoms, and that their cognitive abilities stay intact.

When patients experience anxiety that is channeled into smooth muscles, the defense mechanisms they employ often differ from those used when anxiety is channeled into striated muscles. They mainly turn to *repression* (Abbass, 2015), which results from mental processes that prevent feelings from reaching consciousness. A patient with anxiety channeled into striated muscles who isolates affect will come across as intellectual and argumentative. They can comprehend their feelings intellectually, but they have "isolated" themselves from the actual experience. When repression dominates, intellectual understanding is absent. Instead, other phenomena may be observed: the patient might start to cry in a depressive manner, feel fatigued and lack energy, or experience physical discomfort and pain. Feelings and impulses are pushed away before they reach conscious awareness. The depressive symptoms, along with the corresponding energy deficiency, prevent the physical activation of various feelings. In this state, brain activation is less concentrated on the frontal lobe, leading to a potential decrease in the patient's reflexive abilities.

The Brain Exerciser

The Brain Exerciser reveals that he kept the abuse secret for many years. Given my understanding that he often finds himself overwhelmed by feelings, leading to confusion and difficulty in clear thinking, I encourage him to reflect on his decision to bear the burden of such a challenging experience alone. Understanding and thinking serve as tools to regulate anxiety.

T: May I ask why you kept it to yourself?
P: Because he told me to do so.
T: He told you.
P: That's what he said.
T: What exactly did he say?
P: *SIGHS* He said that it was something we should keep just between us. That it was a secret.

Discussing his cousin's call for secrecy stirs up something within him. As I observe his sigh, I deduce that he's feeling anxious. At this moment, the anxiety is being channeled into his striated muscles, prompting me to delve further into the subject.

T: How was it for you to keep secrets with your cousin?
P: That particularly might have been a bit like …. The fact that he wanted us to keep it a secret …. *BITES HIS LIP* *LOOKS AWAY* *SPEAKS SLOWER* It was perhaps … paradoxically … I felt that it gave us a kind of … or like it was a bit like …

The physical demeanor of the Brain Exerciser starts to change. He averts his gaze, his speech slows down, and his sentences become less coherent and more fragmented. This prompts me to be particularly observant. Could this be an indication that the anxiety is transitioning into another channel? He seems less engaged, and his manner of speaking might suggest muddled thoughts. A decrease in muscle tone suggests that the somatic nervous system is not as activated as before, and that the autonomic nervous system is assuming control. I persist in my exploration, all the while closely monitoring his condition.

T: That you shared something special?
P: Yes, in a way.
T: So, was it somewhat nice?
P: Yes, that specific aspect, perhaps.
T: The fact that you had this unique relationship, that you did these things together, was that nice?
P: No, it was very uncomfortable. Yeah. *A FACIAL EXPRESSION OF DISCOMFORT*
T: Okay. So, it was uncomfortable all the time.
P: Yes, I experienced it as very uncomfortable all the time. *FROWNING* *TOUCHES HIS NECK*

The Brain Exerciser's unease seems to be intensifying. His face bears a troubled expression, and he is holding onto his neck. He has stopped sighing and sits more passively in the chair. Several indications imply that the anxiety is no longer being channeled into his striated muscles. It's now essential to explore the degree of his anxiety.

T: How does it feel for you to talk about this right now?
P: It's very .... I've never done it before. I'm feeling a bit nauseous now.
T: A bit nauseous? So, you're becoming quite anxious now, aren't you?
P: Yes ....

The Brain Exerciser starts to feel nauseous; a sign of anxiety being channeled into the smooth muscles. Upon being questioned whether he feels anxious, he answers affirmatively.[1] His appearance becomes limp, the speed of his speech decreases, and his sentences shorten, leading me to a relative certainty: the anxiety has shifted from the striated muscles to the smooth muscles. This serves as a yellow traffic light for further investigation and necessitates vigilant monitoring of the patient's responses.

Anxiety Causing Cognitive and Perceptual Disturbances

Davanloo identified a third channel of anxiety that manifests as *cognitive and perceptual disruptions*. Patients whose anxiety is channeled in this manner undergo changes in their vision, such as blurred or tunnel vision, and hearing, experiencing ringing in their ears. They may also feel dizzy, have trouble focusing, and struggle to articulate their thoughts. Frequently, they report a loss of muscle tone and a sense of weakness. In this anxious state, patients gain little benefit from therapy and find it challenging to comprehend the therapeutic process they are undergoing. A common characteristic of these patients is their struggle to distinguish between anxiety and fear when they become highly anxious. Instead of associating their anxiety with fear of internal feelings and phenomena, they perceive themselves to be in a situation that is objectively dangerous. In other words, they develop para-noia and *project* the source of their fear from their inner psychological world to the external environment (Abbass, 2015). In such a state, the patient may start to fear the therapist and perceive them as a genuine threat. This is an indication that the patient requires immediate assistance to regulate their anxiety.

Patients who suffer from high levels of anxiety and experience *chronic* anxiety in this system are likely to face significant challenges. They may struggle to comprehend their surroundings, or may react in an irrational and paranoid manner, and often find it difficult to function effectively in educational, occupational, and relational contexts. Such individuals are frequently categorized as having problems on the *fragile spectrum* (Frederickson, 2020) and are often diagnosed with personality disorders (WHO, 1992).

Certain patients may encounter this form of anxiety channeling in a more epi-sodic manner, associated with particularly complex emotional triggers. This is not indicative of fragility or personality disorders. Instead, it signifies that the patient is grappling with an especially challenging psychological issue that requires assis-tance for regulation. Such is the case with the Brain Exerciser.

The autonomic nervous system is responsible for cognitive and perceptual dis-ruptions, with the parasympathetic system playing a particularly pivotal role. This system not only regulates alertness but also controls the reduction of heart rate and blood pressure. A decrease in blood flow to the cortex, especially the frontal lobe, will result in the patient experiencing changes in perception and a decline in the functioning of advanced cognitive abilities. As the level of alertness and bodily activation decreases, there is a corresponding decrease in the activation of the somatic nervous system, leading to reduced activation in the striated muscles. This transition moves the individual from an active and responsive state to a state characterized by altered consciousness. In extreme cases, this altered state could culminate in sleep or loss of consciousness.

Patients who experience anxiety in the form of cognitive and perceptual distur-bances typically employ defense mechanisms stemming from a decrease in cortex activation. This is reflected in their decreased cognitive subtlety, as seen through *projection*. This means that patients attribute the source of their anxiety to exter-nal factors, projecting it out into the world. These patients perceive the world and people around them as threats. They fail to realize that their anxiety stems from their inner life, which makes them appear paranoid as they project the cause of their anxiety onto external elements. Another common defense mechanism in this state of anxiety is *splitting*, viewing the world without nuance, and categorizing things in a binary or black-and-white manner (Abbass, 2015). This defense mechanism complicates social relationships significantly, as patients tend to categorize others as either good or bad, resulting in inflexibility in their relationships.

The Brain Exerciser

The Brain Exerciser began to articulate his thoughts in a slower, more fragmented manner. He also reported sensations of nausea, a symptom associated with smooth

muscle anxiety. Knowing his tendency to become disoriented when discussing difficult experiences, I wondered whether he was experiencing other anxiety symptoms.

T: Are there other things you notice as we discuss this? Just to ensure that you're
       able to follow along…
P: *SPEAKS SLOWLY, WITH A HESITANT VOICE* *DRIES TEARS* It feels
       like things are happening somewhat slowly…
T: Mm, so now things are happening somewhat slowly. *SPEAKS IN A GENTLE
       VOICE* Any changes in your head, your vision, or your hearing?
P: Yes. *NODS*
T: Mm, what are you noticing?
P: *CRYING* I need to concentrate intensely to speak.
T: Right. Right … Mm … Any changes in your vision as well? Tunnel vision, or
       is your vision becoming a bit blurry?
P: Yes, perhaps a little.
T: Clogged ears or ringing in the ears?
P: There is a slightly clogged sensation, maybe, yes.

The Brain Exerciser both describes and confirms the typical symptoms of anxiety when it presents as *cognitive and perceptual disturbances* (refer to Table 14.1).
He struggles with cognition, vision, and hearing. Discussing that the abuse he endured was very uncomfortable for him, triggers a level of anxiety so intense that
it impairs his ability to think clearly. In such a state, the potential for learning is
significantly diminished, as the patient is beyond their window of tolerance and
no longer in the optimal zone of development If I persist in probing the abuse
while the Brain Exerciser is in this state, he will, at best, have no recollection of
the session. At worst, he will have a highly negative experience, exhibit symptomatic deterioration, and subsequently drop out of therapy. In this state, the patient's
defense mechanisms, such as *projection*, come into play, triggering potential para-
noia and the conviction that the therapist *genuinely* bears ill will toward them. The
patient needs help to manage their anxiety and transition out of this state. Patients
for whom this is the main channel of anxiety will require substantial assistance
and meticulous regulation in partnership with the therapist. The Brain Exerciser
primarily experienced this type of anxiety in response to triggers associated with
abuse, and was able, with support, to regulate the anxiety relatively quickly. The
principles of anxiety regulation are consistent across both types of patients, and
these principles will be discussed in the following section.

How to Regulate Anxiety When It Is Too High

When a patient's anxiety escalates excessively, similar to the Brain Exerciser's
case, the therapist aims to help the patient regulate and reduce this anxiety. The
patient has to return to their proximal zone of development and stay within their
window of tolerance. If the patient's anxiety is channeled into smooth muscles, or

if it manifests as cognitive and perceptual disruptions, the therapist needs to help them to reroute the anxiety back into the striated muscle. The goal is not to *remove* the patient's anxiety entirely, but to bring it down to a level where learning and change can occur.

During a therapy session, when a patient becomes overwhelmingly anxious, and they do not have the necessary skills to regulate it, it becomes the therapist's duty to intervene. However, it is important to bear in mind that being able to regulate anxiety is a skill the patient must learn for handling anxiety outside of the therapy sessions as well. Therefore, the therapist must always be mindful that this process should be done *in cooperation* with the patient, rather than carried out by the therapist *for* the patient.

In ISTDP, a key technique is the *response to intervention* (Coughlin Della Selva, 2004). This refers to the therapist's moment-to-moment tracking of the patient's reactions to therapeutic interventions. This becomes particularly crucial for patients struggling with high anxiety levels. The aim is to engage the patient within their zone of proximal development to effectively facilitate change. The patient is challenged to operate at the boundaries of this zone, enabling its expansion and enhancing their capacity to manage feelings when they are triggered next. Simultaneously, it is important to help the patient stay within their window of tolerance. This is because learning is limited when they are outside this window, and the process can turn into a distressing experience. Therefore, the therapist continually assesses the patient's responses to interventions, enabling the application of the anxiety regulation principles that will be discussed subsequently.[2]

1. Pause the Exploration!

When the therapist suspects that a patient's anxiety is escalating beyond a manageable level, the immediate response is to pause whatever is being done in therapy session. The onset of anxiety in a patient is a clear sign that the current proceedings are triggering these feelings. To avoid exacerbating the anxiety, the therapist promptly stops the therapeutic process at hand. Simultaneously, they mentally register the topic of discussion that coincided with the anxiety spike, as it offers valuable insight into what triggers the patient's anxiety. Following this, the therapist assists the patient in regulating their anxiety using the principles below. Once the anxiety is back within the window of tolerance, they can revisit the topic that initially caused the heightened anxiety. Alternatively, the therapist might propose shifting to a less complex subject, if deemed suitable.

2. Assist the Patient in Observing Their Anxiety

Once the exploration is put on hold, the patient's focus is directed toward the feelings of anxiety they are experiencing during the session. It seems paradoxical to many therapists that they should make the patient aware of their anxiety when the goal is to regulate it downward. Some therapists, especially those trained in the cognitive tradition, have the notion that concentrating on the symptoms might exacerbate the anxiety, leading to conditions like panic disorder. It is indeed true that catastrophic thoughts, such as, "Oh no, I'm having a heart attack," in response to anxiety symptoms, can escalate the anxiety. However, a neutral, observant, and reflective approach will not intensify the anxiety. The aim is to make the patient become *consciously aware* that they are experiencing anxiety and that they can observe and reflect on this feeling. Many fail to comprehend that what they are feeling is anxiety, and don't take the experience seriously. Until they understand and acknowledge their anxiety, they cannot regulate it effectively (Frederickson, 2020).

Moreover, the mere act of observing one's anxiety has a direct regulatory impact. Anxiety in the smooth muscle and anxiety manifesting as cognitive and perceptual disturbances are controlled by a nervous system that decreases activation in the cortex, favoring underlying brain structures. Therefore, the goal is to actively "drive" the activation and blood flow back to the cortex. The process of observing and reflecting is a complex cognitive task. It requires an active shift of focus toward a specific aspect, articulating what is being observed, and classifying the observation. Assisting the patient in this process will activate the cortex. As a result, the patient transitions from a state dominated by feelings of activation to a state in which there is more space for thought. This is a fundamental concept in the regulation of anxiety.

For we humans, few things are as daunting as the unknown. The Man Who Worried About His Heart—the case discussed in Chapter 12—failed to comprehend that his physical symptoms were indicators of anxiety about feelings. He was not consciously aware of his feeling of anxiety, didn't understand its origin, and interpreted its physical manifestations as signs of a medical condition. Consequently, the Man Who Worried About His Heart was filled with fear. However, if a therapist assists the patient in self-observation and understanding their inner world, complex feelings become less intimidating.

3. Assist the Patient in Understanding What Led to Anxiety

The subsequent stage in regulating anxiety involves assisting the patient in comprehending the events that led to the escalation of their anxiety. Given that the patient's anxiety surfaced during the session, there must have been a trigger. The therapist and patient collaborate to decipher this trigger. The foundation for this exploration is Malan's triangle of conflict, and the therapist's goal is to help the patient become acquainted with each corner of the triangle. The therapist might say, for instance, "Do you notice that as we discuss the abuse you endured *[the situation]*, something is triggered within you *[feelings/impulses]*, making you intensely anxious, manifesting as nausea *[anxiety]*? Can you see this?" This dialogue facilitates the patient's recognition of how these elements are connected.

Assisting the patient in understanding what led to their anxiety is akin to the restructuring process discussed in Chapter 13. A deeper comprehension of one's own mechanisms will elevate the threshold for anxiety activation. If this process is repeated, and the exposure to feelings is gradually amplified, the patient's ability to tolerate these feelings will improve. This process is referred to as the *graded format* of ISTDP (Whittemore, 1996).[3] The therapist aims to challenge the patient at the edge of the zone of proximal development, allowing for the zone to gradually expand. It is vital for the therapist to be viewed as a safe figure and for a robust therapeutic alliance to be formed. This ensures that the patient can securely work in the outer limits of the zone of development, aided by the therapist's *scaffolding* (Vygotsky, 1978).

While the aim is to prevent anxiety from escalating beyond the activation in the striated muscles, there will inevitably be instances where this occurs. In such cases, the goal is to aid the patient in understanding the situation through intellectualization. Despite being a defense mechanism, intellectualization is beneficial in this context as it assists patients with high anxiety levels to calm down. In simple terms, by engaging cognition, one stimulates the prefrontal cortex and decreases the activation in brain structures like the amygdala, which manage anxiety. Once the anxiety is redirected back into the striated muscles, the exploration process can resume. The next steps involve acquainting the patient with their defense mechanisms (as discussed in Chapter 12), enabling them to experience their feelings (Chapter 15).

As the patient is encouraged to observe and comprehend their anxiety, careful attention is given to indications that the patient's anxiety is being redirected back into the striated muscles. For some patients, like the Brain Exerciser, this process happens rather swiftly. However, for others with more severe issues, an entire session might be dedicated to assisting the patient to return to a level of anxiety that allows for change to occur.

4. Continue Exploration or Change Corner on the Triangle of Person

When the patient once again exhibits signs of anxiety channeled into the striated muscles through actions like sighing, fidgeting, or restless movement, and demonstrates clear thinking, it is possible to resume exploring the patient's conflicts. If the anxiety has been relatively simple to regulate, you can pick up from where the discussion was paused. However, if regulating the anxiety proved more challenging, and the initial topic seemed to provoke too much anxiety, you can request examples of similar challenges. Frequently, these will involve situations with a person who holds less significance for the patient, or you can examine the same issue if it arises with the therapist. In this kind of work, it is advisable to alternate between different episodes at the C and T corners of the triangle of person. Such transitions gradually enhance the patient's capacity to fully experience their feelings.

A Robust Alliance Is Inherently Anxiety-Regulating

Let's not forget the significance of trust in another person as a means of managing anxiety. The investment of sufficient resources in forging an alliance (refer to Part 2), coupled with a shared comprehension of the goals and therapeutic tasks, as well as a strong bond, all contribute to anxiety regulation. Once the patient grasps the therapist's actions and their reasons, this elevates the threshold for triggering anxiety. A sturdy conscious alliance not only regulates anxiety but also enhances the patient's capacity to undertake challenging tasks in therapy.

The Brain Exerciser

How does this form of anxiety regulation manifest in a therapeutic setting? The Brain Exerciser once more serves as our guide. To provide a comprehensive view, let's revisit portions of the dialogue previously used to depict the different anxiety channels.

In the course of the session, he talks about how the abuse was kept as a mutual secret between him and his cousin. The act of sharing a secret had a certain appeal, yet it was the lone positive element among the circumstances.

P: Yes, I experienced that as very uncomfortable all the time. *FROWNING* *TOUCHES HIS NECK*
T: How does it feel for you to talk about this right now?

Discussing the discomfort he experienced from *past* abuse triggers uncomfortable feelings in the *present*. His physical demeanor alters, his face contorts in agony, and he clutches his neck. I choose to halt the exploration (1) and then encourage him to observe and articulate his anxiety symptoms (2). I bear in mind the symptoms characteristic of the three anxiety channels (Table 14.1) during my examination.

P: It's very …. I've never done it before. I'm feeling a bit nauseous now.
T: A bit nauseous? So, you're becoming quite anxious now, aren't you?
P: Yes … uh …. *TEARS UP* *LOOKS AWAY*
T: Are there other things you notice as we discuss this? Just to ensure that you're able to follow along ….
P: *SPEAKS SLOWLY, WITH A HESITANT VOICE* *DRIES TEARS* It feels like things are happening somewhat slowly ….
T: Mm, so now things are happening somewhat slowly. *SPEAKS IN A GENTLE VOICE* Any changes in your head, your vision, or your hearing?
P: Yes. *NODS*
T: Mm, what are you noticing?
P: *ALMOST CRYING* I need to concentrate intensely to speak.
T: Right. Right …. Mm …. Any changes in your vision as well? Tunnel vision, or is your vision becoming a bit blurry?
P: *SIGHING SOFTLY* Yes, perhaps a little. *FIDGETING WITH A KLEENEX*

As the Brain Exerciser articulates and confirms his symptoms, he remains still in his seat. The earlier energy and gestures that were evident during the session have subsided. However, upon observing his anxiety symptoms, he starts to exhibit signs of anxiety reverting to the striated muscles. He lets out a soft sigh and begins to fidget with the Kleenex he is holding. These are the initial indications that his anxiety is starting to abate and shift back to striated muscles.

T: Clogged ears or ringing in the ears?
P: There is a slightly clogged sensation, maybe, yes.
T: How would you label the feeling we're discussing now? What term would you assign to it?
P: Is it anxiety?
T: I would refer to this as anxiety, yes, I would. Does that resonate with you?
P: Yes.
T: Speaking about what your cousin did to you, which was quite distressing at the time....
P: *SIGHS DEEPLY*
T: ... and which comes to mind when you discuss your patient... Yet, it was also a pleasant experience for the young boy to share such a significant secret with his cousin.
P: *SIGHS* *LOOKS DOWN* *WIPES AWAY TEARS*

His sighs grow deeper, and he wipes away his tears. As I recap and encourage him to reflect on his present experience, his anxiety diminishes. Articulating that this is anxiety helps him understand better. I closely monitor his body language, noticing that our actions are alleviating his anxiety. If signs of striated anxiety are still absent at this point, it is necessary to pause and explain things in a more straightforward and serene manner.

T: And we observe that you get really anxious when we discuss it. You start to feel nauseous, it becomes difficult to think clearly.
P: *MUMBLING* It does.
T: Your vision alters slightly ....
P: *SIGHS* *LOOKS DOWN*
T: Mmm .... It appears that a lot of feelings are surfacing within you.
P: Yes!
T: Lots of conflicting feelings. And we notice ... both, this positive bond with your cousin, you mention the significance of preserving a relationship with ... um ... your family.
P: *LOOKS UP* Yes!
T: The intricate facets of this, it's not that simple.
P: *MOVES UPPER BODY* *DISPOSES OF THE KLEENEX IN THE TRASH* Yes!
T: When someone turns this into black and white, when a colleague views it in black and white and is unaware of its complexity for you.
P: Yes. *SIGHS*

T: And you become highly anxious as we inquire into this. Was that how you felt *back then*? Did you get nauseous *back then*?

P: Yes, I did feel somewhat nauseous at times.

T: So now, you're having a somewhat similar experience here, and I presume you're having flashes of mental images or memories or something of that sort?

P: *LOOKS AT ME* Yes. Yes, I am.

T: And they make you nauseous and anxious.

P: Yes. Yes. *SIGHS* *LOOKS RESOLUTE* *LOOKS UP*

T: Does it make sense to you why you're feeling anxious? Can you understand that?

P: Yes.

T: Right. Can you acknowledge that you find it complicated, and how your colleague's remark was complicated, considering your history?

P: Yes. Yes .... *SIGHS DEEPLY*

The Brain Exerciser has let out several sighs; his voice now carries a distinct energy, and his body movements have returned. The anxiety has returned to the striated muscles after numerous cycles of observation, intellectualization, and therapist's summaries. In the passage at the beginning of this chapter, he was actively moving, making eye contact with me, using his hands to gesture, and speaking in a clear and distinct voice. This was in sharp contrast to his demeanor when he expressed feeling nauseous and having difficulty speaking. At that moment, he was completely still, appeared limp and distressed, and the vigor and engagement in his voice had vanished. In the above excerpt, the vigor and engagement gradually reappear, in tandem with the recurrence of the sighs. This method of interpreting body language offers a chance to assist our patients in understanding what triggers their anxiety, how it is experienced, and learning how it can be regulated.

T: Are you aware of any feelings within you, right now? Apart from anxiety? Like, underneath the anxiety?

P: *LOOKS UP*

T: As we discuss this, and you somehow come back .... It looks like your nausea is lessening slightly.

P: Yes, I'm feeling better now. Mmm.

T: *SPEAKING IN A SOFT TONE* Are you aware of any feelings now, as your anxiety eases a little?

P: I might be feeling somewhat relieved now.

T: Relieved about what?

P: Having expressed it, perhaps. Mm. *NODS*

T: Does it feel good to articulate it?

P: Yes, in a sense. But it's also a little uncomfortable.

Even though his anxiety has reached an uncomfortable peak, surpassing his window of tolerance, he finds himself feeling relieved. He has succeeded in discussing something previously unspoken, and has effectively managed his anxiety. This is perceived as a significant advancement for him. However, the process is not yet complete. Enhancing the ability to withstand memories and feelings associated with abuse is commonly a gradual process. In this kind of therapeutic work, multiple cycles are undertaken, each with varying examples of what triggers the patient's symptoms. As a therapist, you reiterate the four steps outlined in the chapter: pausing the exploration, inviting to observe, inviting to understand, followed by either switching examples or resuming the exploration from where it was left off.

P: I really regretted it when it happened to Hans.[4] I still do.

T: Please elaborate ....

P: *SIGHS* Well, I think ... or ... I feel .... It's happening again, I'm feeling somewhat anxious.

T: Okay. It's great that you're aware of it! How are you experiencing your anxiety, right now?

P: It's somewhat similar, I kind of feel like ....

T: Does it feel like it's rising to your head in some way?

P: No, more like my heart is rising to my throat.

T: Okay, right. So, anxiety, but not as intensely as before?

P: Yeah.

T: Mm, it's good that you're noticing this.

P: Yeah.

T: So, what feelings are triggering your anxiety, right now? When we addressed this regret .... I don't know, were there any images that surfaced? What came to mind when you mentioned your regret?

P: Right now, it was when I was talking to Hans.

T: Tell me, what did you visualize?

As he is opening up and sharing the distress of the abuse he endured, it revives the memories of the moment he discovered that his younger brother had also become a victim of their cousin's abuse. Once again, this triggers anxiety within him, which he now recognizes and understands. His anxiety does not manifest as noticeable signs in his smooth muscle or as cognitive and perceptual disruptions, allowing me to proceed with the exploration. He then recounts the incident of discovering his brother in bed with their cousin.

T: Did it dawn on you back then?

P: No. *APPEARS CALM* *FIDDLES WITH THE KLEENEX* *LOOKS AT ME* *SPEAKS IN A NORMAL TONE* That thought didn't cross my mind.

P: *SUDDENLY STARES STRAIGHT AHEAD* *CEASES FIDGETING* *LOOKS SCARED*

T: So, what kind of feelings got triggered when you recalled the memory of finding Gunnar in Hans's bed? That made you anxious, right now?

As is evident from the transcript, there's a sudden shift in his body language. I fail to notice it, and thus continue to inquire about his feelings. However, having been through this scenario several times, the Brain Exerciser takes the initiative to halt the exploration. He notices his anxiety without needing my reminder. He begins to assimilate the concepts we've been working on and starts regulating his anxiety on his own.

P: *SPEAKING IN A SOMEWHAT MONOTONE VOICE* I'm feeling a bit nauseous again, perhaps ….

T: Are you experiencing some nausea again?

P: Yes.

T: Mm.

T: Great that you notice it!

P: *SMILES* Mm! *NODS*

I acknowledge his success in accomplishing this task and applaud him for his efforts. Following this, I encourage him to explore why his anxiety peaked, which is the third step of anxiety regulation.

T: So, there is something here, as we are discussing this and you are allowing these memories to surface.

P: Yeah ….

T: So, it's clear that it triggers something within you that makes you anxious, wouldn't you agree?

P: Yes.

T: And, like … initially, there were palpitations ….

P: Yes.

T: Right. And then it escalates a little more ….

P: Yes. *NODS*

T: … as I probe further into these feelings.

P: *RENEWED POWER IN HIS VOICE* But it's different now, it's much less intense.

T: Right. What is much less intense?

P: The feelings aren't as strong. Last time, I was caught off guard.

The Brain Exerciser listens attentively to me, and appears to agree. He then shares a crucial observation: the anxiety is less intense than it was in the previous instance. His ability to observe and contrast situations implies that he can reflect on and intellectualize his anxiety more profoundly. The theory suggests that this should help reduce the anxiety. He affirms this and mentions that the feelings are not as strong, because he has understood and is therefore ready. This time, he wasn't caught off guard.

As the Brain Exerciser's therapy progressed, we worked through numerous cycles of variations on the themes discussed in this chapter. Our efforts focused on remembering, discussing, and experiencing feelings associated with the abuse. Memories of trying to bring up the abuse with his family and subsequently feeling dismissed also triggered a range of complex feelings that needed to be worked through. An additional crucial concern was his struggle to cope with these memories in a profession where he might come across patients who had also suffered abuse. Eventually, he was able to observe his anxiety and comprehend its triggers. Over time, he was able to discuss his experiences in detail and endure the feelings this triggered without feeling nauseous or dizzy. He had intense feelings toward the perpetrator, as well as feelings of guilt associated with the fact that Hans had also been abused. Managing feelings toward family members who attempted to trivialize and dismiss the abuse was also crucial. By the conclusion of the therapy, he had returned to work. He no longer felt anxious or ashamed when confronted with the memories, but was able to withstand the feelings they elicited.

Notes

1 Experiencing nausea when recalling memories of sexual abuse could also indicate feelings of disgust, rather than anxiety. It is plausible that the Brain Exerciser might also be feeling disgust in this situation.
2 In the realm of psychotherapy, a multitude of techniques exist for the regulation of anxiety. The approach I am introducing here represents the most commonly employed strategy for regulating anxiety within the framework of ISTDP.
3 Within the literature of ISTDP, the terms *restructuring of regressive defenses* and *the graded format* are employed to characterize therapeutic tasks that seem alike. Nat Kuhn's (2014) ISTDP encyclopedia notes that Davanloo utilized the term *restructuring* in his initial works and *graded format* in his subsequent publications.
4 Hans is his younger brother, who was abused by the same cousin a few years later.

Chapter 15

How to Work with Feelings

It was during my psychology studies at NTNU - The Norwegian University of Science and Technology in Trondheim, Norway, that I first came across short-term dynamic therapy. The introduction was made by Leigh McCullough, who held a position as adjunct professor at NTNU through one of her research projects. Once an apprentice under Habib Davanloo, she eventually branched out to create her own form of short-term dynamic therapy, which she termed *affect phobia therapy* (McCullough Vaillant, 1997). McCullough was a dedicated and motivating lecturer, and the therapy recordings she presented left a deep imprint on me. I vividly recall one of the patients she introduced, with whom McCullough interacted in her characteristically warm yet challenging style. This patient permitted himself to experience rage toward a friend who had deceived him, accepted the guilt associated with his aggressive impulses, and grieved the loss of a close companion. The video clearly depicted the patient's sense of relief and liberation following the therapy session. The power of feelings to grant freedom was clearly demonstrated.

Years later, when I revisited my interest in short-term dynamic therapy, my experience was somewhat different. I attended a seminar where a video of a patient, who also had intense feelings, was presented. This time, the emotional breakthrough left me puzzled. I was unable to understand the events in the video, nor could I see any advantage in expressing feelings in such a way. My reaction was adverse, and I perceived what I witnessed as troublesome. The capacity of feelings to induce confusion and unease was evident.

Having learned this method, I now understand what the seminar lecturer was aiming to demonstrate. I've also come to understand that intense feelings can trigger anxiety and unease, not just in patients, but also in students and therapists. It is plausible that this chapter might stir up anxiety and discomfort in you, the reader, as intense feelings are expressed in the example being studied. Therefore, it is crucial to deeply comprehend what feelings are, how they manifest, and what you aim to accomplish when working with feelings in therapy. With this understanding, it becomes less challenging to manage your own feelings when confronted with those of the patient. You can then invite the patient to experience their true feelings, while being assured that you can assist the patient in utilizing them on their journey toward freedom. This chapter discusses what

DOI: 10.4324/9781003516217-19

feelings are, their function, and how to constructively incorporate them into therapy.

What Are Feelings?

Keltner et al. (2019) have formulated a consolidated definition of what constitutes basic feelings. This definition is based on their extensive review of several studies of emotions:

> An emotion is a brief state that arises following appraisals of interpersonal or intrapersonal events, and involves distinct antecedents, signaling, physiology, and action and appraisal tendencies that demonstrate some coherence and are observed in related form in our primate relatives.

> (p. 196)

The definition may seem complex, yet it encapsulates the understanding of emotions, or feelings,[1] in short-term dynamic therapy quite well. Feelings are transient states with a certain duration that arise from specific internal or external antecedents. This implies that feelings come and go, triggered by particular incidents. These incidents could be a thought or memory, or an external event. Thus, feelings are *triggered* by an event or a *situation*.

Moreover, each feeling has distinct triggers, implying that specific triggers lead to the various feelings, such as anger and sadness. Feelings manifest differently, each one with its own unique signals, and the physiological responses vary among different feelings. Each feeling is associated with a unique set of action and appraisal tendencies, referred to in Intensive Short-Term Dynamic Psychotherapy (ISTDP) as impulses. Consequently, different feelings inspire us to respond in specific ways. These characteristics of feelings are also observable in other mammals closely related to humans.

Translated into the language of therapy, feelings are the responses an individual has to specific triggering situations. These feelings present themselves as distinct activations or physiological sensations in the body, experienced similarly across various mammals. Accompanying this activation are action tendencies, or impulses, that are unique to the specific feeling. For instance, the feeling of anger is triggered when one is mistreated or threatened. The physiological activation is marked by power and energy originating from the core and extending to the arms and legs. It results in a characteristic facial expression, and the impulse of the feelings is to physically attack. This is true for bears, chimpanzees, and humans alike.

At the same time, a significant distinction exists between humans and our nearest kin. This distinction is rooted in our ability to use our sophisticated brain to determine whether to act on an impulse. Humans possess the ability to reflect on feelings and evaluate the consequences of acting upon them. We can use *defense mechanisms* that prevent the primitive *impulse* from manifesting into *actions*, in ways other primates cannot.

Unconscious Feelings

Even though humans are creatures of reason, the *feelings* and *impulses* we experience are akin to those in other primates. Feelings do not depend on advanced cognitive processes, such as reflection. This is a perspective strongly held by Antonio Damasio (1999), a respected researcher in the field of feelings. Basic feelings are triggered without the need for reflection or observation. While it is possible to become consciously aware of feelings by focusing on them and reflecting, it is not a prerequisite for a feeling to *emerge* and subsequently influence an individual.

To understand the implications of this, let's consider a few examples. Damasio (1999) discusses the case of "David," who suffered severe damage to both temporal lobes of his brain, including the hippocampus. Following the injury, David was incapable of absorbing new explicit knowledge, such as recent events or people he had encountered. In a week-long controlled experiment, David was made to interact with three different people: one person was directed to behave in a very pleasant and rewarding manner; the second was instructed to act neutrally, and the third was told to behave in a dismissive and uninteresting way. Even though "David" was unable to recall or reflect on what had transpired, he subsequently exhibited distinctly different emotional reactions toward the three individuals. He had no explicit recollections of the events, but responded with *unconscious feelings*.

Unawareness of feelings and physical sensations is a common occurrence. This becomes apparent when a child is so absorbed in playing that they forget to eat or visit the restroom, thus ignoring their basic needs. Similarly, individuals who find themselves in dramatic situations, like being the first to arrive at the scene of a car accident, often become focused and action-driven. It is only after all is sorted out that they acknowledge the fear they experienced. Looking back, they realize that they were indeed scared during the entire incident, but their *awareness* of this feeling only surfaced afterward.

Many can also relate to the experience of only realizing later that they were angry after being mistreated, perhaps by a coworker or a service professional. As time passes, one becomes aware of the clear thoughts and energy characteristic of anger and thinks, "Ah, I wish I had said and done this and that!" In the heat of the moment, one is often so taken aback and focused on adhering to social norms that the underlying feelings are ignored.

Neurological studies back up this understanding. Our experience of feelings is underpinned by multiple independent brain structures. Activation of feelings at the subcortical and brainstem level may—but doesn't have to—result in additional activation and processing at a cortical level (Solms & Panksepp, 2012). Feelings can be triggered in more primitive brain structures without involving the structures that offer reflexive awareness.

Grasping that feelings can be unconscious is crucial to understanding ISTDP. The Man Who Worried About His Heart (Chapter 12) was unconscious of his intense feelings triggered when his chances of finding a girlfriend were dashed due to the COVID-19 pandemic. His conscious perception was that his physical symptoms were the result of an underlying physical illness. He was *unaware* of his *anxiety* about his *feeling of grief*. Consequently, he experienced unconscious grief and unconscious anxiety. In Part I, the Sweet Child was conscious of her complex feelings, but she was unaware of their depth and complexity. By keeping herself busy, she diverted herself from her feelings. When she wasn't able to distract herself, she became numb. In this manner, the experience of the feelings remained unconscious, and she was unable to utilize her excellent cognitive resources to comprehend the situation. The Girl Who Wasn't a Princess (Chapters 8–10 and 13) unconsciously suppressed her anger toward the man she lived with by blindly trusting his evaluation of the situation. In doing so, she kept difficult feelings at bay, but she also lost the strength that could have assisted her in self-care.

Why Do Feelings Exist?

Feelings have been preserved through evolution, as they serve *adaptive functions* and have been crucial to our survival as a species. They offer us essential information about our needs, our boundaries, and our preferences, and assist us in making sense of life (Normann-Eide, 2020). Without feelings, we would be left to cognitively interpret all that occurs around us, basing our actions solely on rational processing. For instance, exposure to violence wouldn't elicit immediate reactions of anger or fear. Instead, we would need to reflect, thinking along the lines of, "Being hit in the face poses a danger to my brain, I should react accordingly." Similarly, upon encountering a large snake, we wouldn't instinctively react with fear. We would have to recall, "I remember reading that this could be dangerous. Perhaps I should flee?" Feelings make the process of information processing more efficient, offering us important insights into suitable courses of action. In addition to providing information, feelings also supply us with the energy and impulses necessary to carry out adaptive actions. Feelings exist to help us.

When Feelings Become Complicated

However, sometimes feelings may provoke anxiety, leading us to resort to defense mechanisms that generate symptoms. Feelings, which are essentially energy and impulses intended to assist us, can become problematic. A child raised by an alcoholic parent often finds their feelings complex. While the child feels a lot of love for their parent, they may also feel anger, even fury, when the parent is drunk. Along with anger come the angry impulses, which are to act out violently. Having violent impulses toward a loved one is a painful and guilt-inducing experience, and is further complicated by the child most likely also being filled with sorrow. When the parent is drunk or suffering from a hangover, they have little capacity to tolerate and assist the child in managing these challenging feelings. Consequently, these children learn to disregard and overlook their feelings, instead attempting to aid the parent in a desperate quest for positive experiences. The child's efforts to express feelings of anger or sadness are often met with poor reception from the parent, leading the child to quickly learn to avoid such expressions. Expressing feelings results in negative experiences, causing the child to develop anxiety about their feelings.

For a child, experiencing anxiety about their feelings and suppressing them can be a healthy adaptation, as this often leads to the child having more positive encounters with their parent. However, as the child transitions into adulthood, these automatic and unconscious strategies for handling feelings can become an issue. When the individual needs to assert themselves, seek help in challenging situations, or establish a close relationship with someone, they feel anxious. These kinds of situations are associated with negative experiences and provoke a whole lot of complex feelings.

Hence, it is not random which situations and feelings become complex; it is those that are closely tied to painful experiences from the past, and that trigger inner psychological conflicts. Thus, when dealing with feelings therapeutically, the focus is not on feelings *in general*. ISTDP is not an emotion-focused therapy that centers on feelings for the sake of feelings. The focus is on the *specific feelings* that are linked to the patient's *unconscious conflicts* and that *lead to problems*. For the individual in the given example to begin standing up for themselves in a healthy manner and seeking help from others, they must have the courage to experience anger when they are mistreated, and love when they are close to someone.

Yet, merely acquainting themselves with the feelings that emerge in their ongoing relationships is not enough. They also need to come to terms with the truth that their childhood needs were neglected, and that their parents, whom they still love, didn't fulfill their responsibilities. As long as the internal conflicts and associated feelings toward their parents are avoided, the patient's issues will continue. Feelings serve as strong triggers for memory. Anger stemming from current injustices brings up more or less conscious memories of similar unfair treatment during childhood, and suddenly, the internal conflict is reignited.

Davanloo's Contribution

Unlocking the Unconscious

Habib Davanloo developed ISTDP based on data from careful examination of his therapy sessions captured on video. Over a span of many years, he identified which therapist interventions triggered specific patient responses, and which ones were linked to significant patient transformation. One of his key findings was that when patients allowed themselves to fully immerse in the physical activation and impulse tied to their feelings, it unveiled substantial therapeutic content. This intense somatic experience of feelings facilitated patients in reconnecting with significant memories, previously unconscious, that were linked to the past events causing their internal conflicts. Thus, experiencing feelings in this manner served as a powerful memory trigger, often leading to experiences that were highly relevant to the psychodynamic project. Davanloo (1990) referred to this process as *unlocking the unconscious*, since *the* somatic experience of feelings *unlocks* memories that were initially inaccessible to the patient. These memories are stored in a manner that allows strong feelings, similar to those experienced in the original situation, to potentially trigger these memories and allow them to resurface into consciousness.

The Three Components of Feeling

Davanloo's studies revealed that having the unconscious unlocked necessitates the patients to be in contact with and understand three components of their feelings. When these three components are present, the patient is deemed to be fully in touch with their feeling (Coughlin Della Selva, 2004). The first element is a conscious cognitive comprehension of the feeling, meaning the ability to *identify and label* the feeling. The second element requires the patient to acknowledge and feel the physiological arousal triggered by the feeling—in other words, to permit themselves to *experience* the feeling physically in their body. The third and final element that needs to be present for the patient to be fully in touch with their feeling is the *impulse* that the feeling induces.

These three components—label, somatic component, and impulse—are the components of emotion the therapist tries to help the patient experience when doing ISTDP. In Chapter 10, the seven emotions most often worked with in this type of therapy were presented with labels, somatic component, impulse, and adaptive function.[2] This table provides information that every ISTDP therapist needs to understand cognitively, and to be able to recognize in both themselves and their patients. For the sake of clarity, Table 15.1 is also presented again here:

The Label

In short-term dynamic psychotherapy, the therapist strives to foster *both* cognitive *understanding* and transformative emotional *experiences*. The goal is to find the balance between the uniquely human ability to rationalize and comprehend, and the more fundamental, primitive aspects we share with other mammals, specifically the emotional and impulsive elements. For potent emotional experiences to lead to substantial change in the patient, understanding of the ongoing process is crucial. As previously discussed in the context of restructuring and the graded format, repeated cognitive summarization of the process plays a significant role. This holds true when working with feelings as well. The initial step toward fostering a sound understanding is for the patient to cognitively recognize the feeling they are experiencing. It is not necessary for identifying and labeling the feeling to be the first achievement in the process. As in psychodynamic therapy in general, the process is dynamic. What is outlined here is not a step-by-step guide, but rather a depiction of the intended outcome. Still, when working with feelings, conscious recognition of the feelings at play often comes early in the process. Sometimes the patient can

Table 15.1 Overview of feelings, associated somatic components and impulses, and their adaptive functions

Feeling	Somatic component	Impulse	Adaptive function
Anger	Energy rising through the body from the stomach reaching the hands, increased pulse, physiological power, heat.	An urge to lash out, potentially violently, manifesting as a desire to strike, kick, bite, etc.	Self-care and self-protection, physically and psychologically.
Grief	Physiological pain, lump in the stomach and throat, pressure behind the eyes, production of tears, increased production of saliva and mucus.	An impulse to cry and sob, to seek solace, and a longing for comfort and support.	Reorganization: Acceptance of loss; ability to reconnect with others.
Guilt	Pain and pressure in the chest and neck. Pain in the stomach. Can be very painful and cause difficulty in speaking.	Crying and sobbing. An impulse to apologize and repair the relationship with the person you have wronged.	Maintain community and connection with important others.
Joy	Warmth and lightness. Energy, vitality, and spontaneity.	Impulse to smile and laugh, and a desire to create more joy. Motivation to facilitate positive experiences in the future.	Appropriate adaptation to the environment, motivation for self-sustaining behaviors.
Love	Experience of calmness, well-being, and often warmth and relaxation (typical for caring relationships). Warmth, excitement, energy, and vitality (typical of romantic relationships—see also sexual feelings).	Impulses to do good for those you love. Desire for closeness and intimacy.	Ensure belonging to the community through the formation of strong emotional bonds.
Sexual feelings	Warmth, tingling, and pleasure in the genitals and erogenous zones. Erect penis or moist vagina. Increased heart rate, heavier breathing, and increased blood pressure.	Desire for sexual stimulation and satisfaction.	Quality of life. Pleasure alone and with others. Attachment to partner and reproduction of the species.

(Continued)

Table 15.1 (Continued)

Feeling	Somatic component	Impulse	Adaptive function
Fear	Tense muscles, increased blood pressure, increased heart rate, nausea, dizziness.	Fight, flight, freeze: Readiness for combat, the impulse to flee from danger, or to freeze and go blank in the face of unavoidable danger.	Ensure survival.

Sources: Normann-Eide (2020), Abbass (2015), McCullough Vaillant (1997), and Grünfeld and Almås (2021).

label it from the beginning, while at other times, this understanding emerges as they start to notice the somatic signals coming from the feeling.

The Somatic Component

Feelings possess distinct physiology and signals (Keltner et al., 2019). A clear indication that a patient allows themselves to fully immerse in a feeling without any defense is that they distinctly experience the feeling's physiological or somatic component. For instance, an angry person is energized and strong, a grieving individual feels a lump in their throat and pressure behind their eyes, and a joyful person experiences energy and vitality. These are internal experiences, and only the patient can truly confirm its existence. At the same time, patients often exhibit clear signs when they are emotionally aroused. Anger frequently presents itself as a clenched fist or bared teeth, grief is noticeable through sobbing and tears, and joy is expressed through smiles and laughter. If the therapist clearly observes these signs and the patient can also label the feeling they are experiencing, it can be confidently concluded that the patient is indeed experiencing that feeling.

Certain patients find it challenging to differentiate between the corners of the triangle of conflict (refer to Chapter 13). For instance, it is common for people to confuse anger and anxiety. If the therapist suspects this, they inquire about the patient's experience of their feeling. The therapist then attentively listens to discern if the sensation the patient experiences in their chest is marked by power and an urge to act, indicative of anger, or by tension and an inclination to retreat, indicative of anxiety.

A common confusion among many patients is the conflation of the *somatic experience* of a feeling with the accompanying *impulse*. For instance, when a patient is asked about their experience of anger, and they respond that they feel a desire to lash out, it exemplifies this confusion. The somatic experience refers to the *energy and power* that is mobilized within an angry individual, which is distinct from the *impulse to lash out*. This distinction is particularly crucial for patients with a history of acting out their feelings. These individuals require assistance to comprehend and manage the somatic energy without succumbing to the impulse to lash out. While lashing out might have been a viable solution for Stone Age man, in our contemporary society, violence predominantly leads to significant repercussions for both the victim and the individual who lashes out.

The Impulse

The final component of feelings, according to Davanloo, is the *impulse*. This impulse is the action tendency that comes with each distinct feeling (Keltner et al., 2019). Acknowledging and managing the reality of having primitive, feeling-driven impulses can be challenging. This is particularly true for impulses associated with anger. After all, we share these impulses with other primates. The aftermath of a bear or chimpanzee attacking in a fit of rage is well known to all—it is primitive violence, often leading to the victim's death. Navigating these impulses, especially when they are directed toward those we care for, can be complex.

Many patients fear that discussing and experiencing these impulses could lead them to enact them in real life. This fear is also shared by many therapists, leading them to avoid such discussions. Consider a mother of a young child who feels the urge to shake her child when his crying keeps her awake for several consecutive nights. For her, acknowledging this impulse and understanding the distinction between *feeling* the urge and *acting on it* would be really helpful, easing her fear of harming her baby. Similarly, a young man vividly recalls the urge he felt as a sixteen-year-old to grab a knife when he witnessed his father assaulting his mother. For him, comprehending the vast difference between *actually* stabbing his father to protect his mother, and merely having the urge or desire to do so, would also be helpful.

Davanloo emphasized that the primary reason patients often defend and keep their anger unconscious is the very impulse of anger itself. When one experiences impulses to harm loved ones, it stirs up feelings of guilt. Guilt is among the most painful feelings we encounter, and we frequently go to great lengths to avoid this feeling. By keeping guilt unconscious, the patient avoids the emotional discomfort it brings. However, guilt is also a feeling that can instigate significant change when genuinely felt. A patient who has feared their aggressive impulses and then comes into contact with the guilt associated with these impulses will discover that there are potent forces in play to deter them from *acting* on them. This realization is comforting for many. To experience guilt, one must also harbor feelings of love for the person they are angry with. Consequently, through this process, the patient gains a profound understanding that they can fully endure their anger, and that they also possess a range of feelings that seek to protect the one they love. The conscious awareness of all these feelings makes the anger much less fear-inducing.

Portraying the Impulse

In his efforts to assist patients understand and tolerate their emotional impulses, Davanloo (1990) invited patients to *portray* these impulses. This means encouraging patients to picture, in their thoughts and imaginations, what these impulses would lead them to do to the individual toward whom the feeling was directed. This approach allows patients to explore the primitive aspects of their feelings in a safe environment where no one gets hurt. It opens up a space for reflection and discussion about mental phenomena that the patient has previously evaded, and can thus bring unconscious impulses into consciousness. Moreover, it creates a pathway for directing the feeling outward, offering an alternative to the defensive mechanism of internal discharge. Consequently, it provides a suitable method for accessing intense feelings.

A common pitfall when utilizing this technique is inadvertently prompting the patient to imagine *random* angry impulses. This would constitute a misunderstanding of the method. It is of utmost importance to work with impulses that are *already* activated within the patient, and which are connected to the feelings that have been kept unconscious, resulting in symptoms. This is particularly important for patients who have a tendency to act so as to please others. If the therapist starts probing for impulses, these patients might provide fitting responses in an effort to appease the therapist. Nor is the portrayal of impulses intended to serve as a venting mechanism through which the emotional pressure is alleviated; rather, it is an integral part of the process to bring previously unconscious feelings and impulses, associated with unconscious conflicts, to consciousness.

A vivid portrayal that allows patients to clearly visualize their impulses and the harmful impact these would have on the individual toward whom they harbor anger frequently stirs up feelings of guilt. Assisting patients in experiencing the guilt over their angry impulses, without resorting to defense mechanisms such as self-punishment, is a crucial element in their recovery process (Abbass, 2015).

The Pancake Maker

The Pancake Maker, a young man in his twenties, turned to therapy following periods of self-isolation in his apartment that spanned almost a year. Despite maintaining his professional responsibilities, his once flourishing social life was now nearly non-existent. He reported experiencing several symptoms of depression, including a lack of energy, an absence of joy, and feelings of guilt. The onset of his difficulties was traced back to ending a romantic relationship with a woman he lived with, a breakup that he initiated. Currently recovering, he had met a new woman. However, the prospect of a new relationship evoked strong negative feelings within him. Thus, he found himself in a quandary, being attracted to this woman and rationally identifying no obstacles to their relationship.

The Pancake Maker and his girlfriend had a passionate beginning to their relationship, and swiftly found a shared living space. He soon realized that cohabitation stirred anxiety within him, and he was uncomfortable with her steering the relationship toward a more serious path, such as investing in costly furniture. Being his first partner, he felt it was premature to make such a commitment, and over time, he acknowledged his desire to exit the relationship. However, for over two years, he kept this realization to himself. During this time, she also withdrew from her social circle, spending most of her time alone with him. He yearned to start a life without her, but was simultaneously worried that she might become depressed and isolated if he ended things. When he finally found the courage to break free, it didn't bring the relief he had anticipated. He was consumed by shame, guilt, and fell into a state of depression and isolation. In contrast, his ex-girlfriend managed to move on with her life quite smoothly.

Labeling the Feeling

The Pancake Maker provides a candid account of his symptoms and the circumstances in which they first emerged. As I delve into his feelings about these experiences, he exhibits clear signs of anxiety. He becomes fidgety, experiences dryness in his mouth, and sighs deeply multiple times. His speech becomes less detailed, he avoids eye contact, and he conveys a strong ambivalence to reveal more. He soon realizes that he is feeling irritated with me for encouraging him to examine these defense mechanisms, and he notices his fists are clenched. Reflecting on this realization, he spontaneously suggests that it has to be related to his mother. The annoyance he feels toward me, coupled with the urge to withdraw and remain closed off, brings back memories of his mother and how she used to control his time with his father:

T: What do you feel toward her for controlling you and your father like that?
P: I was very angry!
T: And now, right here, right now?
P: Now, there is a feeling again!
T: Do you experience that anger in your body, right now?
P: Yes, I do. *GESTURES*

Experiencing the Somatic Component

The Pancake Maker can label his feeling of anger, marking the first of Davanloo's three components associated with feelings. Yet, *identifying* a feeling doesn't necessarily mean genuinely *experiencing* it. This brings us to question whether he is able to notice his anger physically. According to Davanloo, the physical experience constitutes the second component, indicating that a person is in touch with their feelings.

T: How do you experience the anger?
P: I feel a bit more .... *WAVING HIS HANDS* The tightness in my chest is gone.

The Pancake Maker appears angry, his hands gesturing passionately. He also realizes that his chest tightness, previously identified as a sign of anxiety, has gone. He labels his feeling as anger, his appearance aligns with this feeling, and his anxiety is no longer present. All signs point to him being in touch with his anger. Yet, I still inquire if he is able to reflect on his physical arousal.

T: So how do you feel this, how do you notice …. How do you experience your anger on the inside, as you're allowing yourself to feel it, right now?
P: I am full of energy! *LEANING FORWARD, GESTURING*
T: Where do you feel this energy? Could you describe what it is like to feel this anger in your body?
P: I notice, like, *MAKING CIRCULAR MOVEMENTS IN FRONT OF HIS CHEST* a wave, a kind of … shhh ….
T: Mmm.
P: Water flowing quickly through my body. *MAKING CIRCULAR MOVEMENTS*
T: Like, hot water?
P: Yes, right, like hot water. Like radiant, red-hot water, actually.

Portrayal of Impulse

He expresses his anger through both verbal and non-verbal cues. His active demeanor, forward-leaning posture, energetic hands, and warmth in his chest all serve as physical indicators of his anger (refer to Table 15.1). According to Davanloo, the next step is to establish a connection with the impulse. Emotional impulses, shared by humans and other primates, are motoric in nature and have deep evolutionary roots. To help the Pancake Maker acquaint himself with this aspect of his feeling, I invite him to *portray* the impulse (Davanloo, 1990).

T: So, if this anger had come out on your mom?
P: *SIGHS DEEPLY*
T: What would you do, like, physically, with this anger in your body? What does it want to do to your mom?
P: In what way I would be angry with her?
T: How would this anger come out on your mom?
P: *SIGHS DEEPLY*
T: If given the opportunity to take over control. Not in reality, but what it brings with it—this anger, this energy, the warm water.
P: I would tell her what I'm telling you now, from MY point of view.

When I invite him to portray his angry impulse, he lets out a deep sigh. As discussed in Chapter 14, these sighs indicate anxiety in the striated muscles. This suggests that he is within his window of tolerance and is grappling with some internal conflict. It is not surprising that there's a conflict: I encourage him to acknowledge his aggressive impulses toward his mother by visualizing them. There are multiple signs that he has an internal conflict related to his mother, and that feelings of anger are intertwined with this conflict.

For many who are learning ISTDP, this particular aspect of the method can be both challenging and uncomfortable: What can be gained from engaging in anger fantasies? At this point, it is crucial to remember that, according to the definition of basic feelings (Keltner et al., 2019), we share these emotional impulses with our primate relatives. Consider an angry bear or chimpanzee, filled with energy and experiencing a radiant, red heat in its chest. What would it do to the object of its anger? We humans possess these same primitive impulses, which can be quite complex for someone with love and empathy to handle. A key principle in all psychodynamic therapy is the notion that discussing experiences that are seen as frightening and taboo aids in resolving inner conflicts. Therefore, discussing these frightening and taboo impulses is an integral part of this process.

Differentiating Rationality and Impulses

The Pancake Maker continues to express what he would like to *tell* her. He elaborates on the events that have transpired in their relationship and contemplates potential future scenarios. These are *words* and a relatively *complex cognitive analysis* of his relationship with his mother, and are not characteristics we share with bears or chimpanzees. Nor are they his basic, emotional impulses. This way of reflecting on his mother serves as a form of rationalization, acting as a defense mechanism. As the topic at hand is impulses, it becomes a defense against experiencing them.

T: So, that is somehow your words, the rational part of you that wants to sort this out. But on the more emotional.... This anger of yours.... What is its impulse? What does it motivate you to do? What do your hands want to do? We saw them rise like this *MAKING FISTS*, we see them getting activated *MAKING GESTURES AS HE DID*.

P: *SIGHS DEEPLY*

T: What is the animalistic side, in a way?

P: I want to get it out, in a way. But I don't want to take it out on her either. Actually.

The Pancake Maker does not want to take it out on her; not *actually*. He does not want to unleash his anger on his mother, not in reality. His recognition of this is crucial, as when portraying feelings, it doesn't concern portraying potential real-world actions. Instead, it involves utilizing a *mental* space to *acquaint oneself* with complex emotional impulses.

The Mobilization of Motoric Impulses

T: No, not in reality.

P: No, no, not really.

T: But if it *had* been taken out on her, what would the anger have done to her?

P: *SIGHS* I don't know. *MAKING GESTURES* I want, I must make gestures, I must, I must….

T: What would those hands want to do to her? If this anger had been unleashed on her? Not in reality, but if we create a space here *POINTING TO MY HEAD*, where we can become acquainted with these really complicated feelings.

P: *TOUCHING HIS SHOULDERS* Then I would shout at her! *MAKING A THROWING MOVEMENT WITH HIS HANDS* Then I would show her physically! *ANOTHER THROWING MOVEMENT AND STOMPING ON THE FLOOR* Then I would have shown her how much I feel! *ANOTHER THROWING MOVEMENT*

T: Mm! Stomping on floor.

P: I wouldn't touch her, I would be standing up, showing her *GESTURES*.

The Pancake Maker is becoming more and more in touch with his anger. A careful examination of the transcript reveals that his body language displays aggressive impulses *before* he verbalizes them, and prior to their conscious realization.

This is crucial to note: I don't want him to *fabricate* anything, but to assist him in recognizing these *pre-existing motoric impulses*.

However, the Pancake Maker remains in a state of conflict. He asserts that he wouldn't touch her, but instead, would stand up, showing his feelings to her. This might be a viable strategy in everyday life. Yet, consider this: Would a bear or a chimpanzee be content with merely expressing their anger through their physical demeanor alone? To provide him with a chance to face what he has previously avoided, I encourage him to confront the more primitive facets.

T: If this anger had been given the opportunity to come out, out of control, what would it have done to her?

P: That is a line of thinking I haven't followed before ….

T: That makes sense.

P: Hmm ….

T: And we know that your anger against your mom is quite complicated for you ….

P: *MOVING HIS HEAD QUICKLY FORWARD AND STOMPING ON THE FLOOR*

An impulse is activated in his body.

T: Just by us approaching it, you get a pretty guilty conscience.

P: Yes. I had … headbutt! *LOOKS SURPRISED*

Slightly taken aback, he realizes how his body has been activated.

P: *REPEATEDLY THRUSTS HIS HEAD FORWARD AS IF HE IS HEADBUT-TING SOMEONE* I would use my head! Would, sort of, thump.

T: Yeah. Right.

P: *SMILES* *HANDS TWITCHING* Because this … I feel … uh …. *DROPS HANDS LIMPLY* It feels like my hands are not a tool that I would find … satisfying to use at all.

T: So what would be satisfying?

P: *THRUSTS HIS BODY QUICKLY FORWARD IN THE CHAIR AS HE STOMPS* Using my body, just …. *REPEATS THE MOVEMENT*

T: Right! Where would you hit her?

P: *HITS HIS CHEST* Directly to the chest! *THRUSTS QUICKLY FORWARD* Body to body! Feel me, sort of. *THRUSTS FORWARD ONCE MORE* Feel me!

Systematically, I have encouraged him to allow his impulses to enter his consciousness and be released into his imagination. Eventually, they surface as impulses to headbutt and throw his body into hers. It is important to note that these impulses are expressed through his body language before he articulates them verbally. He does not invent random acts of violence. His body signals its intentions in reaction to his anger, and all he needs to do is simply to observe and become aware of what is occurring.

P: I'm sitting on top of her. She's lying on the ground and then … no …. *LAUGHS*

T: If we don't laugh away your anger. Don't laugh away your rage. It's just a feeling. If we don't laugh at your feelings. Take you seriously, shall we?

P: *SIGHS DEEPLY*

T: What would this anger do to your mom? You're sitting on top of her?

P: I'm sitting on top of her. And I thump her. Punching my fist …. *PUNCHING MOTION* and my fist *PUNCHING MOTION* and my fist *PUNCHING MOTION* and my fist … *PUNCHING MOTION* in her face. *SLAPS HIS THIGH* *APPEARS CALM*

T: A lot of punches?

P: Yes … a lot of punches….

Turning Angry Impulses Toward Oneself

Redirecting aggressive impulses toward oneself is a common defense mechanism that results in symptoms of depression. This defense frequently takes the form of self-critical thoughts, which excuse the individual who is the actual target of the patient's anger from any responsibility for the events that have transpired. The following section illustrates how this phenomenon can manifest in a portrait, in a tangible and physical manner.

P: *SIGHS* Yes, I'm still angry!

T: Still angry. So, if all the anger came out, once and for all?

P: I can't do any more to her. She is ….

T: So, what do you do to her? What would this anger do to her body? Is she dead?

P: *PUNCHES HIS THIGH WITH HIS FIST* I would have to punch the ground next to her.

T: But now you're beating yourself up.

P: Yes.

T: And if you punch the ground next to her ....

P: *PUNCHES HIS THIGH AGAIN*

T: Who gets hurt?

P: *POINTS TO HIMSELF* It's me.

T: And now you're beating yourself up. We see how you attack yourself.

The Pancake Maker sought therapy due to a self-imposed isolation that lasted a year following a breakup. The breakup was his own decision and initiative, but as soon as he expressed his desires and impulses toward his girlfriend, he was overwhelmed by guilt, became self-destructive and depressed, and ceased socializing with friends. During the therapy session, he permitted himself to acknowledge and discuss his aggressive impulses toward his mother. Suddenly, he exhibits self-destructive behavior by actually punching his thigh forcefully and experiencing an urge to punch the ground. This is the same pattern that led to his problems. Once he took his desire to end his relationship with his girlfriend seriously, he turned self-destructive. Similarly, when he takes his anger toward his mother seriously, he is once again consumed by guilt and becomes self-destructive. A clear connection can be seen between his impulses, how he handles them in the portrait, and the issues he brought to therapy.

Guilt and Positive Feelings

The Pancake Maker appears calmer in his chair, with no visible signs of angry impulses. Davanloo (1990) observed that once anger had broken into consciousness through a portrait, feelings of guilt and grief often followed. He further noted that bringing this previously unconscious guilt to consciousness played a significant role in healing. Consequently, I inquire about the Pancake Maker's experience when he visualizes the result of his actions and how his mother's eyes appear. The act of looking into someone's eyes is intimate, and stirs up feelings associated with closeness and intimacy.

T: How does she look, how does her face look, how do her eyes look?

P: She has no eyes left. There is nothing left of her. She barely has a face. It is red. It's just red and dark red and .... *RUBS HIS FOREHEAD*

T: How does it feel to look at this bloody, bruised, dark red face?

P: It is not good at all.

T: It hurts.

P: It hurts to look at it. *SIGHS* ... I don't want to look at it.

The Pancake Maker finds it painful to look at this internal image. Observing her eyes and face triggers feelings of intimacy. He realizes that he has harbored impulses to harm someone he loves hurts, and he shields himself from the painful feeling of guilt by avoiding the image. However, given our agreement to confront these complex feelings, I encourage him to face it, nonetheless.

T: Let's take a closer look. If we don't avoid these feelings? Because it seems far from uncomplicated to have this violent rage toward your mom.

P: *NODS* *APPEARS RELAXED*

T: It seems like there is something else there too, which hurts.

P: *NODS* *APPEARS SAD* *SIGHS* Mom ... yes, no, I don't know.

T: Mom ....

P: She ....

T: What is coming up?

P: She's a kind person .... She, like, cares! *APPEARS TOUCHED*

T: What do you remember? How do you know she cares?

P: She makes time. For me.

T: What do you remember?

P: She .... We make pancakes together. *LAUGHS* We make pancakes together and it's nice!

T: When did you do this?

P: We did it a lot when I was little. From when I was very small until I was a bit older. *TEARS UP*

T: Please tell me more ....

P: She taught me the recipe. And I know it by heart. Two to three eggs. Some flour. 500 grams. Lots of milk.

The Pancake Maker vividly describes how they made pancakes together.

T: How does it feel when you recall these pleasant memories? This is a nice memory, isn't it?

P: It's a nice memory. It feels good. Yet, there's a tinge of sadness because ... it's such a nice memory; I wish there had been more of it.

T: So, you've been desiring more of this, haven't you? More connection?

P: I wish that when I think of my mother, I would think of this. Not any other distressing matter.

The Pancake Maker permits his angry impulses to surface into his consciousness, also experiencing the pain and guilt associated with these feelings. This experience paves the way for the resurgence of pleasant memories. During the session, it's a deeply moving experience for me when he explains about the pancakes. It is evident that this is a cherished memory. The positive feelings, previously obscured by anger and guilt, only emerge after he allows himself to confront these complicated feelings.

The Link Between the Mother and the Ex—the Link Between P and C

Again, as the Pancake Maker reconnects with his positive memories, he encounters complex feelings. The warmth and closeness he felt with his mother during his childhood were comforting, but as he matured, their relationship dynamics evolved into something more complex. His mother, having neglected her social network and not found a new partner, relies on her son for conversation and companionship. This has led him to sense that she is becoming overly reliant on him. When he expresses these experiences, a new wave of anger washes over him, accompanied by a fantasy of severing all connections with her.

P: I can send her a message stating ... uh ... I don't want to talk to you again. Then, I can remove her from my contacts, and then I can block her number ... *APPEARS UNCOMFORTABLE* and then I instantly feel a very uncomfortable feeling.

T: Indeed, facing that impulse to sever all ties....

P: Yes.

T: Essentially, to get rid of her, once and for all.

P: Yes.

T: What do you feel? What is stirred up inside you, right now, in your feelings? Facing that impulse?

P: That she is a very fragile person. I know this won't ... I don't want her to ....

T: What do you foresee? How do you imagine her when she reads the message?

P: I worry she might fall into a depression. She can ... I feel like I'm the most important person in her life. And that's something .... Everything would have been much simpler for me if I wasn't the most important person in her life. I wish I wasn't the most important person in her life.

The patient sought therapy because of his relationship with a girl who had neglected her own social network while steering their relationship in a more serious direction. She positioned the Pancake Maker as the most important person in her life. It made him uneasy, but he hesitated to end the relationship for two years, fearing that his girlfriend might fall into depression. The parallel between the girlfriend and his mother is evident. Just as he has been apprehensive about his mother's potential depression if he set boundaries for her, he harbored similar fears about his girlfriend's reaction. When he eventually ended the relationship, she moved on with her life, leaving *him* feeling depressed and burdened with guilt. In psychodynamic therapy, a central understanding is that psychological difficulties arise when the patient reverts to defense mechanisms developed in childhood. The defense mechanisms that the Pancake Maker employs, when confronted with anger toward women he perceives as overly reliant on him, and the guilt he experiences for wanting to distance himself from them, are leading to problems.

Anger, Guilt, Love, and Grief

The Pancake Maker feels a renewed wave of rage, picturing himself stabbing his mother with kitchen knives. The mental picture of his mother lifeless before him naturally stirs up feelings of pain and guilt. He also mourns the unfortunate turn of events, the lack of the motherly presence he needed and longed for during his childhood. Once again, anger and guilt reignite his love and longing for his mother.

P: It's a shame, I wish things were different. But this is how it turned out.

T: So, if you were to honor these positive feelings, this longing. Bringing closure to this chapter, somehow. What would you do to her body? If you were somehow permitted to, okay .... It's such a shame that it turned out like this.

P: Yeah. *NODS*

T: Intensely, desiring more of it. If you were to honor these feelings ....

P: *SIGHS*

T: If you wouldn't let the guilt, and your actions, fuel the destructive, but were given the chance to ....

P: *MOVES HIS HAND UPWARD REPEATEDLY* I would remove the knives from her. I would pull them out of her and .... *SIGHS DEEPLY*

T: *SPEAKING IN A GENTLE VOICE* What would you do to her? To her body?

P: I would bury her ....

T: Where? Can you describe what that funeral would look like?

When experiencing grief and loss, rituals like funerals serve to underscore the grief and loss. These rituals form an integral part of healthy grief management, facilitating the process of moving forward. In his mind's eye, the Pancake Maker does precisely this, and he is deeply moved as he explains:

P: *SIGHS DEEPLY* Ah ... *SMILES* I would make.... I would make ... a tombstone that resembles a stack of pancakes.

T: *LAUGHS* Mm!

P: It would be bright and sunny, and it would be a peaceful burial site .... And there would be other gravestones around. It would be just me who was there, laying her to rest.

T: What would you express to her?

P: *SIGHS* *TEARS UP*

T: What would be your final words to her, as she lies in her grave?

P: "Thank you," I suppose.

T: Thank you?

P: Thank you. *SIGHS* *TEARS UP*

T: Mm ....

P: *CRYING* It's sad. It is sad!

Studying a transcript where an individual imagines ending their mother's life can be a potent experience. If you, the reader, find your feelings agitated by this example, it's quite normal. You might feel uneasy or irate, and question the suitability of this therapeutic approach.

In such a scenario, I encourage you to remember the purpose of these therapeutic strategies. The Pancake Maker has perceived his mother as domineering and intrusive for most of his life. He has not been able to live his life freely. Through his interactions with his mother, he has come to understand that intimacy and a sense of confinement are inextricably linked. This understanding complicates his efforts to form loving relationships in adulthood. For years, he has resented his mother's controlling behavior and for treating him as an equal partner. His anger has induced anxiety in him, as it drives an impulse to sever ties with his mother. In reality, this would mean completely cutting off contact with her. This fantasy has been with him for a long time, and he has been afraid that it would have catastrophic consequences for her. His wish to distance himself from his mother is also connected to a deeper rage that he has feared, felt immense guilt over, and for which he has self-punished. These feelings and impulses are not whimsically conceived and fabricated during the sessions. They have been with him for a long time, and he has finally found someone to share them with. After experiencing these feelings, he feels love for his mother and grief over losing her. The mother he has yearned for does not exist. At long last, allowing himself to express all these feelings brings a sense of relief.

T: She has been laid to rest. She is dead. But there is also something good about it.
P: It's a relief! It's a relief. *SMILES* And it's a shame things couldn't be different, but in a way, it feels good too. It feels as if a burden has been lifted off my shoulders.
T: But there's a stack of pancakes that you can revisit, and that's comforting, too.
P: It is. *SMILES* *HIS VOICE BREAKS* That's the way I want to remember her.
T: Mmm. Right. That is how you would like her to be represented.
P: That's how I want her memory to live on for the rest of my life.

The Pancake Maker employed the same strategies in his adult relationships with women as those he had used to prevent causing harm to his mother. He refrained from expressing his true feelings, grappling with a sense of being entrapped. However, as he began to separate the feelings tied to his mother from those connected to the women he met in his adult life, he found it progressively simpler to establish intimate relationships with women. He realized that the women he met were not the same as his mother, and the fear that they would be destroyed was unfounded.

Summary

The ISTDP therapist aims to assist their patients in permitting themselves to experience their feelings. This is accomplished by collaboratively identifying and labeling the feelings, followed by connecting with the somatic component of the feelings and the impulses associated with them. The therapist also seeks to aid the patient in understanding how they have managed challenging feelings in the past, and the reasons behind their specific coping strategies. Consequently, the patient obtains a coherent narrative about their feelings and experiential knowledge that feelings can be experienced without causing harm to anyone.

This chapter has been specifically dedicated to working with feelings, and I have demonstrated how I dealt with anger, guilt, and grief in the case of the Pancake Maker. Every case presented in this book has had a focus on feelings. The Sweet Child from Part I found it challenging to do healthy things for herself, as the anger, guilt, and grief related to her parents' illnesses were too overpowering. The Girl Who Wasn't a Princess had a hard time handling her anger toward the man who mistreated her. The Man Who Worried About His Heart didn't permit himself to grieve the loss of a potential girlfriend, and the Brain Exerciser was overwhelmed by anxiety when confronted with memories and feelings associated with sexual abuse. In all these therapies, my work involved helping the patient to become conscious of previously unconscious feelings and to allow both the bodily experience and the motoric impulse connected to the feelings to be processed.

In each of these cases, I have also discussed anxiety and defense mechanisms, and the emphasis has varied depending on the focus of the different chapters. It is crucial to remember that even though these various phenomena have their own dedicated chapters, they are all interconnected. The triangle of conflict and the triangle of person (Malan, 1979) are inseparably intertwined, and the specific corners represent phenomena that are interdependent. In short-term dynamic therapy, there is a dynamic movement between the feelings, anxiety, and defense mechanisms that are triggered in the face of situations in the patient's present, with the therapist, and from the past. Therapy is about offering corrective experiences (Alexander & French, 1946) that demonstrate that feelings can be experienced and tolerated. Simultaneously, the unconscious inner conflicts that have led to the avoidance of feelings must be brought to light and made conscious. As a result, the patient can effectively manage situations in their everyday life that remind them of past difficult experiences, without resorting to old and destructive strategies to cope with them.

Notes

1 While there may be arguments made to differentiate between the terms *emotion* and *feeling* (Frederickson, 2013), for the purpose of this text, I will be using the terms interchangeably.
2 By *adaptive function*, I refer to the crucial and healthy role that feelings are designed to play in human lives, a role so significant that they have been conserved throughout the course of evolution.

Chapter 16

Connecting the Dots

How can we link these dots to form a comprehensive therapy? How can we establish a strong therapeutic alliance and a psychodynamic case formulation that allows us to dynamically work with the various corners of the triangles, thereby resolving the underlying conflicts? There are, in fact, slightly differing perspectives on this within the Intensive Short-Term Dynamic Psychotherapy (ISTDP) community. Habib Davanloo, the founder of the method, adjusted his approach throughout his career. His early works (Davanloo, 1980) depict a different approach to ISTDP than his later works (Davanloo, 2000). Current leaders in the field, such as Patricia Coughlin, Jon Frederickson, and Allan Abbass, each highlight different aspects of the method. Additionally, ISTDP is a method that aims to assist a wide spectrum of patients, with different challenges and functional outcomes, in need of different interventions. Due to these variations, regular discussions arise on the IEDTA mailing list (IEDTA, 2024) about the *true nature* of ISTDP. Here are key ISTDP figures Allan Abbass and John Frederickson's contributions to one such discussion in the spring of 2022:

> [...] ISTDP treatment is not a single treatment. [...] So in my view ISTDP is a comprehensive psychodynamic psychotherapeutic system for diverse populations with avoided unconscious feelings manifested as unconscious anxiety and defenses of various types.
>
> (Abbass, 2022a)

> [...] People sometimes refer to ISTDP as "the method," but I think of it as a group of overarching principles of assessment that yield a variety of treatments tailored to patient capacities. That is part of what makes this model of therapy so difficult to learn. It is not "one size fits all."
>
> (Frederickson, 2022a)

There is a growing body of literature on how ISTDP can be tailored to suit various patient groups. While this book does not delve into these specifics, those interested are encouraged to explore further.[1] The key points to remember from Abbass

DOI: 10.4324/9781003516217-20

and Frederickson's insights are that ISTDP provides a framework for understanding, a psychotherapeutic system, and various principles of assessment. It is not a technique-driven, manual-based therapy.

By grasping and applying the various principles outlined in this book, you can significantly aid a substantial number of your patients. Naturally, these principles should be employed with curiosity, respect, and empathy. Such a compassionate approach is not only pertinent to your interactions with patients but also to how you interact with yourself, given the challenges that come with being a therapist. By adopting this approach, you set the stage for utilizing the framework of understanding presented in this book to foster creative partnerships with your patients, leading to profound understanding and liberation. If a mutual understanding is established on how to achieve the patients' goals from a psychodynamic perspective, and if you alternate adeptly between working with feelings, anxiety, and defense, you will achieve considerable progress.

Sub-Goals over Technique

Books on ISTDP often include authentic dialogues from therapy sessions, and this book is no exception. Attending an ISTDP conference provides the opportunity to view video recordings of actual therapy sessions. As a student of ISTDP, this gives you valuable access to examples of how ISTDP is implemented by experienced therapists. While this is a tremendous resource, meaning that as a novice therapist you don't have to invent all the techniques for yourself, it also poses certain challenges. Learners often tend to try to remember specific phrases from the seminar and then strive to say the *right* things at the *right* time. This can lead to the therapist becoming rigid, focusing more on getting things right than truly listening to their patient.

Instead of attempting to apply specific techniques, I recommend concentrating on accomplishing sub-goals. The chapters in Parts II and III provide a summary of the sub-goals that need to be met:

- Develop a shared understanding of the therapy's goal (Chapter 9).
- Develop a shared understanding of the therapeutic tasks (Chapter 10).
- Develop a solid therapeutic bond (Chapter 11).
- Develop a psychodynamic case formulation based on Malan's triangles (Part II).
- Develop a shared understanding of the defense mechanisms used, including their function and consequence (Chapters 12 and 13).
- Help the patient turn against their defense mechanisms (Chapters 12 and 13).
- Help the patient regulate their anxiety to an optimal level (Chapter 14).
- Help the patient to fully experience their true feelings (Chapter 15).

Certainly acquiring techniques or recalling others' words in similar circumstances can be beneficial. Every proficient jazz musician hones their technique, practices scales, and transcribes other accomplished musicians' improvisations.

However, these efforts are futile unless the musician attentively listens to the music and comprehends the chordal progression. In ISTDP, understanding the overarching principles and focusing on achieving goals fosters improvisation and flexibility. Concentrating on what is right or wrong often leads more toward wrong than right. The jazz musician applies their theoretical knowledge and practiced techniques to make music; similarly, the ISTDP therapist employs their theoretical and technical comprehension, along with ISTDP-specific sub-goals, to resolve the patient's underlying, unconscious conflicts.

Stone by Stone, or a Spiral-Shaped Process?

This book, in some respects, adheres to a principle akin to building a structure stone by stone. The sub-goals of ISTDP, which align with the book's chapters, serve as interlocking building blocks. This concept can be visually represented as follows (see Figure 16.1):

The foundation of ISTDP is rooted in the understanding of psychodynamic theory, as introduced in Part I. The subsequent four stones are placed upon this foundation, creating a solid base. This process ensures a shared understanding of the presenting problem, and the relevant therapeutic tasks to address it. Once this understanding is established, it is crucial that the patient clearly sees their defense mechanisms and chooses to put them aside. Concurrently, the patient should remain within the optimal zone of development, ensuring that anxiety does not escalate excessively. This sets the stage for the patient to safely experience their feelings, allowing these feelings to trigger new memories (*unlocking the unconscious*) that contribute to resolving underlying conflicts. Stone by stone, each contributes to the formation of a stack, collectively representing ISTDP. Each stone builds on top of the previous one, and progression to the next level is dependent upon the successful establishment of the preceding one.

However, this understanding is overly simplistic. In a perfect world, one could accomplish each sub-goal and then progress to the next. However, as reiterated multiple times, in ISTDP the dialogue is both dynamic and flexible. The various

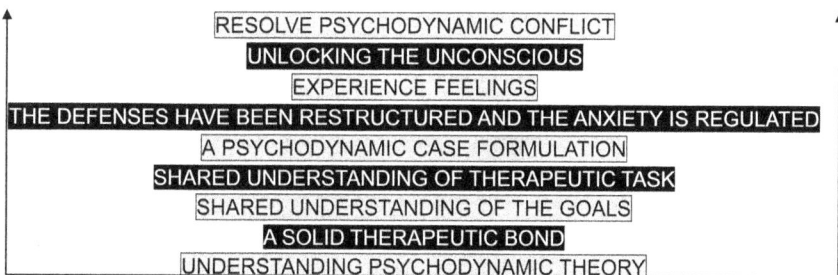

RESOLVE PSYCHODYNAMIC CONFLICT
UNLOCKING THE UNCONSCIOUS
EXPERIENCE FEELINGS
THE DEFENSES HAVE BEEN RESTRUCTURED AND THE ANXIETY IS REGULATED
A PSYCHODYNAMIC CASE FORMULATION
SHARED UNDERSTANDING OF THERAPEUTIC TASK
SHARED UNDERSTANDING OF THE GOALS
A SOLID THERAPEUTIC BOND
UNDERSTANDING PSYCHODYNAMIC THEORY

Figure 16.1 A Stone-by-Stone Progression Through ISTDP's Sub-Goals

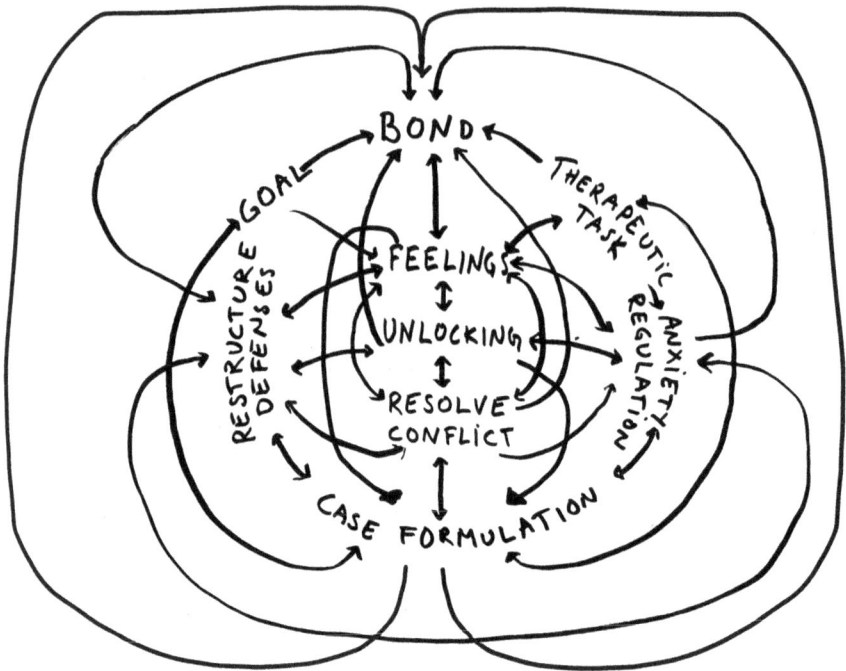

Figure 16.2 A Spiral-Shaped Process of Working Through ISTDP's Sub-Goals

"phases tend to overlap and most interviews of necessity contain a good deal of repetition and thus proceed in a spiral rather than a straight line" (Davanloo, 1990, p. 103). This concept is illustrated in Figure 16.2.

In reality, psychotherapy does not follow a linear path. Instead, it involves oscillating between different sub-goals. Misunderstandings can occur, necessitating the repair of the therapeutic *bond*. Being in the presence of someone who is willing to mend a broken bond can be a corrective emotional experience (Alexander & French, 1946). This experience can awaken *feelings* and trigger the recall of *significant memories*, assisting in *resolving the unconscious conflict*. At times, misunderstandings may require a change in the *goals* and *therapeutic tasks*, or even a revision of the *psychodynamic case formulation*. There may also be instances where the patient's capacity to tolerate feelings has been overestimated, necessitating a step back to *regulate anxiety*. The process, thus, proceeds in a spiral.

Response to Intervention

The spiral progression in psychotherapy, as opposed to a linear one, is driven by the therapist's or patient's perception that certain aspects need to be revisited or reworked. They might find that a consensus on the therapeutic task is still missing, that there are varying understandings of the presenting problems, anxiety levels are too high, or the patient isn't prepared to let go of a certain defense mechanism. To pick up on this, the therapist carefully monitors the patient's response to each therapeutic intervention. Adhering to the central principle of *response to intervention* in ISTDP (Coughlin Della Selva, 2004), the therapist does not assume the effectiveness of their interventions, but rather evaluates their impact based on the patient's response.

The assessment of the patient's response to treatment is exemplified in an excerpt from the therapy of the Girl Who Wasn't a Princess. In this part, she articulates her feelings that arise from her attempts to understand her relationship with a man she was romantically interested in, highlighting his lack of response to her efforts.

T: But what do you feel about that? When you sit here with me and you realize you tried ... you tried to do your best....
P: Just sad. *LOOKING SAD*

I inquire into her feelings (*intervention*), and she reciprocates with a feeling, which aligns with her appearance (*response*). The response is in line with the intervention, and I persist in focusing on feelings.

T: You're sad, right? *SPEAKING GENTLY*
P: Yeah. *NOT LOOKING SAD ANYMORE*

I aim to deepen her experience of sadness by validating her feeling and mirroring the feelings she communicates nonverbally (*intervention*). She answers "yes," albeit without showing any sadness (*response*). Given that her response embodies a contradiction, I opt to clarify and highlight the conflicting aspects within her response.

T: How is that to acknowledge? Because you looked sad for a moment there. And now you don't look that sad anymore.
P: *SMILES*

Following my clarifying *intervention*, she *responds* with a smile. When confronted with something sad, she smiles. Her *response* serves as a defense, and my subsequent *intervention* is designed to inquire into the function of this defense.

T: It's like, it went away like in a flash.
P: Um ... I AM sad about it.

Upon my inquiry into her defense mechanism (*intervention*), she reasserts her sadness (*response*). As she acknowledges this feeling, my attention shifts to the physical experiences of this sadness *(intervention)*.

T: Can you let yourself experience that?
P: Yeah... *SIGHS* *LOOKS AWAY, APPEARING SERIOUS*

The responses of the Girl Who Wasn't a Princess reveal multiple facets. She *verbally* acknowledges her feelings, yet her *demeanor* doesn't reflect sadness. This implies that she can cognitively *identify* her feeling, but it's uncertain if she truly *experiences* it. She sighs, suggesting anxiety in her striated muscles. Her looking away may be a defense mechanism against closeness. Concurrently, her serious expression indicates her commitment to the therapy. In this brief excerpt, it is evident that my interventions are directed toward either feelings or defense mechanisms, depending on her responses. Simultaneously, I monitor signs of anxiety, such as sighs and restlessness, to ensure she remains within the zone of proximal development (Vygotsky, 1978). Throughout five interventions, I have incorporated elements from Chapters 12–15. This exemplifies the concept of *response to intervention*, demonstrating that therapy progresses in a spiral through various phases, rather than linearly.

What Are the Mechanisms of Change in ISTDP?

Just as knowing the patient's goal is crucial in setting the course of therapy, it is equally important for the therapist to grasp what elements incite change in the patient. One of the primary responsibilities of a therapist is to facilitate the processes that promote healing and recovery. So, what are these processes that are believed to instigate change in ISTDP?

The Working Alliance

A strong working alliance, as outlined in the second part of this book, is linked to therapeutic progress (Laska et al., 2014). Forming a solid alliance at the onset of therapy also correlates with positive therapeutic outcomes, more so than an alliance formed later on (Horvath & Symonds, 1991). There are likely multiple reasons why the working alliance is connected to the therapy's outcome. One reason is that when there is agreement on the goals and tasks of therapy, the process becomes more focused, and more time is spent on aspects believed to bring about change. A strong therapeutic bond also facilitates this process.

Restructuring of Defenses and Channeling of Anxiety

Research indicates that getting help to become acquainted with defenses (Chapters 12 and 13), along with help in regulating anxiety (Chapter 14), is linked to recovery. In a study conducted at Viken DPS in Drammen, Norway, ISTDP was the main therapeutic approach. Even though many patients did not experience huge breakthroughs to feelings, leading to subsequent *unlocking of the unconscious*, they still demonstrated substantial improvement (O. A. Solbakken, personal communication, June 24, 2022). The systematic work made by the therapists on Malan's (1979) two triangles contributed to this enhancement.

Affect Exposure

Leigh McCullough and her colleagues (McCullough et al., 2003) developed their unique version of short-term dynamic therapy, termed affect phobia therapy. Drawing inspiration from exposure therapy used for specific phobias, they perceive anxiety responses to feelings as phobic reactions. Consequently, they advocate for systematic exposure to feelings, aiming to reduce the anxiety response. Being gradually challenged to experience one's feelings, leading to a subsequent decrease in associated anxiety, is a pivotal change mechanism in ISTDP. As anxiety lessens in response to feelings, there is a diminished need for symptom-generating defense mechanisms. The gradual exposure to feelings is a crucial component of restructuring (Chapter 13) and the graded format of ISTDP (Whittemore, 1996), which are significant techniques within ISTDP.

Insight

Håvard Kallestad and colleagues (2010) studied the relationship between insight and the effect of short-term dynamic therapy. This research employed the Achievement of Therapeutic Objective Scale (ATOS) (McCullough et al., 2002) to examine the psychotherapy process. In this context, insight was defined as a patient's comprehension of (1) maladaptive behaviors, including awareness of unconscious motivation and feelings, (2) the how, why, and with whom the maladaptive behavior originated, and (3) the how, why, and with whom the behavior is upheld in the present. Kallestad and his team discovered that this kind of insight at the end of therapy was linked with improvement measured two years post-termination. In ISTDP, particularly when restructuring defenses and regulating anxiety, it is crucial for the patient to have a clear cognitive understanding of the corners of the triangles of conflict and person (Malan, 1979). This type of understanding, which ATOS measures as insight, contributes to long-term improvement.

Unlocking the Unconscious

Unlocking the Unconscious, Habib Davanloo's classic book from 1990, is named after a phenomenon he noticed in several of his patients. When they deeply connected with the somatic component and impulses of their feelings, it frequently led to a resurfacing of important memories. These memories, which seemed to shed light on the roots of the patient's issues, were ones that the patient had not consciously recalled before. Davanloo referred to this phenomenon as *unlocking the unconscious*.

For a memory to surface into consciousness, it requires a trigger. Certain childhood memories have limited triggers that can bring them to the forefront. For instance, for me, a specific soap scent brings back memories of my grandparents' bathroom. Absent this trigger, I seldom consciously recall this bathroom. When it comes to memories of traumatic childhood events, the experience of corresponding feelings one had during the event is a powerful trigger for such memories. As the child has kept the challenging and painful memories out of conscious awareness using defense mechanisms, these memories often have limited triggers. Hence, the intense experience of feelings becomes one of the scarce triggers available for these memories, serving as a key to *unlocking* such memories.

Abbass and colleagues (2017) studied the relationship between the *unlocking of the unconscious* and the effect of therapy. They discovered a distinct correlation between unlocking and improvement of both symptoms and interpersonal functioning. The facilitation of strong emotional experiences, with subsequent unlocking of the unconscious, amplifies the therapeutic effect.

On Resolving Unconscious Conflicts

The concept of unconscious conflicts has been a recurring topic in this book since the initial chapters. But what exactly does it mean to resolve unconscious conflicts? And how can one ascertain when an unconscious conflict has been resolved? To shed light on this, let's consider a hypothetical scenario.

Imagine a child who is raised by a mother battling depression. The mother, on medical leave, spends a significant amount of time in bed. Her spirits lift when her daughter returns from school, and she manages to maintain a relatively cheerful demeanor as long as her daughter is home, caring for her. However, if the daughter expresses a wish to socialize with friends or participate in recreational activities, the mother becomes visibly upset, even though she verbally assures her daughter that it's fine. Torn by conflicting feelings, the daughter sometimes opts to stay home, while at other times, she decides to go out. Regardless of her choice, it never feels quite right.

As an adult, the daughter seeks therapy as she experiences feelings of depression following her move into her boyfriend's apartment. She articulates significant challenges in pursuing her own desires, expressing a tendency to comply with her partner's preferences instead. While she harbors some vague thoughts about her mother's influence, she perceives the primary issue to be the discomfort she feels when witnessing her partner's disappointment. Now an adult, the daughter grapples with an internal conflict, struggling to act on her own desires when they contradict those of others. This conflict stirs a cascade of conflicting feelings within her, which she sidesteps by conforming to the wishes of those around her.

To help her resolve the underlying conflict through therapy, all the change mechanisms discussed earlier in this chapter play a crucial role. Her first step is to set a personal goal of treating herself on par with others. She would need help understanding that she must face her avoided emotions and needs in order to achieve this. By doing this, she may feel anger toward her partner for not considering her needs, a feeling that will bring back memories of her self-centered mother. She resorts to the defense mechanism she learned through interacting with her mother, which is to adapt to the needs of others. When she realizes that employing this mechanism is detrimental to her and that her mother didn't assist her in this regard, it triggers further anger. This anger stirs feelings of guilt as she reconnects with the long-held fantasies of her life being better if her mother were no longer alive. She suddenly recalls, with vivid clarity, her walks home from school when she would imagine her mother having ended her life, allowing her to live with a kind aunt. These were memories she hadn't accessed for a very long time, which got *unlocked* in the wake of strong feelings. Along with this revelation comes the grief of never having the mother she yearned for.

Hence, she needs a clear goal, help in letting go of her defense mechanisms, and exposure to the underlying feelings. When she experiences these feelings, they evoke memories that she hasn't processed before. Simultaneously, as she gains these new experiences, she develops cognitive *insight* into the mechanisms that cause her difficulties, their origins, and how they manifest and are upheld in her daily life (Kallestad et al., 2010). Consequently, the patient gains both the experience of feeling painful feelings and an understanding of the mechanisms that cause her difficulties. She also develops a coherent narrative that elucidates why she faces these challenges. In this way, she understands, experiences, and integrates new knowledge.

After therapy, when she finds herself in a situation where she must choose between her own desires or her partner's, she no longer unconsciously opts for the latter. She can freely contemplate her wishes, but simultaneously, memories of her mother surface, accompanied by feelings of anger, guilt, and sorrow. She is now conscious of her conflict, the feelings associated with it, and her habitual solution when confronted with them. The conflict no longer triggers anxiety in her; thus, there is no need for her to resort to defenses. The memories and the feelings persist, but they are no longer overwhelmingly complex. They are familiar and, while clearly painful, she can manage them without automatically acquiescing to her partner's wishes.

She no longer relies on outdated defense mechanisms to manage her desires, and can make decisions freely based on her own feelings. This doesn't mean she has forgotten past events or that recalling them is painless. However, she can *bear* the pain and connect with the memories, much as she does with other memories and feelings in her life. The collective impact of the various change mechanisms that ISTDP strives to effectuate will eventually resolve the patient's underlying conflict.

Common Struggles for a New ISTDP Therapist

This introduction to ISTDP is coming to a close. Whether you are a student or a beginner therapist about to put the knowledge from this book into practice for the first time, or an experienced therapist planning to merge your newfound comprehension of ISTDP with your current expertise, it is wise to be aware of the typical challenges and pitfalls that come with learning to employ this method.

Taking on Undue Responsibility

For many novice therapists, acknowledging the limits to what can be accomplished in therapy poses a significant hurdle. Numerous aspiring therapists step into the field of therapy with the notion that they should independently resolve all of the patient's issues: the therapist treats the sick patient, and the sick patient is the passive receiver of help. This perspective on treatment might be applicable to a surgeon tasked with removing a tumor, but it doesn't hold true for a psychotherapist assisting a patient who is struggling with psychological challenges. A key emphasis of this book is to illustrate that therapy is a collaborative endeavor between the therapist and the patient, through which they *work together* toward a shared goal. In such a partnership, the achievement of the goal relies on both parties contributing their utmost effort.

During therapy, there will inevitably be moments when the patient feels ambivalent about facing what is painful and challenging for them. If the therapist responds to such situations by attempting to *compel* the patient to experience feelings and to *break down* defenses, it quickly leads to a misalliance. The only person who can experience the patient's feelings and tear down their defense mechanisms is the patient themselves. The therapist can act as a cooperative ally, aiding the patient in recognizing their ambivalence and the options available to them. However, the final decision rests solely with the patient. The therapist can assist the patient in understanding how they turn to defense mechanisms that result in symptoms. Yet, the therapist cannot decide whether the patient should lay down their defenses. That decision can only be made by the patient. Being a therapist can be challenging, especially when there is a genuine desire to help, and yet the patient persists in behaviors that ultimately cause them harm. But bear in mind: what may seem like a straightforward choice for the therapist can be complex and difficult for the patient.

A therapist must deeply respect a patient's responsibility for their own life, their right to make their own choices, and even their prerogative to make decisions that may not be in their best interest. Forcing a patient toward an action they are reluctant to undertake can inadvertently amplify their resistance to change. The therapist's eagerness to speed up the patient's recovery and the sense of responsibility they feel toward the patient's healing can, paradoxically, impede the therapeutic process. If, however, the therapist assists the patient in recognizing their self-destructive tendencies, empathizes with the patient's pain and struggles, and respects their freedom to choose their path, it has been my experience that patients most often assume responsibility, paving the way for change.

The subsequent excerpt from the therapy with the Sweet Child, also discussed in Part I, exemplifies the respect a therapist must hold for a patient's autonomy and responsibility for their own life. Up until this stage of therapy, we had observed how she avoided complex feelings by employing a range of defense mechanisms.

T: Right. We see that two of your main ways of dealing with things … one is directed *outward*, taking care of others. Taking care of me, even! Just like your mom did. Then we see the other way, when you bypass the first. Because you come back here and start doing good things for yourself. Then you become numb….

P: Mmm. There are some days where it's just easier not to think than to think.

T: Right.

P: Escape into a book or Netflix or something, to not have to decide what you really feel.

T: So now we are beginning to understand this. We see the pattern. So, what will be our next task? Yours and mine?

P: Well, I don't know!

T: We're beginning to understand this. You can see it, you're a smart young woman. What's the next step after you understand?

P: *LAUGHS* Might have to start practicing, then.

T: Do you want to do that?

P: *NODS*

T: And so we're up against how many years of experience? Twenty? We're up against something that's your identity.

P: Yes. I think it's pretty solidly built in.

T: I wonder what you can do to start opening up, here with me? To take control and put yourself in the driver's seat. Allow yourself to do good things for yourself. What can you do right now?

P: *SIGHS* If you ask me, I'll ask you!

So far, I've taken an active role in assisting her to identify her mechanisms. This is part of my job, and a position I can assume as a therapist. However, she must walk the path ahead on her own, and only if she truly is willing to do so.

T: Right. *SPEAKING SLOWLY AND IN A GENTLE VOICE* And I'm here. And I really want to help you. But at some point, there is a switch you have to flip on your own.

P: Mmm.

T: And I would love to get inside your head and help you and turn things around.

P: *LAUGHS, TEARING UP*

T: *TALKS GENTLY* All I can do is to help you see what it is, but then you have to turn things around on your own.

P: Mmm.

T: That's the harsh reality.

P: *NODS* *TEARING UP*

T: *SPEAKING SOFTLY* But I'd really like to be here with you while you do it. And look at whatever comes from that.

P: *SIGHS*

T: So that you don't have to be there all alone!

P: *WHISPERS* Yes ….

T: *SPEAKING SOFTLY* Because that specific task is yours, but then the success can be yours too. And then freedom can be yours.

P: *WHISPERS* I'd really like to have that!

T: Yes, I understand that.

P: *CRYING INTENSELY*

The Assertion that ISTDP Is Superior to All Other Therapies for All Patients

A common perception among those studying ISTDP is that this method, if only applied correctly, should be capable of resolving *all* a patient's issues. The ISTDP community traditionally presents cases where patients undergo intense emotional experiences and significant transformations. This is great, as it demonstrates the therapy's potential. However, it also presents a challenge. Novice therapists may often presume that they can achieve similar results if they just *adhere* to the method *correctly*. It seems as though the portrayal of ISTDP in literature and seminars can sometimes create an impression that an ISTDP therapist has omnipotence, meaning they possess power that exceeds what is realistically possible.

Undoubtedly, ISTDP stands as an effective therapeutic method. It is versatile and adaptable, proving effective for a wide spectrum of patients (Abbass et al., 2012). However, research indicates that the difference between therapists often outweighs the difference between methods (Wampold, 2017). Striving too hard to implement a specific therapy model "correctly," because you "know" that the method is "superior," can lead to the loss of the fundamental elements that make a therapist effective. These elements include warmth, empathy, verbal fluency, ability to manage feelings, instill hope, form alliances, and maintain a problem focus (Anderson et al., 2009). If these elements are incorporated while practicing ISTDP, it will be an effective therapy and may sometimes lead to tremendous changes in a patient's life. Conversely, if ISTDP is forced upon a patient, it will end up being ineffective.

Technique over Understanding

One appealing aspect of learning ISTDP lies in the vast array of techniques available, which greatly facilitates the implementation of the therapy. Jon Frederickson's 2023 book, *Healing Through Relating*, offers a range of techniques, each accompanied by skill-building exercises. Additionally, Frederickson has developed numerous audio-recorded exercises for practicing central ISTDP techniques (Frederickson, 2022b). However, a common pitfall for novice ISTDP therapists is an overemphasis on mastering the techniques, often at the expense of losing sight of their purpose. Just as a jazz musician's technical skills are futile without the intent to create music, a therapist's technical skill is of no value unless it contributes to achieving therapeutic goals. Therefore, technique and understanding should be viewed as two equal partners.

This issue may appear to affect not only ISTDP students, but also seems to be widespread in the broader field of psychotherapy. It is crucial to recall that the pioneers of today's technique-based therapies had a comprehensive theoretical foundation. Both Aron Beck, the founder of cognitive therapy, and Habib Davanloo, the developer of ISTDP, were trained psychoanalysts. Their shared frustration with the slow pace of change in psychoanalysis, and the method's limited guidance on implementation, led them to devise powerful techniques for quicker transformations.

However, when today's students learn these techniques without the extensive theoretical understanding that both Beck and Davanloo had, there's a risk of the pendulum swinging to the other extreme: from theorists lacking technique, we now face the prospect of technicians lacking theory.

In this book, I have tried to balance this trend by not only elucidating the theoretical underpinnings of the method, but also explaining the rationale behind the use of the various techniques. I urge all those trying to learn ISTDP to concentrate on finding the balance between technique and comprehension.

Can Feelings Simply Be Felt?

Many novice ISTDP therapists struggle with the concept that the alternative to defending against a feeling is simply to *feel* and *experience* it. My students have repeatedly raised the question, "What should we do with the feeling, then?" during our supervisions. As discussed in Chapter 15, feelings are defined as physical arousal accompanied by specific motoric impulses. They are an inevitable part of the human experience and can be consciously recognized. Since feelings linked to a conflict induce anxiety, there is an internal pressure within the patient to manage the feeling in a way that reduces the anxiety it causes. However, this kind of management will necessitate the use of defense mechanisms. If feelings are to inspire self-preservation—which is their ultimate purpose—they must be endured. Healthy self-care seldom involves impulsive actions, but rather planned responses at the right moment. For instance, if a partner behaves in a manner you dislike in front of mutual friends, making you angry, immediately acting on the anger is seldom the most self-caring action. A more effective approach would be to observe and remember what your partner did that angered you, and then address it at a suitable time. This way, the conflict can be resolved effectively. However, it also implies that you must tolerate your anger and still retain the ability to function. Thus, the feeling must be experienced without resorting to defense mechanisms that create symptoms.

Pushing Through Feelings

Given that feelings can seem dramatic and thrilling, some novice ISTDP therapists are eager to have the patient confront their feelings as quickly as possible. The fact that conflicting feelings trigger anxiety, which in turn makes the patient use defense mechanisms, is soon overlooked. The focus on defense work (Chapters 12 and 13) and regulating anxiety (Chapter 14) is downgraded in favor of work on feelings (Chapter 15), thereby forgetting that feelings constitute only one of the three corners of the triangle of conflict. For feelings to be expressed healthily, contributing to enduring change and a profound comprehension of the mechanisms that are causing issues, the patient needs a solid understanding of their defenses, and the anxiety must be channeled in a way that makes learning possible. Therefore, equal attention must be given to all three corners of the triangle of conflict.

The Fear of Being Specific

For many beginner ISTDP therapists, one of the significant hurdles is maintaining clarity and specificity. Specificity is crucial both when building the alliance (Part II) and when dealing with defenses, anxiety, and feelings (Part III). It also holds importance as the initial focus in ISTDP is on specific situations that generate symptoms. A specific episode refers to an event that can, in theory, be timed precisely, occurring at a particular place with certain people: "On Monday, at ten past two, by the office coffee machine, Jon told Anne to toughen up, leading me to believe it was all my fault, making me feel stupid." With such clarity and specificity, one can understand the nature of the triggering situation, identify which feelings were triggered and toward whom, assess the level of anxiety, and determine the defense mechanisms employed. This leads to a clear comprehension of the patient's internal mechanisms. A common pitfall is asking broad questions about general phenomena, such as asking, "What do you typically feel in such situations?" This kind of inquiry prompts the patient to contemplate feelings that are *generally* experienced in *various* situations, leading to a response that is a summary of the patient's existing understanding. To discover what is yet unknown, the therapist and patient must revisit the specifics of particular episodes and examine the patient's precise reactions. Given that *vagueness* serves as a defense mechanism, being specific will evoke feelings and anxiety. This holds true for the therapist as well, and at times, it is the therapist's own anxiety that results in the *vagueness*. The therapist must manage this anxiety, either independently or by seeking assistance.

When the Therapist's Own Conflicts Interfere

Practicing ISTDP can be challenging because it puts the therapist's emotional capacity to the test. It becomes particularly difficult to assist the patient in navigating conflicting feelings toward their attachment figures if the therapist is grappling with similar issues. The patient's emotional experiences will inevitably elicit feelings in the therapist. If these feelings give rise to anxiety, the therapist may unconsciously resort to defensive mechanisms. For instance, if the therapist's defense mechanism involves diverting the patient away from their feelings, it would pose significant challenges to the therapy process.

Another common challenge is that the therapist, like the patient, mixes up the corners of Malan's triangles. Assisting the patient in differentiating between feelings such as anger and anxiety becomes challenging if the therapist themselves confuses these feelings. Obviously, every psychological struggle described in this book represents potential difficulties that the therapist might also encounter. If the therapist grapples with the same issues as the patient, their ability to provide help can be compromised.

Often, supervision from a colleague or mentor is enough, helping you to better manage your challenges. However, sometimes the difficulties are so extensive that the therapist needs to seek therapy themselves. For the majority, learning ISTDP is a journey of both personal and professional growth, and many ISTDP therapists choose to undergo their own ISTDP therapy while learning the method. This can be helpful in several ways: You will, hopefully, experience the method's potential in alleviating symptoms and enhancing relationships. It also provides an insight into the patient's perspective of the therapeutic dyad, fostering a respect for its challenges. Furthermore, you will hopefully gain a deeper insight into your own challenges, thereby enabling you to more effectively assist the patient in confronting their own conflicts.

Good Luck!

As we approach the end of this book, I'd like to extend my best wishes for your future endeavors. Whether you decide to explore this remarkable method in depth, or you incorporate the elements that resonate with you, I hope you found the book engaging. My aspiration is that it has enriched your understanding of psychodynamic theory, the formation of robust therapeutic alliances grounded in this theory, and how to work with feelings, anxiety, and defense mechanisms to help the patient resolve their underlying conflicts.

Writing this book has been incredibly rewarding, and I have learned a great deal in the process. I hope that you have sensed this, and that it has positively influenced your learning and growth as well.

Note

1 Recommended readings are Davanloo (1990), Coughlin Della Selva (2004), Abbass (2015), Frederickson (2013), Frederickson (2020), and Coughlin (2022b).

Bibliography

Abbass, A. (2002). Office Based Research in Intensive Short-term Dynamic Psychotherapy (ISTDP): Data From the First 6 Years of Practice. *Ad Hoc Bulletin of Short-term Dynamic Psychotherapy* 6(2); 5–14, December 2002

Abbass, A. (2015). *Reaching Through Resistance: Advanced Psychotherapy Techniques.* Seven Leaves Press.

Abbass, A. (2021). Intensive Short-Term Dynamic Psychotherapy: Methods, Evidence, Indications and Limitations. *Tidsskrift for Norsk Psykologforening, 58*(10), 874–879.

Abbass, A. (2022a, June 16). Posting at IEDTA's listserv edt@lists.iedta.net. *[EDT-List] interview with Niall Geoghegan.* IEDTA.

Abbass, A. (2022b, December 9). *Allan Abbass: Reaching Through Resistance.* Retrieved from Publications – Research updates. http://reachingthroughresistance.com/wp-content/uploads/2021/04/Cost-Effectiveness-July-2020.docx

Abbass, A., Bernier, D., Kisely, S., Town, J., & Johansson, R. (2015). Sustained Reduction in Health Care Costs After Adjunctive Treatment of Graded Intensive Short-Term Dynamic Psychotherapy in Patients with Psychotic Disorders. *Psychiatry Research, 228*(3), 538–543.

Abbass, A., Lumley, M. A., Town, J., Holmes, H., Luytende, P., Cooper, A., Russel, L., Schubiner, H., De Meulemeester, C., & Kisely, S. (2021). Short-Term Psychodynamic Psychotherapy for Functional Somatic Disorders: A Systematic Review and Meta-Analysis of Within-Treatment Effects. *Journal of Psychosomatic Research, 145*, 1–9.

Abbass, A., Town, J., & Driessen, M. (2012). Intensive Short-Term Dynamic Psychotherapy: A Systematic Review and Meta-Analysis of Outcome Research. *Harv Rev Psychiatry, 20*, 97–108.

Abbass, A., Town, J., Johansson, R., Lahti, M., & Kisely, S. (2019). Sustained Reduction in Health Care Service Usage after Adjunctive Treatment of Intensive Short-Term Dynamic Psychotherapy in Patients With Bipolar Disorder. *Psychodynamic Psychiatry, 47*(1), 99–112.

Abbass, A., Town, J., Ogrodniczuk, J. M., Joffres, M., & Lilliengren, P. (2017). Intensive Short-Term Dynamic Psychotherapy Trial Therapy: Effectiveness and Role of "Unlocking the Unconscious." *The Journal of Nervous and Mental Disease, 205*(6), 453–457.

Abbate-Daga, G., Marzola, E., Amianto, F., & Fassino, S. (2016). A Comprehensive Review of Psychodynamic Treatments for Eating Disorders. *Eating and Weight Disorders, 21,* 553–580.

Ainsworth, M. D., Blehar, M. C., Waters, E., & Wall, S. (1978). *Patterns of Attachment: A Psychological Study of the Strange Situation.* Psychology Press.

Alexander, F., & French, T. M. (1946). *Psychoanalytic Therapy: Principles and Application.* Ronald Press.

Anderson, T., Ogles, B. M., Patterson, C. L., & Lambert, M. (2009). Therapist Effects: Facilitative Interpersonal Skills as a Predictor of Therapist Success. *Journal of Clinical Psychology*, *65*(7), 755–768.

Aron, L. (1990). One Person and Two Person Psychologies and the Method of Psychoanalysis. *Psychoanalytic Psychology*, *7*(4), 475–485.

Bazaz, R., Killingberg, K., Tjørhom, V., & Misje, T. S. (2021, April 26). *Studentundersøkelse: Nær halvparten svarer at de har alvorlige psykiske plager*. nrk.no https://www.nrk.no/norge/studentundersokelse_-naer-halvparten-svarer-at-de-har-alvorlige-psykiske-plager-1.15464686

Betts, J. G., Desaix, P., Johnson, E., Johnson, J. E., Korol, O., Kruse, D., Poe, B., Wise, J. A., Womble, M., & Young, K. A. (2022). *Anatomy and Physiology* (2nd ed.). OpenStax. https://assets.openstax.org/oscms-prodcms/media/documents/Anatomy_and_Physiology_2e_-_WEB_c9nD9QL.pdf

Bienvenu, O., Davydow, D., & Kendler, K. S. (2011). Psychiatric 'Diseases' Versus Behavioral Disorders and Degree of Genetic Influence. *Psychol Med*, *41*(1), 33–40.

Blackman, J. (2004). *101 Defenses: How the Mind Shields Itself*. Brunner-Routledge.

Blagys, M. D., & Hilsenroth, M. J. (2000). Distinctive Features of Short-Term Psychodynamic-Interpersonal Psychotherapy: A Review of the Comparative Psychotherapy Process Literature. *Clinical Psychology: Science and Practice*, *7*(2), 167–188.

Bordin, E. S. (1979). The Generalizability of the Psychoanalytic Concept of the Working Alliance. *Psychotherapy: Theory, Research and Practice*, *16*, 252–260.

Borkovec, T. D., Robinson, E., Pruzinsky, T., & DePree, J. A. (1983). Preliminary Exploration of Worry: Some Characteristics and Processes. *Behaviour Research and Therapy*, *21*(1), 9–16.

Bratko, D., Butkovic, A., & Hlupic, T. V. (2017). Heritability of Personality. *Psychological Topics*, *26*(1), 1–24.

Brody, G. H., Yu, T., Chen, Y., Kogan, S. M., Evans, G. W., Beach, S. R., Windle, M., Simons, R. L., Gerrard, M., Gibbons, F. X., & Philibert, R. A. (2013). Cumulative Socioeconomic Status Risk, Allostatic Load, and Adjustment: A Prospective Latent Profile Analysis With Contextual and Genetic Protective Factors. *Developmental Psychology*, *49*(5), 913–927.

Carveth, D. (2013). *The Still Small Voice: Psychoanalytic Reflections on Guilt and Conscience*. Karnac.

Casement, P. (1985). *Learning from the Patient*. Guilford Press.

Cipriani, A., Furukawa, T. A., Salanti, G., Chaimani, A., Atkinson, L. Z., Ogawa, Y., Leucth, S., Ruhe, H. G., Turner, E. H., Higgins, J. P. T., Egger, M., Takeshima, N., Hayasaka, Y., Imai, H., Shinohara, K., Tajika, A., Ioannidis, J. P. A., & Geddes, J. R. (2018). Comparative Efficacy and Acceptability of 21 Antidepressant Drugs for the Acute Treatment of Adults With Major Depressive Disorder: A Systematic Review and Network Meta-Analysis. *The Lancet*, *391*(10127), 1357–1366.

Collins, A. M., & Loftus, E. F. (1975). A Spreading-Activation Theory of Semantic Processing. *Psychological Review*, *82*(6), 407–428.

Coughlin, P. (2017). *Maximizing Effectiveness in Dynamic Psychotherapy*. Routledge.

Coughlin, P. (2022b). *Facilitating the Process of Working Through in Psychotherapy: Mastering the Middle Game*. Routledge.

Coughlin Della Selva, P. (2004). *Intensive Short-Term Dynamic Psychotherapy*. Karnac Books.

Damasio, A. R. (1999). *The Feeling of What Happens*. Harcourt Brace & Company.

Davanloo, H. (1980). *Short-Term Dynamic Psychotherapy*. Aronson.

Davanloo, H. (1990). *Unlocking the Unconscious – Selected Papers of Habib Davanloo*. Wiley & sons.

Davanloo, H. (2000). *Intensive Short-Term Dynamic Psychotherapy*. Wiley & Sons.

Ecker, B., Ticic, R., & Hulley, L. (2013). A Primer on Memory Reconsolidation and Its Psychotherapeutic Use as a Core Process of Profound Change. *The Neuropsychotherapist*, *1*, 82–99.

Erikson, E. H. (1950). *Childhood and Society*. Norton.

Ezriel, H. (1952). Notes on Psychoanalytic Group Therapy: Interpretation and Research. *Psychiatry*, *15*, 119–126.

Fitzgerald, F. S. (1945). *The Crack-Up (Ed. Edmund Wilson)*. New Directions Book. https://www.pbs.org/wnet/americanmasters/f-scott-fitzgerald-essay-the-crack-up/1028/. (Original work published 1936)

Flåten, C. B., & Thomsen, H. (2021). Ett år Med ISTDP: En Bekymringsmelding. *Tidsskrift for Norsk Psykologforening*, *58*(6), 510–512.

Fonagy, P. (2015). The Effectiveness of Psychodynamic Psychotherapies: An Update. *World Psychiatry*, *14*(2), 137–150.

Fosha, D. (1988). Restructuring in the Treatment of Depressive Disorders With Davanloo's Intensive Short-Term Dynamic Psychotherapy. *International Journal of Short-Term Psychotherapy*, *3*, 189–212.

Frederickson, J. (2013). *Co-Creating Change: Effective Dynamic Therapy Techniques*. Seven Leaves Press.

Frederickson, J. (2020). *Co-Creating Safety: Healing the Fragile Patient*. Seven Leaves Press.

Frederickson, J. (2022a, June 16). Posting at IEDTAs listserv edt@lists.iedta.net. *EDT-List] interview with Niall Geoghegan*. IEDTA.

Frederickson, J. (2022b, June 23). *Skill-Building Series of Audio Courses*. ISTDP Institute. https://istdpinstitute.com/resources/skill-building-series-of-audio-courses/

Frederickson, J. (2023). *Healing Through Relating. A Skill-Building Book for Therapists*. Seven Leaves Press.

Freud, S. (1936). Inhibitions, Symptoms and Anxiety. *The Psychoanalytic Quarterly*, *5*(1), 1–28.

Freud, A. (1937). *The Ego and the Mechanisms of Defense (The International Psycho-Analytical Library, No. 30)*. Hogarth Press.

Freud, S. (1938). *Psychopathology of Everyday Life*. Penguin Books. (Original work published 1901)

Freud, S. (1962). The Neuro-Psychoses of Defense. In J. Strachey (Ed.), *The Standard Edition of the Complete Psychological Works of Sigmund Freud* (book 3, pp. 26–62). Hogarth Press. (Original work published 1894)

Freud, S., & Jones, E. (1922). *Beyond the Pleasure Principle* (C. J. M. Hubback, Trans.). The International Psycho-Analytical Press.

Gabbard, G. O. (2017). *Long-Term Psychodynamic Psychotherapy: A Basic Text, Third Edition*. American Psychiatric Association Publishing.

Geddes, J. R., & Miklowitz, D. J. (2013). Treatment of Bipolar Disorder. *The Lancet*, *381*(9878), 1672–1682.

General Social Survey. (2012, July 9). *Investigating Infidelity in America, with General Social Survey Data and Findings*. https://gss.norc.org/Lists/gssNewsArticles/DispForm.aspx?ID=101&ContentTypeId=0x010097F51E04B6E29A4DA5088910B198C118001E89468CD12E6047A9101BE0A48227BC

Gjerde, H. (2021). Faren Ved Tolkende Intervensjoner. *Tidsskrift for Norsk Psykologforening*, *58*(8), 704–705.

Greenberg, J. R. (1986). The Problem of Analytic Neutrality. *Contemporary Psychoanalysis*, *22*, 76–86.

Gullestad, S., & Killingmo, B. (2019). *The Theory and Practice of Psychoanalytic Therapy: Listening for the Subtext*. Taylor & Francis.

Health Professions Regulatory Advisory Council (2011). *Sexual Relationships between Patients and Health Professionals: A Literature Review*. HPRAC.

Horowitz, A. V. (2002). *Creating Mental Illness*. The University of Chicago Press.

Horvath, A. O., & Greenberg, L. S. (1986). The Development of the Working Alliance Inventory. In L. S. Greenberg & W. M. Pinsof (Eds.), *The Psychotherapeutic Process: A Research Handbook* (pp. 529–556). Guilford Press.

Horvath, A. O., & Symonds, B. D. (1991). Relation Between Working Alliance and Outcome in Psychotherapy: A Meta-Analysis. *Journal of Counseling Psychology*, *38*(2), 139–149.

Huda, A. S. (2019). *The Medical Model in Mental Health: An Explanation and Evaluation.* Oxford University Press.

Hughes, K., Bellis, M. A., Hardcastle, K. A., Sethi, D., Butchart, A., Mikton, C., Jones, L., & Dunne, M. P. (2017). The Effect of Multiple Adverse Childhood Experiences on Health: a Systematic Review and Meta-Analysis. *The Lancet*, *2(*8), 356–366.

IEDTA. (2024, August 7). *EDT-List information.* International Experiantial Dynamic Therapy Association. https://iedta.net/iedta/iedta-online/edt-list-info/

Infurna, R., Reichl, C., Parzer, P., Schimmenti, A., Bifulco, A., & Kaess, M. (2016). Associations Between Depression and Specific Childhood Experiences of Abuse and Neglect: A Meta-Analysis. *Journal of Affective Disorders*, *190*, 47–55.

Kallestad, H., Valen, J., McCullough, L., Svartberg, M., Høglend, P., & Stiles, T. C. (2010). The Relationship Between Insight Gained During Therapy and Long-Term Outcome in Short-Term Dynamic Psychotherapy and Cognitive Therapy for Cluster C Personality Disorders. *Psychother Res*, *20*(5), 526–534.

Kardong, K. (2012). *Vertebrates: Comparative Anatomy, Function, Evolution (6. utg.).* McGraw-Hill.

Keefe, J. R., McCarthy, K. S., Dinger, U., Zilcha-Mano, S., & Barber, J. P. (2014). A Meta-Analytic Review of Psychodynamic Therapies for Anxiety Disorders. *Clinical Psychology Review*, *34*(4), 309–323.

Keltner, D., Tracy, J. L., Sauter, D., & Cowen, A. (2019). What Basic Emotion Theory Really Says for the Twenty-First Century Study of Emotion. *Journal of Nonverbal Behavior*, *43*, 195–201.

Killingmo, B. (1989). Conflict and Deficit: Implications for Technique. *The International Journal of Psychoanalysis*, *70*(1), 65–79.

Killingmo, B. (1997). The So-Called Rule of Abstinence Revisited. *The Scandinavian Psychoanalytic Review*, *20*, 144–159.

Klein, M. (1960). *The Psychoanalysis of Children.* Grove Press.

Kuhn, N. (2014). *Intensive Short-Term Dynamic Psychotherapy: A Reference.* Experient Publications.

Laska, K. M., Gurman, A. S., & Wampold, B. E. (2014). Expanding the Lens of Evidence-Based Practice in Psychotherapy: A Common Factors Perspective. *Psychotherapy*, *51*(4), 467–481.

Leichsenring, F., Luyten, P., Hilsenroth, M. A., Barber, J., Keefe, J. R., Leweke, F., Rabung, S., & Steinert, C. (2015). Psychodynamic Therapy Meets Evidence-Based Medicine: a Systematic Review Using Updated Criteria. *Psychodynamic Therapy Meets Evidence-Based Medicine: A Systematic Review Using Updated Criteria*, *2*, 648–660.

Levy, K. N., Ellison, W. D., Scott, L. N., & Bernecker, S. L. (2011). Attachment Style. *Journal of Clinical Psychology*, *67*(2), 193–203.

Lum, J. A., Conti-Ramsden, G., Page, D., & Ullman, M. T. (2012). Working, Declarative and Procedural Memory in Specific Language Impairment. *Cortex*, *48*(9), 1138–1154.

Mahler, M. (1968). *On Human Symbiosis and the Vicissitudes of Individuation. Vol. 1. Infantile Psychosis.* Basic Books.

Malan, D. H. (1963). *A Study of Brief Psychotherapy.* Plenum Publishing Corporation.

Malan, D. H. (1979). *Individual Psychotherapy and the Science of Psychodynamics.* Butterworth.

Malan, D. H., & Coughlin Della Selva, P. (2007). *Lives Transformed: A Revolutionary Method of Dynamic Psychotherapy.* Karnac Books.

Masten, A. S. (2015). *Ordinary Magic: Resilience in Development.* Guilford Press.

McCullough, L., Kuhn, N., Andrews, S., Kaplan, A., & Wolf, J. (2003). *Treating Affect Phobia: A Manual for Short-Term Dynamic Psychotherapy.* Guilford Publications.

McCullough, L., Kuhn, N., Andrews, S., Valen, J., Hatch, D., & Osimo, F. (2002). The Reliability of the Achievement of Therapeutic Objectives Scale: A Research and Teaching Tool for Brief Psychotherapy. *Journal of Brief Therapy*, *2*(2), 72–90.

McCullough Vaillant, L. (1997). *Changing Character: Short-Term Anxiety-Regulating Psychotherapy for Restructuring Defenses, Affects, and Attachments*. Basic Books.

Menninger, K. (1958). *Theory of Psychoanalytic Technique*. Basic Books.

Mitchel, S., & Black, M. (2016). *Freud and Beyond: A History of Modern Psychoanalytic Thought*. Basic Books.

Molnos, A. (1986). The Process of Short-Term Dynamic Psychotherapy and the Four Triangels. *International Journal of Short-Term Psychotherapy*, *1*, 112–125.

Nordanger, D., & Braarud, H. (2014). Regulering som nøkkelbegrep og toleransevinduet som modell i en ny traumepsykologi. *Tidsskrift for Norsk Psykologforening*, *51*(7), 530–536.

Nordland, J. B., Stensvold, E. A., Kildal, E. S.-M., Larsen, A., Mallaug, L. F., Hjort, S., Riiser, K. F., Bergaust, M. W. M., Tunstad, P., Ivanova, R., Skjærseth, K., Røvik, F. M. G., Haakestad, G., Støver, I. E. A., Igesund, G. H., & Sæter, S. (2022). Vi har knapt begynt, men har behov for å rope varsko. *Tidsskrift for Norsk Psykologforening*, *59*(5), 400–403.

Normann-Eide, T. (2020). *Følelser: Kjennetegn, funksjon og vrangsider*. Cappelen Damm Akademisk.

Norwegian Psychological Association. (2022, March 30). *Fakta om psykiske lidelser*. psykologforeningen.no. https://www.psykologforeningen.no/publikum/fakta-om-psykiske-lidelser

Ogden, P., Minton, K., & Pain, C. (2006). *Trauma and the Body: Examining a Neglected Perspective*. W.W. Norton & Company Inc.

Ossimo, F. (2022, October 13). David Malan Tribute. Presentation at the IEDTA conference, Venice, Italy. IEDTA.

Petterson, E., Lichtenstein, P., Larsson, H., & Song, J. (2019). Genetic Influences on Eight Psychiatric Disorders Based on Family Data of 4 408 646 Full and Half-Siblings, and Genetic Data of 333 748 Cases and Controls. *Psychological Medicine*, *49*(7), 1166–1173.

Piaget, J. (1952). *The Origins of Intelligence in Children*. International University Press.

Plomin, R., & Deary, I. (2015). Genetics and Intelligence Differences: Five Special Findings. *Molecular Psychiatry*, *20*(1), 98–108.

Practice Guideline for the Assessment and Treatment of Patients with Suicidal Behaviors. (2003). *The American Journal of Psychiatry*, *160*(11 Suppl), 1–60.

Proudfoot, J., Whitton, A., Parker, G., Doran, J., Manicavasagar, V., & Delmas, K. (2012). Triggers of Mania and Depression in Young Adults With Bipolar Disorder. *Journal of Affective Disorders*, *143*(1–3), 196–202.

Rognes, W. (2002, September 24). Presentation on the Therapeutic Relation. Trondheim, Norge: NTNU.

Rothbart, M. K., Ellis, L. K., & Posner, M. I. (2011). Temperament and Self-Regulation. In K. Vohs, & R. F. Baumeister (Eds.), *Handbook of Self-Regulation: Research, Theory, and Applications*. Guilford Press.

Sehmi, R., Maughan, B., Matthews, T., & Arseneault, L. (2020). No Man Is an Island: Social Resources, Stress and Mental Health at Mid-Life. *Br J Psychiatry*, *217*(5), 638–644.

Shedler, J. (2006). *That Was Then, This Is Now: Psychoanalytic Psychotherapy for the Rest of Us*. Retrieved December 14, 2023, from https://jonathanshedler.com/writings/

Shedler, J. (2010). The Efficacy of Psychodynamic Psychotherapy. *American Psychologist*, *65*, 98–109.

Sheldon, E., Simmonds-Buckley, M., Bone, C., Mascarenhas, T., Chan, N., Wincott, M., Gleeson, H., Sow, K., Hind, D., & Barkham, M. (2021). Prevalence and Risk Factors for Mental Health Problems in University Undergraduate Students: A Systematic Review With Meta-Analysis. *Journal of Affective Disorders*, *287*, 282–292.

Smedslund, J. (1988). *Psycho-Logic*. Springer Verlag.

Smedslund, J. (1997). *The Structure of Psychological Common Sense*. Lawrence Erlbaum Associates.

Solms, M., & Panksepp, J. (2012). The "Id" Knows More than the "Ego" Admits: Neuropsychoanalytic and Primal Consciousness Perspectives on the Interface Between Affective and Cognitive Neuroscience. *Brain Sciences, 2*, 147–175.

Stänicke, E., & Stänicke, L. I. (2014). Psykoanalytisk Terapi. In L. E. Kennair, & R. Hagen (Eds.), *Psykoterapi: Tilnærminger Og Metoder* (pp. 73–91). Gyldendal Akademisk.

Steinert, C., Munder, T., Rabund, S., Hoyer, J., & Leichsenring, F. (2017). Psychodynamic Therapy: As Efficacious as Other Empirically Supported Treatments? A Meta-Analysis Testing Equivalence of Outcomes. *American Journal of Psychiatry, 174*, 945–953.

Ten Have-de Labije, J., & Neborsky, R. J. (2012). *Mastering Intensive Short-Term Dynamic Psychotherapy*. Karnac Books Ltd.

Torgersen, S., Myers, J., Reichborn-Kjennerud, T., Røysamb, E., Kubarych, T. S., & Kendler, K. S. (2012). The Heritability of Cluster B Personality Disorders Assessed Both by Personal Interview and Questionnaire. *Journal of Personality Disorders, 26*(6), 848–866.

Town, J. M., Falkenström, F., Abbass, A., & Stride, C. (2022). The Anger-Depression Mechanism in Dynamic Therapy: Experiencing Previously Avoided Anger Positively Predicts Reduction in Depression via Working Alliance and Insight. *Journal of Counseling Psychology, 69*(3), 326–336.

Vaillant, G. E. (1992). *Ego Mechanisms of Defense: A Guide for Clinicians and Researchers* (1st ed.). American Psychiatric Association Publishing.

Vygotsky, L. S. (1978). *Mind in Society: The Development of Higher Psychological Processes*. Harvard University Press.

Wachtel, P. L. (1981). Transference, Schema, and Assimilation: The Relevance of Piaget to the Psychoanalytic Theory of Transference. *The Annual of Psychoanalysis, 8*, 59–76.

Wampold, B. E. (2017). What Should We Practice? A Contextual Model for How Psychotherapy Works. In T. Rousmaniere, R. K. Goodyear, S. D. Miller, & B. E. Wampold (Eds.), *The Cycle of Excellence: Using Deliberate Practice to Improve Supervision and Training* (pp. 49–65). Wiley & Sons.

Warshaw, D. (2022). The Effectiveness of Psychodynamic Psychotherapy for the Treatment of Substance Use Problems: A Systematic Review and Meta-Analysis. *Selected Full Text Dissertations, 2011.* 39. https://digitalcommons.liu.edu/post_fulltext_dis/39

Wechsler, D. (2008). *Wechsler Adult Intelligence Scale* (4th ed., WAIS-IV) [Database record]. APA PsycTests.

Weinberger, J., & Stoycheva, V. (2019). *The Unconscious: Theory, Research, and Clinical Implications*. Guilford Press.

Wenzel, A. (2021). *Handbook of Cognitive Behavioral Therapy*. American Psychological Association.

Whittemore, J. W. (1996). Paving the Royal Road: An Overview of Conceptual and Technical Features in the Graded Format of Davanloo's Intensive Short-Term Dynamic Psychotherapy. *International Journal of Short-Term Psychotherapy, 11*, 21–39.

WHO (1992). *ICD-10: The ICD-10 Classification of Mental and Behavioural Disorder: Clinical Descriptions and Diagnostic Guidelines*. World Health Organization.

Winnicott, D. W. (1971). *Playing and Reality*. Penguin.

Winnicott, D. W. (1990). *The Maturational Processes and the Facilitating Environment: Studies in the Theory of Emotional Development*. Routledge.

Yalom, I. D. (1980). *Existential Psychotherapy*. Basic Books.

Index

For Product Safety Concerns and Information please contact our EU
representative GPSR@taylorandfrancis.com
Taylor & Francis Verlag GmbH, Kaufingerstraße 24, 80331 München, Germany

www.ingramcontent.com/pod-product-compliance
Lightning Source LLC
Chambersburg PA
CBHW050635280326
41932CB00015B/2658

9 781032 850375